THE ESSENTIAL CONCEPTS OF NURSING

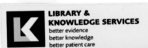

Commissioning Editor: Susan Young
Development Editor: Catherine Jackson
Project Manager: Morven Dean
Designer: Judith Wright

The Essential Concepts of Nursing

BUILDING BLOCKS FOR PRACTICE

Editors

John R. Cutcliffe

PhD, BSc(Hons)Nursing, RMN, RGN, RPN

Senior Administration/Faculty position within the College of Nursing, University of Tennessee (Knoxville), USA
Research Consultant, Mental Health, Interior Health Authority (Penticton), British Columbia, Canada
Adjunct Professor, Community Health, University of Northern British Columbia, Canada
Director of 'Cutcliffe Consulting'

Hugh P. McKenna

PhD BSc(Hons) RMN RGN RNT DipN(Lond) AdvDipEd FFN FRCSI FEANS FRCN

Dean of the Faculty of Life and Health Sciences, University of Ulster, UK
Visiting Professor in Nursing Research, University of Northumbria, and University of Wales, Bangor, UK

Forewords by

Peggy Chinn

RN PhD FAAN
Professor Emerita, University of Connecticut; Editor, Advances in Nursing

Afaf I. Meleis

PhD DrPS (Hons) FAAN
Professor of Nursing and Sociology, Margaret Bond, Simon Dean of Nursing, University of Pennsylvania, USA

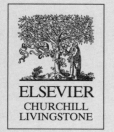

ELSEVIER
CHURCHILL
LIVINGSTONE

EDINBURGH   LONDON   NEW YORK   OXFORD   PHILADELPHIA   ST LOUIS   SYDNEY   TORONTO   2005

ELSEVIER
CHURCHILL
LIVINGSTONE

First published 2005

ISBN 0 443 07372 4

British Library Cataloguing in Publication Data
A catalogue record for this book is available from the British Library

Library of Congress Cataloging in Publication Data
A catalog record for this book is available from the Library of Congress

Notice
Medical knowledge and best practice in this field are constantly changing. As new research and experience broaden our knowledge, changes in practice, treatment and drug therapy may become necessary or appropriate. Readers are advised to check the most current information provided (i) on procedures featured or (ii) by the manufacturer of each product to be administered, to verify the recommended dose or formula, the method and duration of administration, and contraindications. It is the responsibility of the practitioner, relying on their own experience and knowledge of the patient, to make diagnoses, to determine dosages and the best treatment for each individual patient, and to take all appropriate safety precautions. To the fullest extent of the law, neither the publisher nor the editors assumes any liability for any injury and/or damage.

The Publisher

Printed in China

Contents

Foreword

This book and its collection of concepts significantly illustrates the amazing diversity and complexity of nursing's domain, and the richness of nursing's methodologic resources. This book provides a resource for each of the concepts addressed. It also provides an important methodologic resource for those who undertake the task of doing a concept analysis.

Rather than subscribing to a limited description of a single nursing paradigm, the editors and the authors of this volume assume a stance that acknowledges the richness of nursing as a healing and caring science and art. Not only is there a wide range of concepts addressed in this volume, but the analysis of each concept reveals the complexity inherent within each concept, defying a singular or a simplified definition. The substantive concepts that are included here defy a simple answer to the question "what is nursing?" Instead, these concepts paint a rich mental image that addresses the question of nursing's domain, building a clear picture of the depth and breadth of "what is nursing."

As a methodologic resource, the editors provide a succinct, critical and well-balanced assessment of the many approaches to concept analysis that are described in the literature. They discuss the limitations and the strengths of each approach, suggesting an eclectic and pragmatic choice of method. In their editorial commentary, they provide guideposts for the reader in understanding the significance of each chapter, and set the stage for a critical reading of the chapter. The authors in turn build on this methodologic stance; they do not uniformly use a particular method, and their purposes are diverse. Each author has selected methods that are best suited to the analysis of their chosen concept and to their own purpose for attempting the analysis. The authors acknowledge the complexity of their chosen concept, and through their analysis provide a clearer picture of what is possible for the development of knowledge.

Nekolaichuk eloquently addresses the issue of the complexity of the concept of hope, and the need for diverse definitions and perspectives on a concept. Her point applies aptly to each of the concepts that are included here, as well as other concepts that are part of nursing's domain. Abstract concepts take on a wide range of meaning in general, but become quite specific within a given context or used in a specific way, for a specific purpose. Concept analyses can reveal broad meanings inherent in a concept; they can also make specific meanings more clear. Each analysis of the concept adds to the richness of understanding of human possibility, but also serves to clarify a specific meaning and the context in which this meaning becomes significant.

The purposes for undertaking a concept analysis are fundamental to the enterprise. Unless there is a clear purpose, concept analysis remains as an interesting intellectual exercise, lacking significant meaning for the discipline. The fundamental purpose of conceptual clarity is laudable, but for practicing nurses who deal with the realities of practice day in and day out, such an exercise lacks meaning. The authors of the analyses in this volume explicitly or implicitly point to their purpose, usually leading to further theoretical, empirical, or philosophic undertakings. What follows concept analysis is the work that substantively deepens nursing's knowledge, and brings to the discipline new insights and new possibilities. Some of the authors have already published their further work, and we can anticipate significant contributions from all. As readers, we can all look for their further accomplishments with great anticipation.

Peggy Chinn
Connecticut, USA
October 2004

Foreword

This book is a reminder of how far we have progressed in developing concepts that are vital for developing evidence-based practice in nursing. We started thinking about theoretical nursing in the USA in the mid-60s, at which time the major question was "How do we know whether nursing makes a difference?" Reviewing this book reminded me that we have truly moved forward in advancing the discipline of nursing internationally. There are three characteristics of this book that make it unique and a significant milestone in the progress of nursing scholarship.

First, it reflects international thinking and collaboration, establishes our discipline across national divides, uses shared languages and defines innovative problems and partnerships in devising strategies and solutions to enhance understanding and knowing. This book is the result of international collaboration and, as such, it provides the reader with opportunities to witness the dialogues on shared perspectives about nursing and, simultaneously, the styles and approaches in concept development that reflect diversity in gender and cultures.

A second reason for this book being considered a milestone in knowledge development is the scholarly approach by which the various authors combine structure and substance to present their findings. There are excellent books in print about theory that discuss the syntax of a discipline and others equally as profound that provide the substance, the evidence and the outcomes of science. This book provides the reader with central nursing concepts that are presented with the different strategies the authors selected for a analysing and developing the concepts. Students of theory will find the integration of syntax and substance refreshing and illuminating. The chapters model a new wave in developing nursing knowledge.

The third reason this book represents a milestone and a turning point in knowledge development is that it provides an effective example of synthesis and interpretation of knowledge related to some key concepts in nursing that could promote critical thinking about further development. It is a book that should propel clinicians and researchers to ask more cogent questions about nursing practice.

This is a book that will become a vital resource for those who teach, study or practise nursing and, more importantly, it will stimulate robust dialogues about strategies for concept development and analysis, as well as the nature and dimensions of important nursing concepts. Since concepts are the fundamental building blocks of any discipline, they are the basis for the theoretical development that helps in advancing the research. Therefore, the editors and authors of this book have provided the discipline with the tools to advance science.

Afaf I. Meleis
Pennsylvania, USA

Preface

Epistemologists have long purported that theory grows from practice and research, and in turn, returns to inform practice. All credible disciplines, to a greater or lesser extent, value the contribution that theory has to their development. For many nurses, the pursuit of nursing science is perceived as a valuable goal and it is recognized that science equals theory plus research. To try and build or use a theory without having a clear understanding of the conceptual 'building blocks' would be to lay faulty theoretical foundations for the discipline of nursing, for nursing practice and ultimately for patient care.

Many of the concepts used everyday in nursing, such as 'hope', 'caring', and 'empathy' are abstract and nebulous. Nonetheless, nurses have to use them to underpin their thinking and practice. Such a situation leads Morse (1995) to assert that there is a vast amount of conceptual exploration yet to be accomplished. Thus, there is an urgent requirement to build the unique knowledge base of nurses through a clarification of our theoretical building blocks.

In addition to this, a parallel argument needs to be made which centres on the role and value of concepts for the practising nurse. Each day nurses think about or use the concepts within this text, to a greater or lesser extent. More often than not, these concepts are used both implicitly (for example, consideration of a client's dignity) and explicitly (e.g. maintaining a client's comfort as an outcome/aim of care in the care plan.) The danger is, particularly in these days of evidence-based practice, that to use if such terms are used without a full understanding of the concept, the resulting practice may be ambiguous, unfocused, and ill-thought through. Thus, it is incumbent upon practising nurses to understand what they mean when they attempt to 'promote a person's dignity', 'to form a therapeutic relationship', 'to be empathic', or 'to care'. Indeed, it is difficult to imagine any other health-related discipline arguing for a lack of conceptual clarity about the key concepts that underpin and inform their practice. While some practising nurses may feel that some theory may be regarded as removed or distant from the 'real world' of clinical practice, it has been argued that all nursing practice is underpinned by theory (McKenna 1997). Indeed, in his seminal work, Kuhn (1962) declared that theory, be it explicit or implicit, plays a key role in understanding any behaviour, and that there is nothing so useful as a good theory.

Accordingly, in the view of the editors, there are least five reasons for why there is a need for this book on concepts:

1. Concepts are the building blocks of theory and as such need to be analysed to clarify their meaning.
2. The large number of ways concepts are used in practice, education and research leads to confusion and therefore we require greater understanding of the essential concepts of nursing.
3. There are a number of approaches used to analyse concepts, some more well known than others; some more systemtic than others. Nurses concerned with obtaining a deeper understanding of concepts then would benefit from a greater familiarity of these different approaches to concept analysis.
4. The practice of concept analysis itself is an evolutionary or developmental phenomenon. Accordingly, it behoves nurses, particularly those interested in advancing the substantive knowledge base of the discipline, to be familiar with the latest developments in the practice of concept analysis.
5. In these days of evidence-based practice, practitioners do not accept empirical reports at 'face value'; they critique and question and are thus better able to make judicious judgmements about the quality and usefulness of the research findings. Similarly, the same processes and dynamics of critiquing research reports need to be applied to concept analysis papers.

Consequently, we feel that having read this book readers should have a deeper understanding of the twenty concepts featured herein. They should be more familiar with a range of approaches to concept analysis. They should be better positioned to underpin their practice with a firmer conceptual footing and thus, ultimately, enhance the precision and specificity of the care they provide. Also, they should be better placed to undertake further empirical work; work based on a more solid understanding of these key concepts.

In putting together a book that focuses on exploring concepts that are critical to the discipline of nursing, and recognizing and operating within word/space limits, the editors need to point out that difficult choices had to made around which concepts to include and which not to. Crucially, readers should not regard the concepts included in this text as some form of conceptual hierarchial taxonomy for nurses. Understandably, the choice of these concepts reflects, at least in part, the views and values of the editors. The featured concepts might be regarded as a collection of twenty of the essential concepts of nursing. Additional concepts that we considered to be featured in the book include:
euthanasia, suicide, compassion, autonomy, consent, independence, primary nursing, deceit, helplessness, aggression, violence, love, warmth, genuineness, duty, professionalism, spirituality, holism, wellness, and health to name but a few. It is the hope of the editors that these concepts may form the cadre of a second volume.

In order to provide some additional preliminary justification for certain choices we have made in constructing this book (and at the same time, perhaps offsetting potential criticism) the editors would like to offer the following explanations. Readers will note that throughout the book the term 'patient' has been used to refer to the person who is in receipt of nursing care. The use of this term is a purposeful, though contentious choice. The editors acknowledge the extensive debate about the most appropriate term to describe a person who receives care from a nurse (e.g. client, service user, customer). Rather than be drawn into semantic discussions about the 'most appropriate' term in contemporary parlance, the editors opted for pragmatism over political correctness. The sometimes-pejorative nature of this term notwithstanding, the editors believe that this term will be immediately recognizable for the significant majority of our readers.

On a similar note, where assigning gender to a nurse and/or a patient is required in the book, the editors have chosen to stay with the established practice of assigning feminine gender to the term 'nurse' and masculine gender to the term 'patient'. Again, the editors acknowledge that male nurses very much exist (indeed, as both the editors are male nurses themselves, this would be hard to ignore!). It is simply a matter of not wishing to be drawn into discussions about political correctness.

John R. Cutcliffe and
Hugh P. McKenna
April 2005

Contributors

Wendy Austin BScN MEd PhD
*Canada Research Chair, Relational Ethics in Health Care and
Professor, Faculty of Nursing, University of Alberta, Edmonton, Alberta, Canada*

Catherine Black RGN RNT BA(Hons)Nursing Studies MA(Education for Health and Social Care Practice) Dip(Health Services Management)
Nurse Tutor, Centre of Nurse Education, Douglas, Isle of Man, UK

Robert Brown RGN BSc(Hons) PGDip DipSocPsych AdvDipEd RNT
Lecturer in Practice Development and Nursing, Facilitator, University of Ulster, Newtownabbey, and Practice Development Facilitator, Southern Health and Social Services Board, Northern Ireland, UK

Richard Byrt RMN RNLD RGN PhD BSc(Hons)
Clinical/Education Facilitator, Arnold Lodge Medium Secure Unit, and School of Nursing and Midwifery, De Montfort University, Leicester, UK

Jim Campbell MA(Psychology) ITECDiploma in Therapeutic Massage, RN(Mental Health)
Research Fellow, University of Teesside, Middlesbrough, UK

Mary Chambers BEd(Hons) DPhil RMN RGN Cert Ed RNT DN(Lond)
Professor, Mental Health Nursing and Chief Nurse, Kingston University, St George's Hospital Medical School, South West London and St George's Mental Health Trust, London, UK

Peggy L. Chinn RN, PhD, FAAN
Professor Emerita, University of Connecticut, Storrs, CT; Editor, Advances in Nursing Science

John R. Cutcliffe PhD BSc(Hons)Nursing RMN RGN RPN
Senior Administration/Faculty position within the College of Nursing, University of Tennessee (Knoxville), USA; Research Consultant, Mental Health, Interior Health Authority (Penticton), British Columbia, Canada; Adjunct Professor, Community Health, University of Northern British Columbia, Canada, and Director of 'Cutcliffe Consulting'

James Dooher RMN MA CertEd(FHE) DipHCR ILTM
Principal Lecturer, Academic Lead(Mental Health), De Montfort University, Leicester, UK

Dianne Ellis MSc RMN
Senior Lecturer, School of Health, University of Teesside, Middlesbrough, UK

Mary Haase RN PhD
Program Manager, Alberta Hospital, Edmonton, Alberta, Canada

Kristiina Hyrkäs RN MNSc LicNSc PhD
Director, Center for Nursing Research and Quality Outcomes, Maine Medical Center, Portland, Maine, USA

Sue Jackson RGN BSc(Hons) MPhil
Research Fellow, University of Teesside, Middlesbrough, UK

Linda Marie Lowe RN SCM BSc(N) MAHCE MPH
Assistant Professor, University of Northern British Columbia, Prince George, Canada

Lanny Magnussen BA BSW RSW
Social worker; Program Manager, Alberta Hospital, Edmonton, Alberta, Canada

Jerome Marley BSc(Hons) RGN PGDip(Advanced Nursing) PGDip(Nurse Education)
Lecturer-Practitioner in Urological Nursing, School of Nursing, University of Ulster, Newtownabbey and Craigavon Area Hospital Group Trust, UK

Tanya McCance RGN BSc(Hons) MSc DPhil
Senior Professional Officer, Northern Ireland Practice and Education Council for Nursing and Midwifery, UK

Carole McIlrath RMN Dip(Management) Dip(Community Mental Health Nursing) BSc(Hons) PGDip(Primary Health Care/General Practice)
Senior Practice Development Fellow, Royal College of Nursing (Northern Ireland), UK

Hugh P. McKenna PhD BSc(Hons) RMN RGN RNT DipN(Lond) AdvDipEd FFN FRCSI FEANS FRCN
Dean of the Faculty of Life and Health Sciences, University of Ulster, Coleraine, UK; Visiting Professor in Nursing Research, University of Northumbria, Newcastle, and University of Wales, Bangor, UK

Afaf I. Meleis PhD DrPS (Hons) FAAN
Professor of Nursing and Sociology, Margaret Bond, Simon Dean of Nursing, University of Pennsylvania, PA, USA

Janice Morse RN BS MS MA PhD(Nurs) PhD(Anthro) DNurs(Honorary) FAAN
Professor, Faculty of Nursing, Scientific Director, International Institute for Qualitative Methodology Adjunct Professor, Department of Anthropology, Center for Health Promotion, Department of Human Ecology, University of Alberta, Adjunct Professor, The Pennsylvania State University, PA, USA

Cheryl L. M. Nekolaichuk BSc(Pharm) MEd PhD
Senior Research Associate, Palliative Care Research Initiative, Alberta Cancer Board, Edmonton, Alberta, Canada

Karin Olson RN PhD
Associate Professor, Faculty of Nursing and International Institute for Qualitative Methodology, Edmonton, Alberta, Canada

Judee E. Onyskiw RN PhD
Canada Research Chair in Family Violence and Health, Associate Professor, Faculty of Nursing, University of New Brunswick, Fredericton, Canada

William Reynolds PhD MPhil RN
Reader, University of Stirling, UK, and Reader, Turku Polytechnic, Turku, Finland

Jude A. Spiers RN PhD
Canadian Institute for Health Research and Izack Walton Killam (Honorary) Post-Doctoral Fellow, IIQM Assistant Professor, Faculty of Nursing, University of Alberta, Edmonton, Canada

Chris Stevenson RMN BA(Hons) MSc(Dist) PhD
Professor, Mental Health Nursing, Dublin City University, Dublin, Ireland

Kate Sullivan DPhil BSc(Hons) RGN RCNT RNT AdDipEd DN(London)
Professor and Head of the School of Health and Social Care, North East Wales Institute of Higher Education, Wrexham, Wales, UK

Acknowledgements

This book is dedicated to our families; without their support and understanding, it would not have been possible.

For Maryla, Ryan and Tate
and
for Trish, Gowain and Saoirse

We thank you.
Also, to each of the contributors, this book is testament to your efforts.

John Cutcliffe and Hugh McKenna, April 2005

An introduction to concepts and their analyses

Hugh P. McKenna and John R. Cutcliffe

INTRODUCTION

Perhaps the best way to begin a book on concept analysis is to start with describing what is meant by a phenomenon (pl: phenomena). Every day nurses encounter and note phenomena. These are things, events or activities that they perceive through their senses. For instance, a nurse may notice a mother of a sick child walking back and forth across a hospital waiting room, biting her nails, wringing her hands and looking pale. The nurse is noting a phenomenon and if you asked her to label what she is observing she might say 'anxiety'.

Similarly, a nurse may notice that people from a different culture invariably arrive late for appointments in a large inner-city hospital. Other co-workers agree that they too have noted this behaviour. When she gets to know these patients better, they tell her of the slow pace of life in their country of origin and how they cannot come to terms with the hustle and bustle of the large city. Once again the nurse is noting a phenomenon. These and many more phenomena are important to nurses and to nursing. They are the 'seedbed' for our developing knowledge base.

Nurse theorists inevitably commenced their theorizing by noting phenomena. For instance, Dorothea Orem (1958) noted that healthy people habitually looked after themselves; got themselves out of bed, washed and fed themselves. It would be a great insult to help healthy, fit persons out of bed in the morning, brush their teeth for them and feed them. Therefore, she noted that people who were encouraged to care for themselves developed high levels of self-esteem and independence. This phenomenon of looking after oneself is universal and valued. In the 1950s, Orem realized the importance of this for nursing.

Sister Callista Roy (1970) observed that throughout their day healthy people adapted to their environment. If it was cold they put on a coat and removed it when warm. Subconsciously, the human body also adapts by making more red blood cells when it experiences a higher altitude, it makes goose bumps when cold and has an autonomic 'fight or flight' response when frightened or threatened. As with Orem, Roy realized the importance of this phenomenon for nursing.

Hildegard Peplau (1952) was an experienced psychiatric nurse when she realized that people who have good mental health often have good interpersonal relationships with others such as their family, friends and work colleagues. Conversely, she noted that people who were psychiatrically unwell often had poor interpersonal skills and had difficulty communicating appropriately with others. She studied this phenomenon over many years and authors such as Harry Stack Sullivan (1953) and her work colleagues supported her observations.

The work of each of these theorists pushed forward the boundaries of nursing knowledge and skills in the late 20th century and continues to do so. As with other nurse theorists, the theories created by Orem, Roy and Peplau first began to form when they experienced a phenomenon. **It is a truism that many thousand of nurses observe phenomena throughout their working life but do not give them sufficient attention.** However, nurses who are interested in developing their knowledge base should be attuned to the phenomena around them. According to Meleis (1985), there are two stages in this process. The first stage is 'attention grabbing'. Here some clinical situation, event or activity attracts a nurse's attention and she develops a hunch about it. This may occur concurrently or retrospectively. This is followed by a more deliberate 'attention giving' stage where the nurse asks questions such as:

- What has attracted my attention?
- When does it occur?
- Why does it happen?
- Does it have a function?
- Can I describe it?
- Is it similar to or different from other happenings? It is related to time or place?
- Under what conditions do I observe it, hear it, touch it? Does it vary? Under what circumstances?

The nurse may also consider whether or not understanding this phenomenon is important to nursing as a discipline. Suppose through observations and questioning, a community nurse notes that people who have urinary incontinence have poor social lives and seldom go on social outings or visit clubs, cinemas and bars. From talking to colleagues, the nurse finds that this is a common trend. To give this phenomenon fuller attention and to ask the questions outlined above provides greater understanding of the patient's condition (and this has obvious implications for patient/client care).

Orem, Roy and Peplau gave phenomena their full attention and realized the implications for nurses and nursing, if practitioners could encourage patients to be self-caring, to adapt to their internal and external environment and to improve their person-to-person communications. What each of them did was to give the phenomenon a label. In the case of Orem this was 'self care', whereas Roy coined the term 'adaptation' and Peplau wrote about 'interpersonal interaction'. **These labels are concepts and they are the 'building blocks' of theory.** In short, when we put a name to a phenomenon we are identifying concepts. It has been agreed that they are normally represented by a concise word or a short phrase. They should also be precise, be used consistently when referring to the phenomenon, contain one cardinal idea and be fundamental to the definition/description of the phenomenon. However, if we accept the view of concepts as dynamic entities, then, as the concept develops and evolves through application, the issues of consistency in use over time and even the notion of containing one cardinal idea are less than sacrosanct.

Most theories, particularly 'grand level' theories, are nebulous, but if you were able to look at one under the microscope it would not be unlike a molecule (Fig. 1.1). First, there would be a boundary around it marking it off as a discrete entity. This boundary would be permeable, making it possible for the theory to link with other similar theories. Further, the boundary is not static, it is 'fluid' over time, making it possible for the content and scope of the theory to evolve and grow. For instance, a theory of adaptation may share some common concepts with a theory of change or a theory of transition. Similarly, as new findings about 'change' are discovered, these can be woven into the theory. Within the boundary of the theory are a number of concepts and what makes the theory work is that these concepts are joined together in pairs or other configurations forming propositions.

Propositions may have several different types of relationship. For instance, in Figure 1.1 there could be a contingent relationship within the proposition A, B, C such as 'if A then B but only in the presence of C' (Dickoff & James 1968). Translating this into a nursing context, it could mean that if you provide preoperative information (A), a patient would recover more quickly and with fewer postoperative complications (B), but only if the information was given by an experienced nurse (C). Similarly, the proposition could signify that if a person was encouraged to be self-caring (A), they would recover (B) but only if they were physically capable of being self-caring (C).

Other propositions within the same theory could have many different types of relationship. Take for instance the proposition between concepts D and E. The relationship could be:

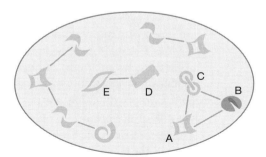

Figure 1.1 Diagrammatic representation of a theory

- a concurrent relationship – if D then also E
- a sequential relationship – if D then later E
- a deterministic relationships – if D then always E, if no interfering conditions
- a probabilistic (stochastic) relationships – if D then probably E.

Another way of conceptualizing a theory is to imagine it as a brick wall. On the wall, the bricks are the concepts and the cement between the bricks is the propositions. The more developed propositions are, the better able they are to define, explain and predict the nature of the relationship between concepts. **There is much written about testing theories but in reality it is the propositions that are tested; the entire theory is seldom tested.** For example, with Orem's theory (1980), a researcher may test what properties a self-care agent (a concept) needs to have to overcome a specific self-care deficit (a concept). Here, it is one proposition within Orem's theory that is being tested, not the whole theory.

Propositions are set up to be tested through research, often with the object of knocking them down. If a proposition survives the testing in a range of settings then it is considered robust, but only until the next testing. One way of viewing a proposition is as a paper boat. The boat is constructed and is tentatively pushed out into a pond to see if it floats. If it does then it has been successfully tested. It may float successfully many times but perhaps on the twentieth occasion a slight gust of wind sinks it. The paper boat has failed and it may be back to the drawing board where a new paper boat is constructed based on what was learned from the previous one. Regardless of whether the boat sinks or floats, learning has occurred and knowledge has increased.

Like a paper boat, a proposition is constructed and is tested and re-tested by research in different settings until it fails. By so doing the boundary of our knowledge base is extended. Therefore, 'theory + research = science' and science should underpin the evidence base for our clinical decisions, our teaching and our management. The important fact is that the cornerstones for all these endeavours are the concepts. Without concepts there would be no scientific body of knowledge and no evidence-based decision-making. Without concepts, there would be nothing for the proposition to link together. Returning to our metaphor, without concepts we have no bricks to build the wall; our raw materials are missing. So it is with theory construction; without the 'raw materials' – the concepts – as a scientific discipline we lack the theoretical raw materials that are necessary for theory construction.

Meleis (1991, p. 12) defined a concept as 'a label used to describe a phenomenon or a group of phenomena'. Therefore, a concept is not a real entity – it merely provides a name for a phenomenon and refers to the phenomenon's properties. Just as the concept 'home' conjures up in our minds the phenomena of being comfortable and secure, it is simply a label representing a range of pleasant phenomena. Concepts therefore are our special vocabulary denoting things, events and activities of importance to our occupation or our lives.

All professions have a number of core concepts that pertain to their work. For example, the concepts of importance to an architect include structure, material and design, while to a clergyman important concepts include devotion, prayer and forgiveness. Throughout their working day, nurses use concepts in a fairly 'cavalier' fashion. For instance, while they use the term 'caring' consistently, they may not have a common understanding of what that concept means. Similarly, comfort, empathy and dignity are some of the many other underlying elements of our discipline, yet nurses interpret them differently. Each day, to a greater or lesser extent, nurses think about or use the concepts featured within this text. More often than not, these concepts are used both implicitly (e.g. consideration of a client's dignity) and explicitly (e.g. maintaining a client's comfort as an outcome/aim of care in the care plan). The danger is, particularly in these days of evidence-based practice, that using such terms without a full understanding of the concept can result in practice that is ambiguous and unfocused. Therefore, it is incumbent upon practising nurses to understand what they mean when they attempt 'to promote a person's dignity', 'to form a therapeutic relationship', 'to be empathic' or 'to care'. Indeed, it is difficult to imagine any other health-related discipline arguing for a lack of conceptual clarity about the key concepts that underpin and inform its practice.

So far we have tried to illustrate how concepts are of central importance to our thinking and to our work as nurses. Because of this, it is incumbent upon us to strive to have a common understanding of these concepts. One way of achieving this is to undertake a concept analysis.

QUANTITATIVE APPROACHES TO CONCEPT ANALYSIS

Formal 'academic' approaches to concept analysis are relatively young; hence it is not entirely surprising that there remains much room for additional methodological development in this area. (We return to this point in Chapter 22.) However, examination of the relevant methodological and epistemological literature shows that there are several different ways to analyse a concept. Nonetheless, the approaches can be categorized as quantitative (Wilson 1969, Chinn & Kramer 1995, Walker & Avant 1995) or qualitative (Rodgers 1994, Morse 1995).

The quantitative approaches tend to involve a series of linear steps or stages. Invariably, these include:

1. Select the concept of interest
2. Clarify why analysis is required
3. Identify uses of the concept
4. Determining the defining attributes
5. Identify a model case
6. Identify alternative cases
7. Identify antecedents and consequences
8. Consider context and values
9. Identify empirical indicators.

We will briefly deal with each of these stages.

1. SELECT THE CONCEPT OF INTEREST

Many of the phenomena of relevance to nursing have already been given labels. For instance, nurses experience on a daily basis a phenomenon called empathy. They realize that much confusion exists around this concept; it is sometimes confused with sympathy. The nurse may decide that it is so important for her practice that she is determined to gain a deeper understanding of empathy through undertaking an analysis.

When selecting a concept to analyse there are three issues that should determine the choice of concept. First, the concept should interest you and be important for your practice. Second, there should be some confusion, lack of clarity or lack of consensus about the concept's meaning. Therefore, concept analyses are most often undertaken with abstract concepts such as comfort or trust rather than with more concrete concepts such as thermometer or computer. Third, you should avoid concepts that have a broad scope. It may be more straightforward to analyse concepts such as shame, humour or hope but it would be more difficult to analyse a concept as broad as communication.

2. CLARIFY WHY ANALYSIS IS REQUIRED

Nurses are busy people and even when they have to undertake concept analysis as part of an educational programme, they have little time to waste on meaningless concepts. Therefore, each concept analysis should be underpinned by a sound rationale. The justification could simply be to obtain greater clarity about an overused but little understood concept. Another justification may relate to an attempt to gain a more in-depth understanding of a concept from a theory (e.g. adaptation). It is also possible that a nurse may be undertaking research and needs to clarify a key concept within the study. For instance, a nurse who was researching loneliness among older people in rural areas would have a difficult task if they did not have a clear understanding of the concept of loneliness.

3. IDENTIFY USES OF THE CONCEPT

This step is normally the most interesting. It entails searching for meanings and examples of the concept in a wide variety of places. The first source is often a dictionary or a thesaurus. Further searching may lead you to explore meanings in the nursing literature, fictional literature, poetry, song, photographs, paintings and film. You could also enquire of colleagues, family and friends as to what is their understanding of the concept. It is also a good idea to see how theorists and researchers have used the concept. You should keep searching until you reach the stage where no new meanings are being uncovered. Once this step is complete you have a greater understanding of how the concept is used in a range of different settings. Whether or not you use all these sources will depend on the concept and the purpose of the analysis as identified in step 2.

4. DETERMINING THE DEFINING ATTRIBUTES

You should read all the uses identified in step 3 and note the particular characteristics of the concept that recur. These represent its hallmarks, or what Walker and Avant (1995) referred to as the 'defining attributes' of the concept. In essence, the defining attributes distinguish the concept from similar or related concepts. It is normal to have a number of defining attributes for any one concept. A note of caution: try not to add extra defining attributes just because you think your list is too short. The 'rule of thumb' is to identify only those attributes that really characterize the concept. (Examples of these attributes are given in many chapters in this book.)

5. IDENTIFY A MODEL CASE

The next step in the concept analysis process involves identifying a model case that represents all the defining attributes of the concept. Normally, a model case is a short story illustrating the concept. It is possible to construct a hypothetical model case but the best ones tend to be drawn from real-life examples. For example, Richmond and McKenna (1998) undertook a concept analysis of homophobia. After a comprehensive exploration of the uses of the concept (step 3) six defining attributes were identified (step 4); these were:

- heterosexuals' persistent dread of confrontation with homosexual individuals
- an overwhelming desire by heterosexuals to avoid physical contact/interaction with homosexual individuals
- heterosexuals' experience of revulsion and aversion when imagining/visualizing homosexual relationships
- preservation of negative/prejudicial attitudes by heterosexuals towards homosexuals
- experience of anxiety when heterosexuals are confronted with homosexuals
- homosexuals' experience of shame and guilt upon discovering their sexual orientation.

From these they constructed a model case (step 5) based on real-life experiences of homophobia.

> *John is admitted to a coronary care unit following an episode of chest pain. A younger male (Henry), who appears to have a very close relationship with John, accompanies him. Henry stays for a while and then goes to leave. He tells Kate (John's named nurse) that he will ring around lunchtime and call in to see John on his way home from work. Kate agrees to this arrangement, even though the ward does not allow visitors outside visiting times, and also says that they will contact Henry if there are any changes in John's condition.*

Upon Henry's departure, Kate says 'John you have a very loving and caring son', and John explains that Henry is his partner, not his son. Kate's attitude suddenly changes. She becomes very anxious about visiting times and suggests that special arrangements will have to be made for visiting. Kate quickly finishes admitting John and goes to the nurses' station and reports to the nursing staff that John is gay. She no longer refers to him by his name but calls him 'the queer man' and tells another nurse to make special arrangements for Henry to visit John, preferably while she is not on duty. Kate goes on to discuss with the nurses how disgusting, abnormal and perverted John must be and states that she will 'stay well clear of him'.

Later that morning John needs to use the bedpan. Kate states that she has been dreading him asking for the bedpan all morning and refuses to assist him. A student nurse says that she will assist him instead and Kate warns her to be very careful as 'he probably has AIDS'. The student apologies to John for the nurses' behaviour, but John says that this is the normal reaction he receives when people find out he is a homosexual. John also says that, although he finds such behaviour hurtful, he can understand it, as he had problems coming to terms with his own sexual orientation and experienced severe shame, guilt and even self-hatred when he discovered he was a homosexual.

(Richmond and McKenna 1998, p. 364)

In this model case all six defining attributes were included. Wilson (1969) maintained that with the model case the reader could say with absolute certainty that if this is not *X* (the concept) then nothing is. In Richmond and McKenna's example the model case reflects exactly what the concept is. There must be no contradictions between the model case and the defining attributes.

6. IDENTIFY ALTERNATIVE CASES

At this stage the person undertaking the concept analysis is beginning to get an understanding of what the concept is and how it is used. While the model case has done much to clarify the concept, Walker and Avant (1995) recommended that clarity could be enhanced further through identifying alternative cases. There are several types of alternative case.

- *Borderline case*: This example is very similar to a model case but some of the defining attributes are missing (e.g. empathy without concern).
- *Related case*: In such an example none of the defining attributes are included but the concept is still similar to the concept being analysed. For instance,

transition is related to change, the concept anxiety is related to burnout and adaptation to coping.

- *Contrary case*: This case does not represent the concept being analysed, and this would be obvious to most people. When examining the concept of caring, a contrary case would be an example of an interaction where a nurse or a midwife consciously harmed a client.
- *Invented case*: This represents a creative case that takes the concept out of its normal context and places it in an invented, out of the ordinary, situation. For instance, Martians floating on a cloud might be an example of the concept comfort.
- *Illegitimate case*: This type of case is a real-life example of the concept being used inappropriately for the purpose of the analysis. For example, if the concept being analysed was nursing, an illegitimate case could be a billiards game where the player nurses the white ball up against a red ball. Similarly, if the concept was attachment an illegitimate case could be an attachment for an electric drill.

7. IDENTIFY ANTECEDENTS AND CONSEQUENCES

When something occurs that prompts or stimulates a concept to be invoked, this a priori stimulation is called an antecedent. Conversely, consequences are those events that happen after the occurrence and as a result of the concept. For example, if the concept was loss, an antecedent might be a death in the family or unemployment. Consequences of loss might be sadness and depression. Identifying antecedents and consequences further clarifies the concept.

8. CONSIDER CONTEXT AND VALUES

Our perception of phenomena and concepts alters depending on the context and our values and beliefs. Concepts have different meanings for different people in different settings. For example, privacy in a hospital unit in England might be perceived differently from privacy in a community day hospital in China. Similarly, abortion is anathema to some societies but is acceptable in others. Some nurses may perceive self-care as a worthwhile goal whereas other nurses may perceive it as a disruptive influence in a well-managed clinical setting.

9. IDENTIFY EMPIRICAL INDICATORS

Empirical indicators sometimes get confused with defining attributes (step 4). However, they are very different – empirical indicators are explicit criteria to show that the concept exists. They can often take the form of measures. For instance, the patient satisfaction questionnaire of LaMonica et al (1986) is an empirical measure containing a number of indicators that, if present, would suggest the presence of patient satisfaction. Such indicators are useful in research and practice because they can provide criteria against which a concept can be measured. It is perhaps logical to intuit that empirical indicators would be easier to identify for concrete concepts than for abstract concepts. However, this is not always the case and many have been identified for abstract concepts such as empathy (Reynolds 2000) or hope (Herth 1992).

QUALITATIVE APPROACHES TO CONCEPT ANALYSIS

There have been many articles published where concepts have been analysed. In the main, most of these have employed the above approach or a version of that approach. One reason for this is that it is an easy stepwise recipe. However, critics have denigrated this approach. It is attributed to the logical positivist movement following the entity view of concepts. Here, concepts are character-ized by rigid boundaries and necessary conditions, which Clarke (1995) asserted is an attempt to permit control and replication. The approach is also perceived as being linear, too superficial and unable to achieve an in-depth understand-ing of the concept being analysed (Rodgers 1994). Rodgers (1994) and more recently Morse (1995) criticize the context stripping inherent in the positivist stance. They suggest that quantitative investigators who bring scientific equa-tions into human relationships inevitably demean them to the extent that human action is lost.

These criticisms have led to the development of qualitative methods for the analysis of concepts. The most common of these are those of Rodgers (1994) and Morse (1995). Rodgers (1989) in particular argues that Walker and Avant (1995) present a static view of the world where concepts do not change with time. In con-trast, she offers an 'evolutionary view' where the process of concept development is a dynamic cycle with three distinct influences: significance, use and application.

In 1989, and again in 1994, Rodgers highlighted the evolutionary nature of con-cepts and addressed current interest in valuing dynamism and interrelationships within reality. Here too critics have been active. They argue that Rodgers' approach is empirical in origin, uses reductionism to detect the constituents of the concept, simplifies the complexity of concept analysis and produces insignificant results (Maben & Macleod Clark 1995, Morse 1995).

Morse's (1995) six approaches to concept analysis are a departure from the stepwise approach adopted by most other authors. One of the main differences is that Morse used qualitative data from real-life situations, incidents and events in an inductive manner. She maintained that a comprehensive review of the lit-erature should be the first phase in concept analysis. This is similar to step 3 in the quantitative approach. However, what follows diverges significantly from the method recommended by Walker and Avant (1995) and Chinn and Kramer (1995). Depending on what is found in the literature, Morse recommends six dif-ferent strategies.

1. UNDERTAKE 'CONCEPT DEVELOPMENT' IF THE CONCEPT REMAINS UNCLEAR AFTER THE LITERATURE REVIEW

This strategy identifies an incident or event that is considered to be a perfect example of the concept. Unlike the 'model case' approach of Walker and Avant (1995), this has to be a real-life event or incident. By closely scrutinizing the example, it should be possible to extract the concept's key attributes. These attributes are then verified by applying them to other situations where the concept is thought to be important. If the attributes from the example do not hold true for these new situations then the analyst must return to the first phase and select another example. If the attributes do hold, then the additional information contributes to the concept analysis. While the attributes of the example may be seen in each of the new situations, they may not be in the same order or pattern. These variations should be identified, as this further develops the concept.

2. UNDERTAKE 'CONCEPT DELINEATION' IF THE LITERATURE REVIEW NOTES THAT THE CONCEPT IS SIMILAR TO ANOTHER

Within the English language there are many concepts that are similar to other concepts: transition – change, anger – rage, etc. According to Morse, when this occurs a literature review must be undertaken so that the two concepts can be separated in terms of meaning, attributes and differences and commonalties.

3. UNDERTAKE 'CONCEPT COMPARISON' IF THE LITERATURE REVIEW SUGGESTS NUMEROUS CONCEPTS TO DENOTE ONE PHENOMENON

When there are many competing concepts to explain a relatively underdeveloped phenomenon, these concepts should be identified and a literature review undertaken. The attributes for each competing concept should be described and compared and the limitations of each concept in explaining the phenomenon should be stated. The result of 'concept comparison' may indicate that, apart from some overlap, each of the concepts is unique. It may also show that none of the concepts, when used alone, accurately explain the phenomenon. A further outcome could be the identification of a need to undertake further research on the phenomenon.

4. UNDERTAKE 'CONCEPT CLARIFICATION' IF, AS A RESULT OF TOO MUCH LITERATURE ON THE TOPIC, THE CONCEPT APPEARS CONFUSING

Concepts such as caring and empathy have been the subject of much theorizing, research and description. This can often lead to confusion rather than clarity. Here, Morse calls again for a literature review to identify, describe and compare the attributes of the concept. This process of concept clarification can add significantly to the understanding of such overused concepts.

5. UNDERTAKE 'CONCEPT CORRECTION' IF THE CONCEPT AS FOUND IN THE LITERATURE DOES NOT ADEQUATELY EXPLAIN THE PHENOMENON

As stated at the outset of this chapter, being a relatively young discipline many of the concepts of importance to nursing have not been adequately explained. Furthermore, the concept as discussed in the literature may not do justice to the clinical phenomenon it is supposed to represent. Morse recommended that data are collected through interviews and observations and are examined for commonalties and differences between them and the concept that purports to represent them.

6. UNDERTAKE 'CONCEPT IDENTIFICATION' IF DATA EXIST FOR WHICH THERE IS NO APPROPRIATE CONCEPT IN THE LITERATURE

When nurses give their attention to what they believe to be a new clinical phenomenon they may label it as a concept. Through 'concept identification' Morse suggested that the nurse should undertake a comprehensive literature review to establish that the concept is indeed unique. This will allow them to identify the concept's attributes, establish if it is present in other contexts and explore its relationship to other related concepts.

Both qualitative and quantitative approaches to concept analysis have strengths and weaknesses. Positivists see their qualitative counterparts such as Rodgers as descriptive, soft and anecdotal (Clarke 1995). Further, and almost paradoxically, Rodgers relies on a model case as advocated by Wilson (1969). Some people may criticize concept analysis by saying that they knew all along what the term meant and that the exercise was futile. This is an erroneous assumption. With the many abstract concepts encountered in 'everyday use' and 'everyday nursing practice', not everyone knows their meaning or may not even share the same understanding of their meaning. **Concept analysis is an intellectual exercise that requires creative and critical thinking.**

CONCLUSION

Concept analysis has an important role to play in the development of nursing as a discipline. Concepts are the 'foundation blocks' of nursing knowledge and, if their characteristics are not well understood, the result will be confusion and conceptual disarray. The most common method for concept analysis emanates from Wilson's original work (1969) and entails a series of steps. More recently, critics have become disenchanted with this approach and called for a more qualitative approach to concept analysis. From the subsequent chapters, the reader will note the benefits from using (and hopefully understanding) a range of approaches to concept analysis.

Readers should be aware that the defining attributes of a concept may alter over time and different analyses on the same concept carried out by different people may produce different defining attributes. Therefore, concept analysis, while worthwhile, is often a tentative business. This key issue is returned to and discussed in detail in Chapter 22.

REFERENCES

Chinn PL, Kramer MK 1995 Theory and nursing: a systematic approach, 4th edn. CV Mosby, St Louis, MO

Clarke L 1995 Nursing research: science, visions and telling stories. Journal of Advanced Nursing 21: 584–593

Dickoff J, James P 1968 A theory of theories: a position paper. Nursing Research 17: 197–203

Herth K 1992 Abbreviated instrument to measure hope: development and psychometric evaluation. Journal of Advanced Nursing 17: 1251–1259

LaMonica EL, Oberst MT, Madea AR, Wolf RM 1986 Development of a patient satisfaction scale. Research in Nursing and Health 9: 43–50

Maben J, Macleod-Clarke J 1995 Health promotion: a concept analysis. Journal of Advanced Nursing 22: 1158–1165

Meleis AI 1985 Theoretical nursing: development and progress. JB Lippincott, Philadelphia, PA

Meleis AI 1991 Theoretical nursing: development and progress, 2nd edn. JB Lippincott, Philadelphia, PA

Morse JM 1995 Exploring the theoretical basis of nursing using advanced techniques of concept analysis. Advances in Nursing Science 17: 31–46

Orem DE 1958, 1980 Nursing: concepts of practice. McGraw-Hill, New York

Peplau HE 1952 Interpersonal relations in nursing. GP Putnam & Sons, New York

Reynolds W 2000 The development and measurement of empathy in nursing. Ashgate, Aldershot

Richmond J, McKenna HP 1998 Homophobia: an evolutionary analysis of the concept as applied to nursing. Journal of Advanced Nursing 23: 362–369

Rodgers BL 1989 Concepts, analysis and the development of nursing knowledge: the evolutionary cycle. Journal of Advanced Nursing 14: 330–335

Rodgers BL 1994 Concepts, analysis and the development of nursing knowledge: the evolutionary cycle. In: Smith JP (ed.) Models, theories and concepts. Blackwell Scientific, Oxford

Roy C 1970 Adaptation – a conceptual framework for nursing. Nursing Outlook 18: 42–45

Sullivan H 1953 The interpersonal theory of psychiatry. WW Norton, New York

Walker LO, Avant KC 1995 Strategies for theory construction in nursing, 3rd edn. Appleton & Lange, Norwalk, CT

Wilson J 1969 Thinking with concepts. Cambridge University Press, London

A concept analysis of abuse

Judee E. Onyskiw

EDITORIAL

All too often, and for a variety of reasons, the nursing care of people in need is limited to the immediate, the acute, the obvious and the observable. Yet as a discipline, nursing makes the claim that it is concerned with holism; moving beyond the immediate and the obvious.

Judee's chapter reminds us of a common underlying and pervasive problem – the concept of abuse. Thankfully, as Judee points out in her chapter, there is an increasing awareness of the holistic manifestations that ignored or 'untreated' abuse can create in the person and his interpersonal relationships. This phenomenon has been well documented in a range of people with various presenting mental-health problems (e.g. depression). Such manifestations, however, are by no means restricted to this population and, given the contemporary epidemiological evidence concerning the incidence of abuse, the likelihood is that all nurses will encounter former abuses at some point in their careers. We will not belabour the obvious need for nurses of all specialities to be conversant with the concept of abuse.

Having said that, this is not to make the case that every nurse must be prepared to help abused patients begin (and hopefully end) the hard work of dealing with their abused background. Such a position is clearly not only unrealistic but could also be counterproductive. In many clinical situations nurses simply would not have the time (or the skill base/experience) to engage in this interpersonal work. Furthermore, to deal with such issues needs to be the choice of the patients – not the nurse. Additionally, such issues often take a long time to address and it is likely to be harmful to the patient to 'open up' and then be unable to reach any sense of closure.

It is more a matter that nurses need to mindful of how previous experience(s) of abuse would be manifest in the present and how they might interfere with the current care/intervention. For example, difficulty with trusting people, problems with intimacy, transference and metaphors of the abuse are all matters that would have to be handled with sensitivity, compassion and tact.

INTRODUCTION

Woman abuse is a pervasive social problem and a global phenomenon. According to the World Health Organization (2002), there is no country, city or community that is immune to this social ill. In population-based surveys from various countries, 10–69% of women reported being physically abused by an intimate partner at some point in their lives. Abuse can affect any woman, irrespective of economic, educational, social, geographical or racial background, and it inevitably results in significant morbidity and mortality.

Nurses and other health providers have long cared for abused women, although they may not have always been aware that the women were abused. Nevertheless, a high proportion of their patients are women who have been or are currently being abused by their intimate partners. As a result of the abuse, women may seek care in hospital emergency departments for serious or life-threatening injuries (Dearwater et al 1998). Women also seek care in other health settings for a wide range of chronic symptoms related to the abuse. Health professionals have begun to realize the serious impact of abuse on women's health and to consider their critical role in the prevention and detection of abuse as well as in the treatment of women, their perpetrators and other family members.

Although the concept of abuse has been widely used in both the scholarly and lay literature, there is actually no clear agreement on how to define it (Cantin 1994, DeKeseredy 2000, Gelles 1980, 2000, Gordon 2000). This absence of agreement leaves the way open for additional questions such as: What does abuse really mean? When is someone considered abused? What behaviours are considered abusive? According to Fawcett (2000), abuse is a concept and a concept is merely a word or phrase that summarizes the essential characteristics or properties of a phenomenon. As a concept, abuse has been poorly defined, which suggests the need for additional conceptual consideration and subsequent analysis. Accordingly, the purpose of this chapter is to analyse the concept of abuse in an attempt to develop a clearer and more useful definition for nursing practice, research and policy. This definition is not meant to be definitive or absolute; rather it is to provide nurses with a better understanding of abuse so that they are more comfortable and competent suspecting, detecting, screening for and reporting abuse as well as intervening effectively with abused women and their perpetrators.

Although abuse can occur in most family relationships and there are similarities in these different forms of victimization, for the purposes of this chapter abuse will be confined to the abuse of women that occurs in the context of their intimate relationships. These include current, dissolving or past intimate relationships with husbands, common-law partners and boyfriends. The approach to concept analysis proposed by Walker and Avant (1995) is followed but not strictly adhered to. The historical foundation of the concept, its derivation and applications in other disciplines are examined. Dictionary and thesaurus sources, as well as selected nursing, sociology, psychology, legal and medical literature, are used to clarify the concept. A model case and additional cases are developed to facilitate understanding of abuse. Finally, the defining attributes, antecedents and consequences of abuse are presented.

EXAMINATION OF DEFINITIONS AND HISTORICAL PERSPECTIVES

DEFINITIONS

The word *abuse* was introduced into the English language during the 12th or 13th century and originated from either the English word *abusen* or the French word *abuser* (Hoad 1996). *Abuso* was a counterpart word in Spanish and Italian (Gove 1986). Another possible source for abuse was the Latin word *abusus*, which means 'wrong use'. *Abusus* is the past participle of *abuti*, which means using up, wasting or wearing out (Simpson 1959). From the Latin word *abusus* two English words were derived, *abuse* and an obsolete word *abusion*. *Abuse* meant to consume or to misuse, whereas *abusion* is defined as abuse of the truth, i.e. deception.

According to the *Concise Oxford Dictionary*, in present-day language abuse means 'to use to bad effect or for a bad purpose' (Pearsall 2001). Synonyms for abuse are maltreatment, mistreatment and misusage (Steinhardt et al 1980). Other terms are perversion, misapplication, degradation, desecration, injury, damage, harm, hurt, wrong, injustice, violation, malevolence, mishandling, mismanagement, pollution, defilement and prostitution (Laird 1974). Allen (1999), an experienced lexicographer, states that in the 20th century abuse developed a sinister, violent meaning, 'maltreatment or (especially sexual) assault of a person'. At the same time, the older meaning, 'misuse or improper use', has been greatly extended in explicit combinations such as alcohol abuse, drug abuse, heroin abuse, solvent abuse, steroid abuse, etc. Allen (1999) maintains that there are few developments in semantics that have such appalling social implications as these.

The *Dictionary of Psychology* (Coleman 2001) defines abuse in the context of spouses as 'any form of physical or mental exploitation or cruelty towards a husband or wife, causing significant harm to its victim'. **It is interesting to note that there are no entries in the *Dictionary of Nursing* (McFerran 2003), the *Concise Medical Dictionary* (Martin 2002) or the *Dictionary of Sociology* (Marshall 1998) for woman abuse, only for child abuse**. Allen (1999) asserts that abuse is most familiar in the context of children.

HISTORICAL PERSPECTIVE

A contextual assessment includes considering how the meaning of the concept has been shaped by dominant social institutions. To understand this contemporary social problem, it is necessary to understand the historical treatment of wives (Dobash & Dobash 1979). Wife abuse is neither a recent nor a rare phenomenon. It has been approved and sanctioned in our cultural, legal, political and religious traditions. Historically, men were the absolute and undisputed heads of the family; women and children were viewed as property. Norms of family privacy, coupled with the sensitive nature of the issue, prohibited public investigation and sanctioned the violence. Abuse has been legitimized by the role of women in society and cultural approval of the mistreatment of women.

There is evidence of wife abuse for centuries in literary works and historical accounts. For example, in Shakespeare's 16th-century play *The Taming of the Shrew*, Katharina is subjected to psychological abuse and physical deprivation in an effort to force her to conform to the standards of her husband, Petruchio. Petruchio refers to his wife as his goods and his chattel (act III, scene II; Shakespeare 1975). It is only current social values that would evaluate the treatment inflicted upon Katharina as abusive. It was not considered abusive then because it did not deviate from the customs prevailing in society at the time. Any concept analysis will reflect, at least in part, the contemporary views and customs regarding abuse.

While it is not surprising that social values have changed dramatically since the 16th century, social norms and values have continued to evolve even in the last century. The change in public tolerance to abuse is reflected in media of our times. For example, in the 1950s, 'The Honeymooners' was a popular comedy on television. Audiences roared when hot-headed, ill-tempered Ralph Kramden shook a fist at his wife issuing a threat to hit her 'right in the kisser' or 'send her to the moon'. It is debatable whether contemporary audiences would have the same reaction. By current social standards, this type of behaviour is less acceptable. Movies about abused women such as *The Burning Bed*, *Sleeping with the Enemy* and *Enough* suggest that there is less tolerance thesedays of abuse in intimate relationships.

The first form of violent behaviour in families to receive recognition, though, was not woman abuse but child abuse. Henry Kempe, a paediatrician, described the abuse as a clinical condition with physical symptoms and named it the 'battered child syndrome' (Kempe et al 1962). Abuse came to be defined by the physical effect on the victim. In spite of the considerable attention that Kempe drew from both the media and the scholarly community, it was still another 10 years before woman abuse was recognized. Feminists made woman abuse public when they called attention to the fact that most violence against women and children did not occur at the hands of strangers or in strange places but in families and at home where people ought to be safe. Their efforts transformed a problem that had been virtually ignored to one that demanded professional, public and policy attention (Yllo 1993). Thus, the static aspect of abuse is that it has existed for centuries and the evolutionary aspect is how society reacts to (and often) tolerates it. It is society that determines what is considered abuse and determines the extent that is tolerable (Campbell 1992). Society only considers actions to be abusive that deviate from current social norms.

The evolution of social norms is reflected in our legal system and in the past, the legal system reinforced an acceptance of woman abuse. There were few laws to discourage abuse, although some limits were imposed on abusive behaviour. For instance, the expression 'rule of thumb', derived from English common-law, was long part of Canadian and American law. This law allowed a husband to beat his wife with a rod that was no thicker than his thumb (Dobash & Dobash 1979). The legal system made a clear distinction between behaviour that threatened public safety and behaviour that occurred in private. Men as heads of households had the responsibility to punish and discipline their wives. Today, men do not have the right to beat their wives and women are no longer legally considered their husband's property. Physical and sexual abuse are criminal offences and are included in the Canadian Criminal Code (Government of Canada 1984).

REVIEW OF THE LITERATURE ON WOMAN ABUSE

Definitions of abuse in the research and lay literature vary widely (Campbell 2000, DeKeseredy 2000, Gelles 2000, Gelles & Straus 1988, Gordon 2000). In the early 1980s, Murray Straus and his colleagues at the University of New Hampshire influenced methodological approaches and terminology in 'violence' research when they conducted the first landmark study of violence in American families (Straus et al 1980). They used the term 'abusive violence' to refer to those acts of violence with a high probability of causing injury drawing attention to the fact that the violent action does not have to result in injury, only that the intent to harm is present. They differentiated 'abusive violence' from 'normal violence', which referred to acts that some people might include as acceptable in a relationship (i.e. grabbing, pushing and shoving). The amount considered acceptable is dependent on cultural values, leading to great variation about what is considered abuse

(Counts et al 1999, Gelles & Cornell 1985). Straus and his colleagues (1980) introduced the notion of a continuum of violent behaviour with abuse as one extreme on the continuum.

In the literature, abuse is still sometimes restricted to acts of physical violence ranging from relatively minor acts such as grabbing or pushing to severe acts that cause injury or death. An advantage of this approach is that it is easier to categorize certain discrete, episodic behaviours/events as abusive and therefore easier to measure. Reliance on specific acts of physical violence continues to be used in some research efforts, in hospital-based surveillance systems and in criminal justice surveillance systems (Gelles 2000). The criticism of this approach is that it identifies only the injurious events and fails to capture the chronicity of women's experience in abusive relationships (Smith et al 1999).

Other definitions of abuse are consistent with legal definitions of physical and sexual assault. For instance, a national survey in Canada (i.e. 1993 Violence Against Women Survey) assessed the prevalence of abuse using definitions that conformed to the criminal code (Johnson 1996). Other researchers and advocates include psychological and emotional abuse, recognizing that the physical or the sexual infliction of harm does not occur in isolation from a psychological component (Finkelhor 1983). Victims of abuse are made to feel worthless, incompetent, unlovable and insignificant. Some scholars acknowledge that psychological abuse often accompanies physical or sexual abuse but continue to define abuse in terms of physical or sexual harm, discerning that the physical safety of women takes priority over concerns of self-esteem and other psychological states (Stacey & Shupe 1983). Others conceptualize psychological abuse as an early warning sign of physical or sexual abuse or impending violence (Kelly 1994, Walker 1979). Indeed, Walker (1979) included emotional abuse as part of the tension building stage in her theory on the cycle of violence.

Other definitions of abuse include any act that is harmful to the victim (Campbell 2000, Gelles 2000). These definitions include actual or threatened physical or sexual abuse, psychological or emotional mistreatment, while other definitions include spiritual or economic deprivation. Some researchers maintain that by combining behaviours that are debatably abusive with what everyone agrees to be seriously abusive serves only to trivialize the latter (Gelles & Cornell 1985). However, from a health perspective this broader definition captures the full range of harm that can impact on women's physical, emotional and social well-being, and therefore is more humanistic and congruent with the holistic orientation of nursing.

THE LACK OF CONSENSUS ON A LABEL FOR ABUSE

In addition to the lack of consensus on what constitutes abuse, there are many different terms used to label the phenomena. These include wife abuse, wife assault, wife battering, spouse abuse, partner abuse, intimate partner violence, conjugal violence, domestic violence, interspousal violence, abusive violence and assaultive violence. Some terms (e.g. spouse abuse, partner abuse, interspousal violence and domestic violence) do not specify the gender of the abused. Efforts to define violence in gender-neutral terms insinuate that there is symmetry of violence perpetrated by men and women, when the overwhelming majority is men using violence against women (Dobash & Dobash 1992, Gelles 2000).

The words violence and abuse are sometimes used synonymously despite the fact that they are not conceptually equivalent (Gelles & Cornell 1985, Gelles 2000). Violence is an act of maltreatment carried out with the intention, or the perceived intention, of causing physical pain or injury to another person (Gelles 1990). It can be perpetrated in a single act. Abuse refers to physical, sexual, psychological or emotional mistreatment, and other controlling tactics such as economic or spiritual deprivation. Abuse begins in subtle forms that are often difficult to detect. There is usually an insidious pattern of abuse already occurring when violence happens (Campbell 2000). Abuse should be conceptualized not as specific acts of physical and sexual violence but rather as a *pattern of behaviour and experiences* used to achieve domination and control in the relationship (Campbell 2000, Campbell & Fishwick 1993, Dobash & Dobash 1979, 1992, Gordon 2000, MacLeod 1987, Walker 1979, Yllo 1993).

While the various terms used to label violence against women are not equivalent conceptually, they share an important, unifying feature. All terms carry strong emotive and visual associations and a powerful pejorative charge (Gelles & Cornell 1985). The concept of abuse, along with all the myriad labels applied to the phenomenon of violence against women, force one to conjure up mental images that provoke strong emotion. Perhaps this is the reason they are used interchangeably, rather than their definitive precision or their conceptual equality.

The lack of agreement on a definition for abuse has been a significant and enduring problem in the field and the cause of considerable debate. Defining abuse is not an exact science but a matter of judgement. There are different conceptions of what constitutes 'appropriate behaviour' in families and what constitutes harm. These conceptions are culturally influenced and change as values and social norms change and evolve over time (World Health Organization 2002). Definitions also vary depending on the purpose. A definition for research purposes may be different from one for nursing, social service or police intervention, further clouding the issue. The lack of consensus is a contentious issue and has serious implications for describing the nature of violence against women, assessing its prevalence in society, comparing across countries and communities, and in formulating research efforts.

ATTRIBUTES OF ABUSE

Attributes are defining characteristics or salient features that help define and differentiate the phenomenon from other similar or related concepts (Walker & Avant 1995). The defining attributes may change as our understanding of the concept improves, and may change over time if the concept changes.

One critical attribute of abuse (in the context of woman abuse) is that it involves some form of mistreatment or harm that compromises a woman's well-being. Abuse can include, but is not limited to, physical, sexual, psychological, spiritual or financial abuse. **Further, the abuse occurs within the context of an intimate relationship between the abuser and the victim**. The relationship may be a current one, a past one or one in the process of dissolving, but at some point in time there was an emotional bond and sexual intimacy. **Intimacy implies trust and abuse is a betrayal of that trust.**

Another essential attribute is the intent to cause harm. Abuse is meant to connote acts that are intended to cause harm by the offender or are perceived to cause harm by the victim. Whether or not the action results in injury is irrelevant, if maleficent intentions are present. This aspect is of particular significance because it means that actions that do not result in physical injury can still be considered abusive. To illustrate the point, if a husband fires a gun at his wife but misses her because his aim is poor, it is still abuse. He had every intention of causing harm.

Implicit in all forms of violence against women is the notion of power, domination and control (Campbell 1992, Dobash & Dobash 1979, Walker 1979, Yllo 1993). Typically, abusers attempt to dominate and control by engaging in actions that threaten or harm women's physical or emotional well-being, sexuality, social life, parenting ability, financial situations, possessions or spiritual life (Campbell 2000). Women's subordination is secured when they become fearful of future abuse, and alter their behaviour to avoid negative reprisals from their abusive partner (Stark & Flitcraft 1996). Abuse is also seen as a response to perceived powerlessness. The abuser perceives that he is powerless and attempts to compensate for this lack or loss of power (Finkelhor 1983). This is the irony of abuse.

In summary, the attributes of abuse are as follows.

- abuse involves physical, sexual or psychological mistreatment and/or economic or spiritual deprivation
- abuse includes the intention or perceived intention of causing harm
- abuse occurs within the context of an intimate relationship
- abuse is intended to achieve domination and control.

CASE EXAMPLES

A MODEL CASE

Walker and Avant (1995) assert that a model case is an example that includes all the critical attributes of the concept. As such, it is a paradigmatic example (Walker & Avant 1995). The story of Anna provides an excellent example of abuse.

Case study

> Mark and Anna have been living together for 6 years. Over the years, Mark has become very controlling and possessive. He chooses Anna's clothes and her hairstyle. He imposes rigid schedules for her to follow – dinner has to be served precisely at 6 o'clock – the children have to be in bed by 8 o'clock. He is obsessive about knowing every detail of her day, even minor ones. Because she talked with a stranger at the grocery store, he got angry and struck her with enough force that she fell and chipped her tooth. He continued to beat her and threatened to hurt her worse 'the next time' it happened. She cried and begged him to stop. Although she wanted to explain the innocence of her talking with the man at the grocery store, she has learned that this only seems to make him more violent. Although Anna is afraid of living with Mark, she is even more afraid of leaving him. She knows he will seriously hurt her or the children when he finds them.

This model case is an unambiguous example of abuse. There is both psychological and physical harm being inflicted. The intent is clearly malicious. The abuse is purposeful behaviour designed to dominate and control.

A BORDERLINE CASE

Walker and Avant (1995) purport that a borderline case may contain some of the critical attributes but other important attributes are missing. It is a case that is inconsistent in some way and therefore highly debatable but used to promote further understanding of the concept under study. The following is an example of a borderline case.

Case study

> Pat and Bob have been married for 11 years. Bob is very traditional in his thinking about roles for women. He is proud that he is the provider and does not want Pat to work outside the home. He pays all the household bills and gives Pat money for household expenses. Although Bob gives her the same amount that he gave her when they were first married, he believes it is enough. Pat knows it is never enough and has to deny herself and the children things that she considers important. When Pat asks for more money, she is told to be more frugal. Although Bob earns a good salary he wants to save as much as they can for their future or for 'a rainy day'. Pat has secretly earned some extra money sewing clothes for other people. She is worried that Bob will find out because he would be upset to learn that she is working.

In this scenario, it can be argued that Pat is economically deprived. It seems clear that the amount of money that she is given for household expenses is unrealistic. Yet, there does not appear to be any malicious intent. Bob is frugal himself. He is restricting money in an effort to save for their future and for things that will ultimately benefit the family, not as a strategy to dominate and control his wife.

A RELATED CASE

Walker and Avant (1995) declare that related cases are similar and in some way connected to the concept being analysed. They help understanding of how a concept fits into the network of concepts surrounding it. Accordingly, here I draw upon the concept of aggression as it is related to abuse.

Case study

Mary decides to return to university to obtain a business degree now that her children are in school. Her husband, Don, overtly commends her for her ambition. Yet, he does not really want her to return to university. He does not have a degree and secretly worries what this will mean to their relationship. He has always made the family decisions and he likes this authority. Mary returns to school but finds many demands on her time. She continues to assume all responsibility for the children and household chores. Her husband continues to make demands on her, insisting that they continue to entertain as they have in the past and often inviting people over when she is studying for exams. He makes her feel guilty about the added expense that a university education entails even though they can afford it. When there is a problem with the children, he blames her for not properly caring for them. After the first year Mary quits university, feeling that it would be better if she spends more time at home.

This is a subtle example of aggression. Aggression is getting what is wanted at the expense of others (Campbell & Fishwick 1993). The husband uses manipulation to achieve what he really wants, a wife who stays at home. He is controlling her, although his methods are subtle and sophisticated. It is not known if his intentions are even conscious. He does not overtly dominate and control his wife but his behaviour is a subtle attempt to sabotage her efforts and control her. This situation is not abuse but is related.

A CONTRARY CASE

According to Walker and Avant (1995), contrary cases are often helpful because it is sometimes easier to demonstrate what the concept is not. The following scenario illustrates a case which is clearly not abuse.

Case study

Claire and Cliff have an egalitarian marriage, sharing household responsibilities, finances and decision-making. Their eldest son, Richard, has been accepted at two universities but is having trouble deciding which university to attend. Since cost is a considerable factor and his parents will be paying, he leaves the final decision to them. Cliff feels strongly about his son attending the university he himself attended. Claire feels that he should attend the university that she attended. They have a lengthy discussion, with each person presenting the factors they consider important in choosing a uni-

Case study—*cont'd*

> versity as well as the financial implications. They discuss the advantages and disadvantages of each university, and all possible alternatives, and together they reach a consensus.

This is a contrary case. There are no attributes of abuse present with the exception that it involves an intimate relationship. Although the couple had a disagreement they used healthy conflict resolution strategies to resolve their disagreement.

AN ILLEGITIMATE CASE

Walker and Avant (1995) assert that an illegitimate case is sometimes included in a concept analysis to illustrate the improper use of a concept. In the following case, the term is used incorrectly in relation to its generally accepted meaning.

Case study

> Ron and Marion have been living together for 8 years. They are driving home late one evening when their car gets a flat tyre. Ron tries to loosen the nuts to change the tyre while Marion shines a flashlight so he can see. Because the nuts are rusty, Ron needs considerable force to loosen them. The spanner suddenly slips and hits Marion on the jaw, fracturing it.

This case includes the attribute of physical mistreatment and it occurs within the context of an intimate relationship; however, the action is accidental, not intentional. This is not abuse and to use the term would be to use it improperly.

ANTECEDENTS AND CONSEQUENCES OF ABUSE

ANTECEDENTS OF ABUSE

Walker and Avant (1995) describe antecedents as behaviours or conditions that must occur before the concept can occur. Identifying such behaviours or conditions that precede abuse is a challenging and daunting task. Abuse is a complex and multifaceted problem that is conceptualized as a violation of human rights, as a social problem and, most recently, as a serious health issue. Several decades of research devoted to understanding and explaining the nature of abuse have led to a multiplicity of explanations for abuse focusing on psychological, sociological and feminist explanations. Explanations with a psychological focus stress individual characteristics of offenders such as certain psychological traits (i.e. low self-esteem), psychological pathology (e.g. substance abuse), exposure to abuse during childhood and certain demographic variables (e.g. low socioeconomic status and education level). Other explanations focus on dysfunction on the marital dyad or the family unit implicating factors such as the way the family unit is organized (e.g. male dominated versus equality between partners), marital satisfaction and communication, family functioning and social isolation. Abusers often prevent women from having contact with family, friends and community, which results in the women losing potential sources of support. This increases women's dependency on the abuser and places women at increased risk for abuse (Dobash & Dobash 1979).

Other explanations focus on societal-level variables such as the social structures and conditions in society that support and sustain abuse, and provide fertile ground for abuse to occur. For example, the socialization of men to have rigid expectations of gender-specific roles, to adopt aggressive and dominant behaviours in interpersonal interactions, and to have attitudes justifying male privilege and domination over women are conditions that contribute to abuse (Gordon 2000). In a patriarchal society, men have special privileges afforded them on the basis of gender that result in men having higher status and authority, in the devaluation and oppression of women and in gender inequality (Code 1993). Notions of oppression, power and gender are central to understanding abuse; structural inequalities due to differences in race and class further contribute to women's oppression (Varcoe 1996).

CONSEQUENCES OF ABUSE

For some women, the consequences of abuse are fatal. In a typical year in Canada, 120 women are killed by their partners or ex-partners (Johnson 1996). For other women, abuse has grave consequences for physical, emotional and social health and well-being (Campbell 2000). Physical injuries range from bruises to permanent disability (Canadian Advisory Council on the Status of Women 1991). In addition to the acute injuries (e.g. fractures, lacerations and internal injuries), women often suffer chronic health problems such as gastrointestinal problems, musculoskeletal pain, headaches, hypertension, irritable bowel syndrome, palpitations and substance abuse. Women who are sexually abused have more chronic pelvic, genital and uterine pain, infections and bruising or tearing of the vagina or anus, as well as frequent and/or unintended pregnancies and sexually transmitted diseases.

Despite the severity of physical injuries and health problems, women often report that the psychological abuse is more difficult to cope with (Campbell 2000). Living with emotional tension, chronic stress, humiliation, degradation and fear leave women with a poor self-image, low self-esteem and low self-worth (Dobash & Dobash 1992, Walker 1979). Psychological effects include fearfulness, acute anxiety, sleeping problems, memory loss and post-traumatic stress disorder. However, the most common mental health response to abuse is depression (Campbell et al 1996). Some women use alcohol or drugs to cope with the abuse, which leads to further health problems. In addition to the health problems, abuse affects other aspects of women's lives such as their ability to work, their relationship with their children, other family members and friends.

There are implications for the children living in violent homes. Children exposed to abuse have similar problems to children who are themselves physically abused. They have more social, emotional and behavioural problems, as well as school-related difficulties than non-exposed children (see Mohr et al 2000, Onyskiw 2003, Wolak & Finkelhor 1998 for recent reviews). Children exposed to violence in their families (not necessarily woman abuse) have lower health status and more conditions or health problems that limited their participation in normal age-related activities than children in non-violent families (Onyskiw 2002).

Children are often inadvertently injured during the abusive episodes and frequently they also are victimized. Woman abuse and child abuse are clearly linked within families (Appel & Holden 1998, Ross 1996). The percentage of overlap ranges from 20% to 100% with a median rate of 40% reported in clinical samples of abused women or children. These children are at risk of repeating the abusive dynamics in their own adult lives (Egeland 1993, Wolak & Finkelhor 1998).

Finally, woman abuse has profound ramifications for all of society. In Canada, the costs associated with woman abuse were estimated at $4.2 billion annually in social services, education, criminal justice, labour and employment as well as health and medical costs (Handivsky & Greaves 1996).

EMPIRICAL REFERENTS

According to Walker and Avant (1995) the final step of a concept analysis is to identify empirical referents. Once identified, empirical referents are meant to provide clear, observable, measurable and verifiable means to measure woman abuse for practice or research purposes. The nature of abuse, although broadly conceptualized as it is in this analysis to include various acts of maltreatment that are intended to cause harm by the abuser or are perceived to cause harm by the victim, seriously complicates measurement efforts. Not all the attributes of abuse identified lend themselves easily to observable, measurable and verifiable phenomena. For example, what indicators measure intent? What indicators could be used to determine if the context for abuse was to dominate and control?

Measuring abuse has long been controversial and hotly debated. The Conflict Tactics Scale (CTS) developed by Straus and his colleagues (1980) to measure reasoning, verbal aggression and physical violence experienced in conflict is the most widely used measure of abuse. Despite its widespread use, it has been seriously criticized for its deficiencies, particularly that it is gender neutral, does not differentiate the severity of certain acts of violence, lacks items to assess sexual abuse and assumes that abuse occurs in the context of conflict (Yllo 1993). Straus and his colleagues attempted to address some criticisms in their revised version of the CTS (Straus et al 1996). Nevertheless, the instrument still assumes that abuse occurs in the context of conflict thereby overlooking the broader social forces that motivate some men to victimize their female partners (Yllo 1993). Smith and her colleagues (1999) discuss how the current approach to conceptualizing and measuring abuse has been inadequate and has hampered knowledge development in violence research. One strategy, long recommended, is to use multiple measures as a method of enhancing the reliability and validity of social variables (Schwartz 2000). In addition, qualitative studies are needed to capture the nuances and subtleties and shed light on contextual issues (Johnson 1996, Smith et al 1999).

To identify abused women in the clinical setting, the Nursing Research Consortium on Violence and Abuse designed the Abuse Assessment Screen (AAS; Parker & McFarlane 1991). This instrument consists of questions to assess the frequency, severity, perpetrator, and the body site of injury that occur within a stated period of time. The AAS was effective in detecting abuse in an ethnically diverse population of women (Soeken et al 1998).

CONCLUSION

There are striking disagreements among authors about definitions of abuse and, more importantly, the values and connotations attached to them. However, abuse is a difficult concept to define because it is dependent on different conceptions of what is considered appropriate behaviour in intimate relationships, what constitutes harm and what purpose the definition serves. Following a critical analysis of the literature, abuse is defined in the context of the woman, as physical, psychological or sexual mistreatment and/or other controlling behaviours such as economic or spiritual deprivation, that are intended by the abuser to cause harm or are perceived by the victim to cause harm. It is purposeful behaviour designed to achieve domination and control in the relationship.

The definition of abuse is offered so that nurses in various health settings will have a clearer understanding of woman abuse in order to identify, detect and assist abused women and to be able to contribute more fully to the interdisciplinary response to violence and abuse. At the same time, a caveat is in order. The definition, given here, is offered in light of current understanding, but abuse like other concepts is not a static entity. Concepts change and evolve over time. Walker and Avant (1995) warn us that the best one can hope for is to capture the critical elements of a concept at the current moment in time. Indeed, our understanding of abuse will change as new insight is gained through research and scholarly discussion. This concept analysis provides the basis for future discussion; the insight and criticisms of others will expand and elucidate the concept further.

REFERENCES

Allen R 1999 Pocket Fowler's modern English usage. Oxford University Press, New York
Appel AE, Holden GW 1998 The co-occurrence of spouse and physical child abuse: a review and appraisal. Journal of Family Psychology 12: 578–599

Campbell JC 1992 Wife-battering: cultural contexts versus western social sciences. In: Counts DA, Brown JK, Campbell JC (eds) Sanctions and sanctuary: cultural perspectives on the beating of wives. Westview Press, Oxford

Campbell JC 2000 Promise and perils of surveillance in addressing violence against women. Violence Against Women 6: 705–727

Campbell J, Fishwick N 1993 Abuse of female partners. In: Campbell JC, Humphreys J (eds) Nursing care of victims of family violence, 2nd edn. Mosby, St Louis, MO, pp. 68–104

Campbell J, Kub J, Rose L 1996 Depression in battered women. Journal of the American Medical Women's Association 51: 106–110

Canadian Advisory Council on the Status of Women 1991 Male violence against women: the brutal face of inequality: a brief to the House of Common subcommittee on the status of women (Publication No. 91–S–175). Canadian Advisory Council on the Status of Women, Ottawa

Cantin S 1994 Is there an abuse in the way violence against women is defined and measured? Available on line at: http://www.asca-caah.ca/pdf/ang/abuseinwayviolencewomen.pdf (retrieved January 2004) (Translated from Informell 4, March 1994)

Code L 1993 Feminist theory. In: Burt S, Code L, Dorney S (eds) Changing patterns: women in Canada, 2nd edn. McClelland & Steward, Toronto, pp. 19–58

Coleman AM 2001 A dictionary of psychology. Oxford University Press, Oxford

Counts DA, Brown JK, Campbell JC (eds) 1999 To have and to hit: cultural analysis of the beating of wives. University of Illinois, Bloomington, IL

Dearwater SR, Coben JH, Campbell JC et al 1998 Prevalence of intimate partner abuse in women treated at community hospital emergency departments. Journal of the American Medical Association 280: 433–438

DeKeseredy WS 2000 Current controversies on defining non-lethal violence against women in intimate heterosexual relationships. Violence Against Women 6: 728–746

Dobash RE, Dobash R 1979 Violence against wives: a case against the patriarchy. Free Press, New York

Dobash RE, Dobash R (eds) 1992 Rethinking violence against women. Sage, London

Egeland B 1993 A history of abuse is a major risk factor for abusing the next generation. In: Gelles R, Loseke DR (eds) Current controversies on family violence. Sage, London, pp. 197–208

Fawcett J 2000 Analysis and evaluation of contemporary nursing knowledge: nursing models and theories. FA Davis, Philadelphia, PA

Finkelhor D 1983 Common features of family abuse. In: Finkelhor D, Gelles RJ, Hotaling GT, Straus MA (eds) The dark side of families: current family violence research. Sage, Beverly Hills, CA, pp. 17–28

Gelles RJ 1980 Violence in the family: a review of research in the seventies. Journal of Marriage and the Family 42: 873–885

Gelles RJ 1990 Methodological issues in the study of family violence. In: Straus MA, Gelles RJ (eds) 1990 Physical violence in American families transaction. New Brunswick, NJ, pp. 17– 28

Gelles RJ 2000 Estimating the incidence and prevalence of violence against women. Violence Against Women 6: 784–804

Gelles RJ, Cornell CP 1985 Intimate violence in families. Sage, Beverly Hills, CA

Gelles RJ, Straus MA 1988 Intimate violence. Simon & Schuster, New York

Gordon M 2000 Definitional issues in violence against women: surveillance research from a violence research perspective. Violence Against Women 6: 747–783

Gove PB 1986 Webster's third new international dictionary of the English language: unabridged. Warner, Springfield, MA

Government of Canada 1984 Law Reform Commission of Canada: working paper 38: Assault. Government of Canada, Ottawa

Handivsky O, Greaves L 1996 The costs of violence: another piece of the puzzle. Vis-à-vis 13

Hoad TF (ed.) 1996 The concise oxford dictionary of English etymology. Oxford University Press, Oxford

Johnson H 1996 Dangerous domains: violence against women in Canada. Nelson, Toronto

Kelly KD 1994 The politics of data. Canadian Journal of Sociology 19: 81–85

Kempe CH, Silverman FN, Steel B, Droegemueller W, Silver HK 1962 The battered child syndrome. Journal of the American Medical Association 181: 17–24

Laird C 1974 Webster's new world thesaurus. Warner Books, New York

McFerran TA (ed.) 2003 A dictionary of nursing, 4th edn. Oxford University Press, Oxford

MacLeod L 1987 Battered but not beaten: preventing wife battering in Canada. Canadian Advisory Council on the Status of Women, Ottawa

Marshall G (ed.) 1998 A dictionary of sociology, 2nd edn. Oxford University Press, New York

Martin EA 2002 Concise medical dictionary, 6th edn. Oxford University Press, Oxford

Mohr WK, Noone-Lutz MJ, Fantuzzo JW, Perry MA 2000 Children exposed to family violence: a review of empirical research from a developmental-ecological perspective. Trauma, Violence, and Abuse 1: 264–283

Onyskiw JE 2002 Health and the use of health services of children exposed to violence in their families. Canadian Journal of Public Health 6: 416–420

Onyskiw JE 2003 Domestic violence and children's adjustment: a review of research. Journal of Emotional Abuse 3: 11–45

Parker B, McFarlane J 1991 Nursing assessment of the battered pregnant woman. Maternity Child Nursing Journal 16: 161–164

Pearsall J (ed) 2001 The concise Oxford dictionary. Oxford University Press, New York

Ross SM 1996 Risk of physical abuse to children of spouse abusing parents. Child Abuse and Neglect 20: 589–598

Schwartz MD 2000 Methodological issues in the use of survey data for measuring and characterizing of violence against women. Violence Against Women 6: 815–838

Shakespeare W 1975 The complete works of William Shakespeare. Avenel Books, New York

Simpson DP 1959 Cassell's Latin English: English Latin dictionary. Cassell & Co., London

Smith PH, Smith JB, Earp JL 1999 Beyond the measurement trap: a reconstructed conceptualization and measurement of women battering. Psychology of Women Quarterly 23: 177–193

Soeken KL, McFarlane J, Parker B, Lominack MC 1998 The abuse assessment screen. A clinical instrument to measure frequency, severity, and perpetrator of abuse against women. In: Campbell J (ed.) Empowering survivors of abuse: health care for women international. Sage, London, pp. 195–203

Stacey W, Shupe A 1983 The family secret: domestic violence in America. Beacon Press, Boston, MA

Stark E, Flitcraft A 1996 Woman at risk: domestic violence and women's health. Sage, Thousand Oaks, CA

Steinhardt A, Soukhanov A, Harris D, Boyer M 1980 Roget's II: The new thesaurus. Houghton Mifflin, Boston, MA

Straus MA, Gelles RJ, Steinmetz SK 1980 Behind closed doors: violence in the American family. Anchor Books, New York

Straus MA, Hamby SL, Boney-McCoy S, Sugarman DB 1996 The Revised Conflict Tactics Scale: development and preliminary psychometric data. Journal of Family Issues 17: 283–316

Varcoe C 1996 Theorizing oppression: implications for nursing research on violence against women. Canadian Journal of Nursing Research 28: 61 –78

Walker LE 1979 The battered woman. Harper & Row, New York

Walker LO, Avant KC 1995 Strategies for theory construction in nursing, 3rd edn. Appleton & Lange, Norwalk, CT

Wolak J, Finkelhor D 1998 Children exposed to partner violence. In: Jasinski JL, Williams LM (eds) Partner violence: a comprehensive review of 20 years of research. Sage, Thousand Oaks, CA, pp. 73–111

World Health Organization 2002 World report on violence and health. WHO, Geneva

Yllo KA 1993 Through a feminist lens: gender, power, and violence. In: Gelles RJ, Loseke DR (eds) Current controversies on family violence. Sage, London, pp. 47–62

A concept analysis of caring

Tanya McCance

EDITORIAL

In many a discourse on the nature of nursing, on what it is to be a nurse and on the defining attributes of the practice of nursing, the concept of care (and caring) features with conspicuous regularity. Tanya's chapter, not surprisingly then, reminds us of the centrality of care to nursing, as this is a 'finding' that reoccurs throughout the empirical and theoretical literature on caring. Tanya's chapter further reminds us that, despite the commonalities in these 'findings', these analyses serve as a heuristic and do not provide the definite answer to the question: What is caring?

Interestingly, an examination of the etymology of the word 'nursing' adds support to the link between nursing and caring. The word is derived from the old French word meaning 'to nourish' and was synonymous with a mother nourishing her infant. Consequently, the palpable relationship and similarity between the practices of nurturing an infant and providing care for/with patients is once more ushered into our consciousness and our subsequent conceptualizations. As a result we are reminded that the roots of nursing can be located in what was (is?), rightly or wrongly, historically regarded as an activity of women (the nurturing and nourishment of an infant).

While we have neither the space nor the scope within this book for a thorough examination of the ramifications of the association between nursing and 'women's work', several key issues emerge. In a world dominated and driven by 'masculine' values, thinking and practice, where 'masculine traits' are valued more highly than 'feminine traits', it should be little surprise that a discipline synonymous with 'women's work' is given little esteem and regard. In healthcare systems driven by 'masculine ideology' it should not be a revelation that nursing is valued less than other, more 'masculine' professions. Similarly, in their perpetual endeavour to achieve equality with their medical colleagues, some nurses can be seen to be turning their backs on their raison d'être, their association with providing care, and acquiring additional status and esteem by becoming nurse/medic hybrids (see, for example, the discourses around the creation of nurse practitioners and the introduction of nurse prescribing).

INTRODUCTION

Caring is a difficult concept to define and the consequent lack of an acceptable definition has been a common theme within the caring literature. Publications dating back to the 1970s identified the problem of obtaining a clear and concise definition of caring and this remained constant during the 1980s, the 1990s and indeed into the 2000s (McFarlane 1976, Watson 1979, Leininger 1981, Morrison 1991, Kyle 1995, Webb 1996, Stockdale & Warelow 2000, Scotto 2003). This is despite the existence of an existing and evolving theoretical base, with key nurse theorists making a significant contribution to nursing knowledge (Roach 1984, 1987, Watson 1985, Leininger 1991, Boykin & Schoenhofer 1993) and a growing number of concept analyses aimed at clarifying the concept within the context of nursing (Morse et al 1990, Buchanan & Ross 1995, Eyles 1995, McCance et al 1997, Sourial 1997). In his own particular style, Paley (2001) levelled heavy criticism at the knowledge development represented within the caring literature for this very reason. He argued that, despite repeated efforts to define caring in nursing, we seem to be no closer to gaining clarification of caring as a concept. Within this chapter the maturity of caring as a concept will be explored, followed by the presentation of a completed concept analysis using the approach developed by Walker and Avant (1995). The concluding section will demonstrate how this preliminary work is being built upon through further research.

CONCEPT DEVELOPMENT AND MATURITY

The lack of a universally accepted definition of caring speaks to the level of maturity of the concept. Morse et al (1996b) describe the maturity of a concept in relation to its anatomy as comprising:

- a definition
- characteristics or attributes that distinguish one concept from another
- boundaries that provide delineation for that concept
- preconditions that identify the similar conditions giving rise to the behaviours that distinguish the concept
- outcomes resulting from the concept.

According to Morse et al (1996b, p. 387) the level of maturity of a concept reflects the degree to which these features have been met and hence Morse et al define a 'mature' concept as that which 'is well-defined, has clearly described characteristics, delineated boundaries, and documented pre-conditions and outcomes'. Concept maturity can be examined and evaluated using the following principles:

- *Epistemological principle*: Is the concept clearly defined and well differentiated from other concepts?
- *Pragmatical principle*: Does the concept fit with the phenomena common to the discipline? Is it useful to the discipline?
- *Linguistical principle*: Is the concept used consistently, appropriately and within context?
- *Logical principle*: Does the concept hold its boundaries through theoretical integration with other concepts? (Morse et al 2002, p. 8).

Applying each of these principles to the concept of caring, one would have to conclude that it is not a mature concept. For example, the point has already been made in the introductory section that it lacks a universally accepted definition. Similarly, the semantic aspects of the concept have been the focus of a number of early analyses on caring (Gaut 1983, Griffin 1983, Blustein 1991), all of which have highlighted several meanings for the term 'caring'; a point also made in a recent article by Stockdale and Warelow (2000). The usefulness of caring as a concept for nursing has also been the subject of much debate, as has its fit with other concepts such as comfort (Morse 1992) and support (O'Berle & Davies 1992).

An alternative view would suggest that, given the complexity of the concept, conceptual differences regarding caring are inevitable. These differences can enrich, yet also complicate, understandings about caring. This debate is explored more fully in Chapter 22.

One could therefore conclude that caring is a concept that could be described as partially developed. This level of maturity, according to Morse et al (2002), has the following characteristics: multiple competing definitions and competing concepts; partial fit with phenomena and partially operationalized; partially linked to context; and has begun to establish linkages with other concepts. However, it is accepted that concepts are refined over time and exist at various levels of development before becoming 'mature'. The evolutionary nature of concept development has been highlighted by Rodgers (2000, p. 82), who comments that 'concepts must be continually refined and variations introduced to achieve a clearer and more useful repertoire'.

Concept analysis is a broad term that refers to 'the process of unfolding, exploring, and understanding concepts for the purposes of concept development, delineation, comparison, clarification, correction, identification, refinement, and validation' (Morse et al 1996a p. 255). Various approaches to concept analysis have been described in the literature. The concept analysis of caring presented in this chapter uses the approach advocated by Walker and Avant (1995) – a Wilson-derived method, i.e. based on the approach initially developed by Wilson (1969). It should be highlighted, however, that Walker and Avant's (1995) approach has been subject to heavy criticism because of its linear approach, positivistic nature and oversimplistic procedures (Morse 1995, Morse et al 1996a). Nevertheless, it should be acknowledged that this is a well-tried and tested approach to concept development, evidenced by the number of concept analyses published in the nursing literature that have used this method.

A CONCEPT ANALYSIS OF CARING

The steps involved in a concept analysis, as described by Walker and Avant (1995, p. 37) are as follows:

1. Select a concept
2. Determine the aims or purposes of the analysis
3. Identify all uses of the concept that you can discover
4. Determine the defining attributes
5. Construct a model case
6. Construct borderline, related, contrary, invented and illegitimate cases
7. Identify antecedents and consequences
8. Define empirical referents.

In relation to this chapter, the selection of the concept (step 1) and the purposes for carrying out the analysis (step 2) were predetermined in that research regarding the concept of caring in nursing practice was ongoing. The remaining steps 3–8 will be discussed in turn.

STAGE 3: IDENTIFY ALL USES OF THE CONCEPT

This step involves the identification of as many uses of the concept as possible. According to Walker and Avant (1995), the various sources that can be used include dictionaries, thesauruses, available literature and discussion with colleagues.

Dictionary definitions

The sixth edition of the *Concise Oxford Dictionary* (Sykes 1976) and the second edition of the *Collins Dictionary of the English Language* (Collins Dictionary 1986) were consulted in order to obtain definitions of care and caring.

Care as a noun

- Trouble, anxiety, serious attention, caution, protection, ensure safety of (*Concise Oxford Dictionary*, p. 149).
- Careful or serious attention, protective or supervisory control, trouble, anxiety, cause for concern, caution (*Collins Dictionary*, p. 239).

Care as a verb

- Feel concern or interest (for, about); feel regard, affection; provide for (*Concise Oxford Dictionary*, p. 149).
- Be concerned; have regard affection or consideration for; provide physical needs, help or comfort (*Collins Dictionary*, p. 239).

Caring as an adjective

- Feeling or showing care and compassion, a caring attitude; of or relating to professional, social or medical care (*Collins Dictionary*, p. 240).

Caring as a noun

- The practice or profession of providing social or medical care (*Collins Dictionary*, p. 240).

Thesauruses

The *Chambers Paperback Thesaurus* (Schwarz et al 1992) and *Roget's Thesaurus* (Kirkpatrick 1987), which provides a detailed explanation of word alternatives, were consulted. The following are a sample of alternative terms used for care and caring:

Care (noun)

- Anxiety, attention, caution, concern, consideration, custody, guardianship, interest, protection, regard, responsibility, solicitude, supervision, trouble, vigilance, ward, watchful, woe, worry (*Chambers Thesaurus* 1992)
- Carefulness, business, function, protection, management, detention, mandate, economy, worry, painfulness, dejection, nervousness, caution (*Roget's Thesaurus*).

Care (verb)

- Be attentive, love, philanthropize (*Roget's Thesaurus*).

Care for

- Look after, safeguard, desire, love, be benevolent (*Roget's Thesaurus*).
- Attend, foster, like, love, nurse, protect, tend, watch over (*Chambers Thesaurus*).

Word usage of the concept

Several authors have examined the common uses of the term 'caring' in an attempt to uncover its meaning. Leininger (1981), focusing mainly on the professional use of the term, attempted to establish the semantic uses of 'care' by nurses, physicians and the public by undertaking a superficial review of the literature. This review relied on samples from a number of major nursing and medical journals. She discovered that very often the term 'care' was not defined but was linked as a suffix to 'nursing', with no differential made between nursing and caring – the terms were often used interchangeably.

Griffin (1983, p. 290) conducted a philosophical analysis on the linguistic uses of 'caring' and identified two clusters of meanings. The first cluster is located along a continuum beginning with 'interest and attention, and moving towards consideration, concern, guidance, protection and serving needs'. The second cluster refers to 'inclination, or liking for a person to attachment, or wanting to be near someone'. Similarly, when analysing the concept of caring, Gaut (1983) examined the common use of the term and found that, although there was no clear-cut rule for usage, there were basically three general meanings: attention to or concern for; responsibility for or providing for; regard, fondness or attachment.

Theoretical definitions

Several nurse theorists have focused on caring, highlighting its centrality to their work. The theoretical definitions presented in these theories are as follows:

- *Leininger (1991, p. 46)*: Care refers to actions and activities directed towards assisting, supporting, or enabling another individual or group with evident or anticipated needs to ameliorate or improve a human condition or life-way, or to face death
- *Watson (1985, p. 32)*: A value and an attitude that has to become a will, an intention or a commitment that manifests itself in concrete acts
- *Roach (1984, p. 2)*: Caring is not simply an emotional or attitudinal response; caring is a total way of being, of relating, of acting; a quality of investment and engagement in the other – person, idea, project, thing, or self
- *Boykin & Schoenhofer (1993, p. 25)*: Caring is the intentional and authentic presence of the nurse with another who is recognized as person living caring and growing in caring.

Definitions from other literature sources

Other literature sources view caring from perspectives consistent with some of those identified by Morse et al (1990). These include caring as a human trait and caring as a moral imperative. Caring as a human trait has its origins in existential philosophy. Heidegger (1962), whose work has greatly influenced the work of Roach (1984) and Boykin and Schoenhofer (1993), described caring as 'being in the world'. This notion of care as a 'mode of being' is also referred to in the writings of the philosopher Mayeroff (1971). Furthermore, philosophers such as Heidegger (1962), Sartre (1972) and Buber (1970) describe ways of being with others that can be 'authentic' or 'inauthentic'. The term 'presence' has often been used in the nursing literature to denote the 'authentic being' with others. **Elements of existentialism are evident in the writings of the nurse theorists discussed above, where caring is considered a human trait: i.e. to care is to be human.**

The ethics of caring have also been addressed within the literature with the focus on caring in nursing as a commitment, placing strong emphasis on the principle of respect for persons (Gadow 1985, Fry 1988). To be committed is defined as to be 'morally dedicated; obliged to adhere to a course of action' (*Concise Oxford Dictionary*, p. 203). In another source, respect for persons involves treating people with consideration, i.e. 'listening to others, understanding them, and responding with appreciation of their intentions' (Jameton 1984, p. 125). Also, respect for persons involves the realization that the person has an autonomous nature: the person is self-determining and self-governing (Downie & Calman 1994).

Studies on caring

Many empirical studies have investigated the concept of caring using both qualitative and quantitative methodologies. A large number of researchers have used formalized tools to measure the importance of certain caring behaviours. A popular example is the CARE-Q instrument, initially developed by Larson (1984, 1986) and since used by several other researchers (Keane et al 1987, Mayer 1987, von Essen & Sjoden 1991, Greenhalgh et al 1998, Larsson et al 1998). This instrument consists of 50 behavioural items ordered in six subscales of caring: accessible; explains and facilitates; comforts; anticipates; trusting relationship; and monitors and follows through. A Q-methodology is used that involves a forced-choice distribution where each participant selects a predetermined number of items in the most important or least important categories.

Much debate has been generated in relation to the most appropriate method for researching the concept of caring, with the qualitative methods advocated as the preferred approach because of the nebulous nature of caring (Leininger 1986). Qualitative studies have largely employed phenomenological or grounded theory approaches, which can obtain a view of caring experienced by those involved in the process or experience. When considering these studies it is important to remember the cultural differences that may exist. Leininger (1991) developed a Theory of Culture Care, which is based on the premise that care meanings and expressions can differ across cultures. Boxes 3.1 and 3.2 summarize several studies that have focused on patients' and nurses' descriptions of caring, and the main themes that emerged from the data. It should be noted that this is not an exhaustive list of the qualitative work in this area; nevertheless, the sample provides a key literature source for the analysis of the concept, as well as incorporating qualitative data, as advocated by Rodgers (1989).

STAGE 4: DETERMINE THE DEFINING ATTRIBUTES

Following identification of as many uses of the concept as possible, it is then necessary to read the information and note the characteristics that appear time and time again. The subsequent list of characteristics are called defining or critical attributes. However, since concepts have many possible meanings, one may be

Box 3.1

Major themes from qualitative studies on caring from the patient's perspective

Themes relating to good/bad caring

Drew 1986

- Sense of energy being expended on their behalf
- Facial expressions, e.g. a smile
- Not being in a hurry
- Open and willing to share their lives
- Touch

*Fosbinder 1994**

- Translating: informing; explaining; instructing; teaching
- Getting to know you
- Establishing trust
- Going the extra mile
- Identifying what is important to the patient

Reiman 1986

Themes identified refer to non-caring interactions:
- Being in a hurry and efficient
- Doing a job
- Being rough and belittling patients
- Not responding

Themes relating to an overview of caring

Brown 1986

- Recognition of individual qualities
- Reassuring presence
- Provision of information
- Demonstration of professional knowledge and skills
- Assistance with pain
- Amount of time spent
- Promotion of autonomy
- Surveillance

*This study involved a sample of both patients and nurses.

selected that is most relevant to the aim of the analysis (Walker & Avant 1995). In the present analysis the meaning of caring most relevant to nursing is the focus. The following are the characteristics consistently cited to illustrate the concept of caring.

- *Serious attention*: Dictionary sources have used the term 'serious attention' when describing care. 'Attention' and 'being attentive' have also been presented

Box 3.2

Major themes from
qualitative studies on
caring from the nurse's
perspective

Themes relating to good caring

Chipman 1991

- Giving of self
- Meeting patients' needs in a timely fashion
- Providing comfort measures for patients and their families

Ford 1990

- Sensing the patient's vulnerability
- Beyond the call of duty
- Being in tune with the patient's world
- Being attentively present
- Centring on the patient
- Being comfortable with the patient

Forrest 1989

- Involvement: being there; respect; feeling with and for; closeness
- Interacting: touching and holding; picking up cues; being firm; teaching; knowing them well

Themes relating to an overview of caring

Clarke and Wheeler 1992

- Being supportive: loving concern; valuing people; respect; trust; giving of self; awareness of patients' needs; prompting independence
- Communicating: talking; information giving; listening; touching and hugging; presence
- Pressures affecting care
- Caring ability

Morrison 1991

- Personal qualities
- Clinical work style
- Interpersonal approach
- Level of motivation
- Concern for others
- Use of time
- Attitudes

as alternatives to the term 'care' in thesauruses and have been consistently identified in the word usage of the concept. The idea of being seriously attentive would appear to be similar to the notion of being 'authentically' present, as indicated in the philosophical literature sources and by theorists such as Boykin and Schoenhofer (1993).

- *Concern*: The term 'concern' has been cited in dictionary sources and as an alternative to the term 'care' in the thesauruses.
- *Providing for*: Both dictionary and common word usage sources include the notion of providing for a person. The *Collins English Dictionary* (1986, p. 239) expands on this idea: 'to provide physical needs, help or comfort (for)'. This notion is reflected in several definitions of nursing, the prime example being Henderson's (1966), which describes nursing's unique function as 'assisting the individual, sick or well, in the performance of those activities, he would perform unaided if he had the necessary strength, will or knowledge' (p. 66).
- *Regard, respect, or liking*: These meanings are consistently cited in all the literature sources examined. It focuses the discussion on caring as a form of love, a view held by several authors (Bevis 1981, Ray 1981, Jacono 1993). **For nurses to like all patients they care for, let alone love, is a difficult idea to comprehend in the reality of professional nursing.** Respect for persons, on the other hand, may be a more apt description of this critical attribute. One does not have to like an individual to care for them, but can respect them as a human being.

Reviewing the themes emerging from the studies on caring reinforces the credibility and authenticity of the above attributes. However, several additional attributes can be identified from these studies:

- *Amount of time involved.*
- *Getting to know the patient*, which would incorporate identifying what is important to the patient and his subsequent needs.

On reflection, two of the attributes could be described as either an antecedent to care taking place or a critical attribute; these are 'respect for persons' and 'amount of time'. It could be argued that to show a person respect is in fact to care, or that one needs to respect a person before caring can take place. It could also be argued that to give time is to care, or that in order to care one first needs time. The possibility of these factors being antecedents to care will be further discussed in stage 7, which deals with the identification of antecedents and consequences.

STAGE 5: CONSTRUCT A MODEL CASE

According to Walker and Avant (1995, p. 40) a model case is 'a "real life" example of the use of the concept that includes all the critical attributes and no attributes of any other concept'. In other words, the model case presents an instance that we are sure is an example of the concept. It is worthy to note that Rodgers (1989) also includes the identification of a model case in her approach to concept analysis. The following case is cited by Ford (1990), who investigated the caring encounters of six nurses working with cardiac patients:

Case study 1

> Mr Cook was in the terminal stages of congestive heart failure. He had two myocardial infarctions. He was alone, his family were out of town. We knew he wasn't doing well... When I touched his hand and introduced myself, he squeezed my hand and began to talk... I sat on his bed, and he reached out and held my hand. He talked to me about his life, about his family, and the things he wanted to do but wasn't able to... I ignored everything else that was going on in the unit at that time: and it was busy. I pulled the curtains around one side of the bed because there was some activity coming from that side. I just sat and listened as he spoke (Ford 1990, p. 160).

The nurse in the case described above has shown concern for the patient who is alone at this critical time in his life. For this reason the nurse is providing comfort to the patient and is seriously attentive to what the patient is trying to say. Additionally, the nurse is getting to know the patient and the things that are, and have been, important to him during his life.

STAGE 6: CONSTRUCT ADDITIONAL, BORDERLINE, RELATED AND CONTRARY CASES

Additional cases

The construction of additional cases serves to provide examples of what the concept is not, thus promoting greater understanding of the concept (Walker & Avant 1995).

Borderline cases

Borderline cases are examples which demonstrate some of the critical attributes, but not all of them. Alternatively, such cases may contain all the attributes, but

Case study 2

> Jim Smith was 45 years old when I met him. ... He was admitted to the cardiopulmonary unit where I was working. The patient had an 8-hour history of slurred speech and blurred vision. The symptoms had cleared up prior to his admission and he was now admitted for a diagnostic workup. ... He was worked up for transitory ischaemic arterial spasm. Four days later he went home with a negative workup. Two days after that he was readmitted after having a seizure at home. I was on holiday at the time, and by the time I had returned he had a diagnosis of metastatic lung cancer.
>
> I do not know how he responded to the initial diagnosis – when I returned, I didn't go in to see him for a couple of days. I was really frightened about seeing him because I did not know what to say or do. He made it easy for me, and I did begin working with him again, concentrating on teaching him about chemotherapy and radiotherapy. I felt I was teaching him a lot, but actually he taught me. One day he said to me, 'You are doing an OK job, Mary, but I can tell that every time you walk in that door you are walking out.'
>
> He was right. He had developed so much meaning in his illness and life that I was not relating to. This man had really expanded the context of his life into areas where I could have been effective, had I had some understanding (Benner & Wrubel 1989, p. 16).

differ for example in intensity of occurrence (Walker & Avant 1995). Case study 2 comes from the work of Benner and Wrubel (1989).

The above example has been categorized as a borderline case because there are two critical attributes missing. The nurse expresses concern for the patient because of his recent diagnosis of metastatic lung cancer. She is providing information through teaching the patient about chemotherapy and radiotherapy. However, despite all her efforts she is not seriously attentive, that is, she is not present with the patient and listening to what he really wants to say, nor has she recognized what has become important to the patient as a result of his illness.

Related cases

Related cases are examples of concepts closely related to the concept under examination, but they do not contain the critical attributes (Walker & Avant 1995). I experienced some difficulty in identifying a concept that is closely related to caring but is not considered part of caring. For example, when discussing the issue of related cases with experienced colleagues, compassion or empathy was suggested as related concepts. However, compassion has been identified by Roach (1984) as one of her 'five Cs' of caring. The critical attributes that were previously identified for caring were examined, and compared to a definition of empathy. Empathy is defined in the *Concise Oxford Dictionary* (Sykes 1976, p. 338) as the 'power of projecting one's personality into (and so fully comprehending) the object of contemplation'. While on initial reflection this concept would appear to be different from caring, it could also be said that to be authentically present requires a significant degree of empathy.

Support was also considered as a related concept to caring, but again the distinction of support as something different from caring is questionable. Following a qualitative study, a model of supportive care was developed by O'Berle and Davies (1990) that focused on one nurse's in-depth descriptions of her palliative nursing role. The model was comprised of six interwoven dimensions: valuing, connecting, empowering, doing for, finding meaning, and preserving own integrity. In a follow-up paper, O'Berle and Davies (1992) examined the concepts of support and caring and concluded that the two concepts were very similar and difficult to differentiate. In support of this, if the dimensions of the supportive caring model were compared with the critical attributes of caring identified from the present concept analysis, there are a number of remarkable similarities. For example 'connecting' would be comparable to 'serious attention' or 'presence', and 'doing for' to 'providing for'.

Contrary cases

Walker and Avant (1995) describe contrary cases as examples that are clearly 'not the concept'. The following example is a description of a nurse given by a 21-year-old nursing student with lupus erythematosus, cited from a study by Reiman (1986), who used a phenomenological approach to examine patients' descriptions of caring and non-caring interactions:

On reflection, the nurse in the above case shows no concern, provides no help or comfort to the patient, is in no way present or attentive and makes no attempt to get to know this young girl or what is important to her. This would be considered a clear example of what caring is not.

Case study 3

> She was always in a hurry, she didn't have time to talk or even if she had time she didn't really seem to want to talk. Her body language let me know she wasn't interested in what I had to say. All she was here to do was to perform her duty and go home. She stood at a distance, she didn't even come close. She made me feel I have some kind of illness and I might rub off on her. When I was talking to her she wouldn't look at me directly. When I would ask her a question she would be snappy, even on the defensive side. She wasn't interested in the person as a whole. She would cut me off short and she talked in such a rush. She never would say when she'd be back. I was not at ease. I was uncomfortable. I became depressed by not being able to talk. I felt I had to keep my mouth shut (Reiman 1986).

STAGE 7: IDENTIFY ANTECEDENTS AND CONSEQUENCES

Antecedents are the event or incidents that must happen before caring takes place, while consequences are those events or incidences that occur as a result of caring. It should be noted that, according to Walker and Avant (1995), a criterion cannot be both an attribute and an antecedent; it is either one or other. On examination of the various uses of the concept and the illustration of these in the cases presented, three themes emerge that could properly be described as antecedents rather than critical attributes. As mentioned earlier, 'respect for persons' and 'amount of time' could be considered as critical attributes or antecedents. Respect for persons must be present in order for caring to take place, and amount of time can influence the extent to which caring can take place. The third antecedent, 'intention to care' stems from the work of theorists such as Watson (1985) and Boykin and Schoenhofer (1993). **Similarly, Leininger (1991, p. 46) describes caring as 'actions and activities directed towards assisting, supporting or enabling another individual'. The use of the words 'directed towards' would also suggest an intentional act.** However, it could be argued that one can care without explicitly intending to do so.

Considering the model, contrary and borderline cases presented above, it would appear that the consequences of caring are not easily identifiable. However, the cases do highlight, to a degree, the effect caring or non-caring can have on the patient. In Case study 3, the young student nurse states that she became depressed because of the actions of the nurse. **Therefore, patients who have experienced caring or non-caring may be the most appropriate persons to inform nurses as to the consequences or outcomes.** One suggested outcome of caring could be well-being, both physical and mental. It could also be argued that comfort is an outcome of caring, especially when one considers the definition provided by Morse (1992, p. 93): 'a state of well-being that may occur during any stage of the illness–health continuum'. However, this definition could be challenged. In the present analysis it is argued that providing comfort is a critical attribute of caring rather than a consequence of caring. In other words the nurse provides comfort and as a result the patient experiences a feeling of well-being.

STAGE 8: DEFINE EMPIRICAL REFERENTS

Defining the empirical referents is the final step in concept analysis. Walker and Avant (1995) point out that very often the critical attributes are the empirical referents. However, if the concept being analysed is highly nebulous then the critical attributes may be equally nebulous. **The abstract nature of the critical attributes of caring identified within this concept analysis reinforces the qualitative nature of caring, and highlights the need to further examine the experience of caring using qualitative methods before measurable empirical referents can be operationalized.**

AN EXPLORATION OF CARING: A QUALITATIVE STUDY

Following on from the above concept analysis, a qualitative research study was conducted aimed at exploring the concept of caring from the perspective of patients and nurses. The research approach used in this study was interpretative phenomenology using a narrative method (McCance 2001). The results from this doctoral research led to the development of a conceptual framework based on Donabedian's (1980) constructs of structure, process and outcome. Structures included nurse attributes, organizational issues and patient attributes. Processes comprised the activities of caring, which included providing for patients' physical and psychological needs, being attentive, getting to know the patient, taking time, being firm, showing respect and the extra touch. The outcomes emanated from the process of caring and included a feeling of well-being, patient satisfaction and effect on the environment (McCance 2003). The conceptual framework emphasizes a potential link between the three constructs, suggesting a positive linear relationship between structures required for the process of caring, which will lead to patient outcomes.

The four critical attributes identified from the concept analysis are evident in the study findings, albeit in a slightly different form. 'Serious attention' can be compared to 'being attentive' but, as McCance (2003) highlights, the level of attention described by study participants was at a more superficial level than would be expected from being 'seriously attentive'. 'Providing for' was represented by two categories within the research study articulated as 'providing for patients' physical needs' and 'providing for patients' psychological needs'. However, the critical attribute of 'concern' was a subcategory under 'providing for patients' psychological needs' along with 'providing for information', 'providing reassurance' and 'communicating'. Finally, 'getting to know the patient' was a critical attribute identified by the concept analysis and also a category identified from the research study, with both presented in a similar context.

The three antecedents identified from the concept analysis included 'respect for persons', 'amount of time' and 'intention to care', which reflect similarities with categories identified under structure. For example, 'time' was identified as an issue that had the potential to impact on the process of caring, and 'commitment to the job' was reflective of a desire and willingness to meet the needs of the patients not dissimilar to the critical attribute of 'intention to care'. As previously highlighted it could be debated as to whether or not 'respect for persons' was a critical attribute or an antecedent, and interestingly, from the research results, it was incorporated in the process of caring and not considered a prerequisite to caring. The outcomes identified from the research study included 'a feeling of well-being' (affective and physical), 'patient satisfaction' and 'effect on the environment', and again could be considered analogous to the consequences of caring, which were more difficult to articulate from the concept analysis.

While it is encouraging to see a degree of congruence between the concept analysis using Walker and Avant's (1995) approach and the qualitative study presented by McCance (2003), it should be highlighted that several additional categories were identified within the study findings that were not identified from the concept analysis. This emphasizes the cyclical nature of concept development, a stance advocated by Rodgers (2000, p. 97), who argues that concept analysis is a continuous and evolutionary process. Furthermore, Rodgers reminds us that using a technique such as concept analysis is not an end in itself:

> *The results of analysis, therefore, do not provide the definitive answer to questions concerning what the concept is. Instead they may be viewed as a powerful heuristic, promoting and giving direction to additional inquiry,. The purpose is not to provide a final solution, a 'crystal clear' notion of what the concept is. Instead the aim is to provide the foundation and clarity necessary to enhance the continuing cycle of concept development.*
>
> *Rodgers 2000, p. 97*

CONCLUSION

Caring as a concept requiring clarification is a consistent theme within the nursing literature, and this is further evidenced by evaluation criteria that highlight it as a 'partially mature' concept. The use of Walker and Avant's (1995) method of concept analysis as a means to explicate the meaning of caring in nursing resulted in the identification of four critical attributes of caring – 'serious attention', 'concern', 'providing for' and 'getting to know the patient'. The antecedents of caring included: 'amount of time', 'respect for persons' and 'an intention to care'. While the consequences of caring were more difficult to ascertain, the effects of non-caring were demonstrated clearly through the contrary case exemplar. Furthermore, the difficulty in identifying empirical referents serves to reinforce the nebulous and qualitative nature of caring and the subsequent need for further development of the concept. A summary of a qualitative study that aimed to build on the completed concept analysis was also presented. The study findings served to reinforce several of the critical attributes but also highlighted some differences, thus emphasizing the nature of concept development as an evolutionary and continuous process.

REFERENCES

Benner P, Wrubel J 1989 The primacy of caring. Addison-Wesley, Menlo Park, CA

Bevis EM 1981 Caring: a life force. In: Leininger MM (ed) Caring: an essential human need. Wayne State University Press, Detroit, MI, pp. 49–59

Blustein J 1991 Care and commitment. Oxford University Press, Oxford

Boykin A, Schoenhofer S 1993 Nursing as caring: a model for transforming nursing. National League of Nursing Press, New York

Brown L 1986 The experience of care: patient perspectives. Topics in Clinical Nursing 8: 56–62

Buber M 1970 I and thou by Martin Buber: a new translation with a prologue 'I and You' and notes by Walter Kaufmann, 3rd edition. T & T Clark, Edinburgh

Buchanan S, Ross K 1995 A concept analysis of caring. Perspectives 9: 3–6

Chipman Y 1991 Caring: its meaning and place in the practice of nursing. Journal of Nursing Education 30: 171–175

Clarke JB, Wheeler SJ 1992 A view of the phenomenon of caring in nursing practice. Journal of Advanced Nursing 17: 1283–1290

Collins Dictionary 1986 Dictionary of the English language, 2nd edn. Collins, London

Donabedian A 1980 The definitions of quality and approaches to its assessment. Health Administration Press, Ann Arbor, MI

Downie RS, Calman KC 1994 Healthy respect: ethics in healthcare. Oxford University Press, Oxford

Drew N 1986 Exclusion and confirmation: a phenomenology of patients' experience with caregivers. IMAGE: Journal of Nursing Scholarship 18: 39–43

Eyles M 1995 Uncovering the knowledge to care. British Journal of Theatre Nursing 5: 22–25

Ford SJ 1990 Caring encounters. Scandinavian Journal of Caring Science 4: 157–162

Forrest D 1989 The experience of caring. Journal of Advanced Nursing 14: 815–823

Fosbinder D 1994 Patient perceptions of nursing care: an emerging theory of interpersonal competence. Journal of Advanced Nursing 20: 1085–1093

Fry ST 1988 The ethic of caring: can it survive in nursing? Nursing Outlook 36: 48

Gadow SA 1985 Nurse and patient: the caring relationship. In: Bishop AH, Scudder JR (ed) Caring, curing and coping. University of Alabama Press, Alabama pp. 31–43

Gaut DA 1983 Development of a theoretically adequate description of caring. Western Journal of Nursing Research 5: 313–324

Greenhalgh J, Vanhanen L, Kyngas H 1998 Nurse caring behaviours. Journal of Advanced Nursing 27: 927–932

Griffin AP 1983 A philosophical analysis of caring in nursing. Journal of Advanced Nursing 8: 289–295

Heidegger M 1962 Being and time. Blackwell, Oxford

Henderson V 1966 The nature of nursing. Macmillan, New York

Jacono BJ 1993 Caring is loving. Journal of Advanced Nursing 18: 192–194

Jameton A 1984 Nursing practice: the ethical issues. Prentice-Hall, Englewood Cliffs, NJ

Keane SM, Chastain B, Rudisill K 1987 Caring: nurse–patient perceptions. Rehabilitation Nursing 12: 182–184

Kirkpatrick B (ed) 1987 Roget's Thesaurus of English words and phrases. Longman, Harlow

Kyle TV 1995 The concept of caring: a review of the literature. Journal of Advanced Nursing 21: 506–514

Larson PJ 1984 Important nurse caring behaviors perceived by patients with cancer. Oncology Nursing Forum 11: 46–50

Larson PJ 1986 Cancer nurses' perceptions of caring. Cancer Nursing 9: 86–91

Larsson G, Peterson VW, Lampic C et al 1998 Cancer patient and staff ratings of the importance of caring behaviours and their relations to patient anxiety and depression. Journal of Advanced Nursing 27: 855–864

Leininger MM 1981 Some philosophical, historical, and taxonomic aspects of nursing and caring in American culture. In: Leininger MM (ed) Caring: an essential human need. Wayne State University Press, Detroit, MI, pp. 133–143

Leininger MM 1986 Care facilitation and resistance factors in the culture of nursing. Topics in Clinical Nursing 8: 1–12

Leininger MM 1991 Culture care diversity and universality: a theory of nursing. National League for Nursing Press, New York

McCance TV 2003 Caring in nursing practice: the development of a conceptual framework. Research and Theory for Nursing Practice 17: 101–116

McCance TV, McKenna HP, Boore JRP 1997 Caring: dealing with a difficult concept. International Journal of Nursing Studies 34: 241–248

McCance TV, McKenna HP, Boore JRP 2001 Exploring caring using a narrative methodology: an analysis of the approach. Journal of Advanced Nursing 33: 350–356

McFarlane JK 1976 A charter for caring. Journal of Advanced Nursing 1: 187–196

Mayer DK 1987 Oncology nurses' versus cancer patients' perceptions of nurse caring behaviors: a replication study. Oncology Nursing Forum 14: 48–52

Mayeroff M 1971 On caring. Harper & Row, London

Morrison P 1991 The caring attitude in nursing practice: a repertory grid study of trained nurses' perceptions. Nurse Education Today 11: 3–12

Morse JM 1992 Comfort: the refocusing of nursing care. Clinical Nursing Research 1: 91–106

Morse JM 1995 Exploring the theoretical basis of nursing using advanced techniques of concept analysis. Advances in Nursing Science 17: 31–46

Morse JM, Solberg SM, Neander WL et al 1990 Concepts of caring and caring as a concept. Advances in Nursing Science 13: 1–14

Morse JM, Hupcey JE, Mitcham C et al 1996a Concept analysis in nursing research: a critical appraisal. Scholarly Inquiry for Nursing Practice 10: 253–277

Morse JM, Mitcham C, Hupcey JE et al 1996b Criteria for concept evaluation. Journal of Advanced Nursing 24: 385–390

Morse JM, Hupcey JE, Penrod J et al 2002 Integrating concepts for the development of qualitatively-derived theory. Research and Theory for Nursing Practice 16: 5–18

O'Berle K, Davies B 1990 Dimensions of the supportive role of the nurse in palliative care. Oncology Nursing Forum 17: 87–94

O'Berle K, Davies B 1992 Support and caring: exploring the concepts. Oncology Nursing Forum 19: 763–767

Paley J 2001 An archaeology of caring knowledge. Journal of Advanced Nursing 36: 188–198

Ray MA 1981 A philosophical analysis of caring within nursing. In: Leininger MM (ed) Caring: an essential human need. Wayne State University Press, Detroit, MI, pp. 25–36

Reiman DJ 1986 Non-caring and caring in the clinical setting: patients' descriptions. Topics in Clinical Nursing 8: 30–36

Roach S 1984 Caring: the human mode of being. University of Toronto, Toronto, Ontario

Roach S 1987 The human act of caring. Canadian Hospital Association, Ottawa

Rodgers BL 1989 Concepts, analysis and the development of nursing knowledge. Journal of Advanced Nursing 14: 330–335

Rodgers BL 2000 Concept analysis: an evolutionary view. In: Rodger BL, Knafl KA (eds) Concept development in nursing, 2nd edn. WB Saunders, Philadelphia, PA, pp. 77–102

Sartre JP 1972 Being and nothingness. Methuen, London

Schwarz C, Seaton A, Davidson G et al (eds) 1992 Chambers paperback thesaurus, new edn. W & R Chambers, Edinburgh

Scotto CJ 2003 A new view of caring. Journal of Nursing Education 42: 289–291

Sourial S 1997 An analysis of caring. Journal of Advanced Nursing 26: 1189–1192

Stockdale M, Warelow PJ 2000 Is the complexity of care a paradox? Journal of Advanced Nursing 31: 1258–1264

Sykes JB (ed) (1976) The concise Oxford dictionary of current English, 6th edn. Clarendon Press, Oxford

von Essen L, Sjoden P 1991 Patient and staff perceptions of caring: review and replication. Journal of Advanced Nursing 16: 1363–1374

Walker K, Avant K 1995 Strategies for theory construction in nursing, 2nd edn. Appleton & Lange, London

Watson J 1979 Nursing: the philosophy and science of caring. Little, Brown & Co., Boston, MA

Watson J 1985 Nursing: human science and human care – a theory of nursing. National League for Nursing, New York

Webb C 1996 Caring, curing, coping: towards an integrated model. Journal of Advanced Nursing 23: 960–968

Wilson J 1969 Thinking with concepts. Cambridge University Press, Cambridge

A concept analysis of comfort

Linda Marie Lowe and John R. Cutcliffe

EDITORIAL

It is heartening to see that the concept of comfort has received attention from nursing scholars, educationalists and practitioners over the years since few would dispute that providing comfort is a key aspect of nursing. As Linda and John point out in this chapter, nurses have been providing comfort since the first formal (academic) records of nursing practice were began. (Perhaps most notably in Nightingale's seminal work.) The many forms that this comfort and comforting can take were less evident, it seems, in these early writings. Again, as Linda and John point out, the historical emphasis has been on providing physical comfort and/or finding ways to minimize a person's physical discomfort. Relieving pain, easing aches and help with physical repositioning are conspicuous in the literature. Perhaps, though, as nursing has moved away (somewhat) from a physiological focus to a more holistic view, then one might expect the focus within the comfort-related literature to mirror this shift. A domain of nursing practice and theory where clear evidence of this movement has occurred is within the chronic illness literature. The work of Rolland, Nolan, Grant and Keady is particularly illuminating and it powerfully reiterates the messages in this chapter. Most notably, that people with chronic conditions can adapt remarkably well, even to severe physical discomfort and debilitation, and yet still achieve a position of (relative) holistic comfort.

While there is evidence of this movement, it still appears that the some of the literature retains this physiological focus. If we can learn anything from the 'comfort within chronic illness literature' it is that we, as nurses, are potentially missing the point if we focus exclusively (or predominantly) on the physical. Consequently, there are important implications here for practitioners about how we ask about comfort and, clearly, how we determine a person's level or degree of comfort.

There are additional issues and questions that are similarly underexplored. For instance, we know that certain nursing situations, certain dynamics and certain practices leave some nurses feeling uncomfortable, mostly (if not exclusively) as a result of their psychological discomfort – for example, dealing with some inebriated patients, dealing with the dying, working with groups who have been socially ostracized and interacting with offenders. In many of these situations it is unlikely to be physical discomfort that causes the nurses problems. Yet, as an academic community, we have much to explore with such nurses around their lived experiences of working in these situations, the processes of reaching a state of discomfort and, importantly, the processes whereby they can feel OK with such situations and how they deal with the psychological discomfort in themselves.

INTRODUCTION

According to Blackstock (1996, p. 3), 'comfort is the business of nursing' and nurses' common uses of the term 'comfort' indicate that it is regarded as a way to describe a desired outcome or state. Wurbach (1996) asserts that comfort can be examined using several varied approaches, such as a dichotomous relational ethic of care (vis-à-vis the greater good), principlism and even job satisfaction in nursing! However, as the term is both personal and contextual in nature, a widely accepted and precise definition is proving elusive. For nursing practice and research, this is frustrating, as comfort per se is considered a fundamental value; a foundation for some nursing theories and a starting point for intervention (Siefert 2002). In order to identify the particular approach and the various components of concept analysis, the seminal work of Rodgers (1989) was used to guide this analysis. That is not to say that this analysis of comfort is either based purely in a positivistic context or blatantly reductionist in nature. It is our belief that, like Rodgers (1989, p. 331), in order to explain or at least identify attributes/components of comfort, we should 'emphasize the use of concepts, the behaviours or capabilities that are possible as a result of an individual having a grasp of particular concepts'.

In addition, like Rodgers, we believe that a dispositional analysis of the concept will possibly provide the rigour for appropriateness in application and that this clarification is necessary in order to develop the concept and add to nursing knowledge.

Having said that, we acknowledge that the application can change over time through 'use' of the concept. Accordingly, the remainder of this chapter looks at the etymological origins of comfort and explores the historical background of the 'use' of the term; definitions are then considered. Following this we make some attempts to explicate the key attributes of comfort before looking at the antecedents and consequences. A model case, based on a 'real case', is included and then we offer some concluding remarks.

ANALYSIS OF THE CONCEPT

> *My comfort is, that old age, that ill layer-up of beauty, can do no more spoil upon my face.*
>
> *William Shakespeare, 1564–1616*

Comfort is a transitive verb finding its roots in the late Latin *comfortare* = 'to strengthen greatly' (*fortis* = 'strong'). Comfort is considered a state, a philosophy, a dynamic, a process and even a goal/outcome. Morse (1983) postulated that comfort is the major instrument for care in the clinical setting and, as nurses, we plan to optimize our client's comfort each day; hence the rigorous attention to comfort-related care plans and nursing interventions. However, the literature is clear in suggesting that the attributes of comfort are fluid as developments in technology, biopsychosocial sciences, even the sophistication of the 'client as consumer' progress. So what is comfort? In order to find appropriate definitions and explore the phenomenological interrelationships that exist within the literature, we searched usage of the term and this brought forth many interpretations, which in itself was surprising as there is an overall assumption in nursing that we *know* what comfort is. The literature search undertaken for this chapter uncovered a phenomenological product, one theoretical notion of holistic comfort, six conceptual analyses, one exploration of vocabulary (with subcomponents of pain analyses), one exposition on emotional comfort and two on the nature of comfort for inpatients.

HISTORICAL BACKGROUND

The *Collins Concise Dictionary* defines comfort as 'a person, thing, or event that brings solace or ease' (*Collins Concise Dictionary* 1988).

Language, not unlike concepts, is constantly changing and adapting to inventions and societal nuances of each successive century, and this view of language is in keeping with the dispositional construction of concepts (Wittgenstein 1968). However, an examination of some ancient works demonstrates that there are elements inherent in the historical use of the term 'comfort' that would perhaps have similarity and/or resonance with our contemporary understanding of the concept. For example, Plato's (327 BC) original Greek writing was translated as, 'The venture is a glorious one, and he ought to comfort himself with words like these, which is the reason why I lengthen out the tale.' By contrast, some historians have concluded that, although the meaning may remain more or less constant, the state, or the achievement of that state, had little importance for some societies and in others it was considered impolite to indulge in such decadent pursuits (Crowley 2001).

Perhaps we can find a more relatively modern and therefore more fitting interpretation in Florence Nightingale's (1860) seminal work *Notes on Nursing: What it is, and what it is not*. Nightingale makes frequent mention of the strenuous and repeated efforts that diligent nurses must make to achieve the state of comfort for their patients. For instance: 'The amount of relief and comfort experienced by the sick after the skin has been carefully washed and dried, is one of the commonest observations made at a sick bed' (Nightingale 1860, p. 115). It is evident from the majority of her publications that Nightingale saw the provision of comfort, whatever form that may take, as the fundamental underpinning guiding the delivery of what was then considered to be premium health care (considering the appalling conditions troops suffered during the Crimean War 1853–1856). Repeatedly, she stressed the importance of keen and constant observation of the patient in order to provide the means for achieving this elusive state (predicated upon the notion that *dis*-ease brings about *dis*-comfort). She made this argument most clearly when she stated: 'In dwelling upon the vital importance of sound observation, it must never be lost sight of what observation is for. It is not for the sake of piling up miscellaneous information or curious facts, but for the sake of saving life and increasing health and comfort' (Nightingale 1860, p. 155).

Nearly one and a half centuries later, we health professionals believe we have a firm understanding of what it means to be comfortable and how we can facilitate such a state for our patients. However, even though the nursing knowledge base has expanded exponentially, and today most nursing associations emphasize the fundamental and intrinsic components of caring in nursing that are found in the provision of comfort and the plethora of subconcepts related to this issue in nursing practice, there is no general consensus about a concrete meaning (Cameron 1993, Siefert 2002).

DEFINITIONS AND USES OF COMFORT

Comfort has many uses: to soothe, to cheer, to provide and to offer protection. It can be considered a state, a condition, an intervention, an outcome/goal, a process and a continuum. As to what application or use the term has in nursing, we again turn to the literature, to find that there is a multitude of opinions. Regardless of its lack of a firm definition, one of the fundamental attributes of human nature is the capacity to provide comfort. Kolcaba and Kolcaba (1991, pp. 1302–1303) identified six meanings (uses) of the word comfort. Drawing on various dictionaries and thesauruses, their six meanings/uses are as follows:

- A cause of relief from discomfort and/or the state of comfort
- The state of ease and peaceful contentment
- Relief from discomfort
- Whatever makes life easy or pleasurable
- Strengthening, encouragement, incitement and succour, support
- Physical refreshment or sustenance, refreshing or invigorating influence.

More recently, a number of authors (e.g. Cameron 1993, Tutton & Seers 2004) have suggested that comfort is considered to be a fundamental principle for nursing and is the desired outcome of comforting. Clearly associated with the notion of comfort as an outcome is the position, asserted by a number of authors, that comfort is a nursing goal (Fleming et al 1987, Hamilton 1989, Arruda et al 1992). Several North American nursing bodies (e.g. the Oncology Nursing Society, the American Nurses Association and North American Nursing Diagnosis Association) formalized their conceptualization of comfort and predicated that comfort is a 'standard of care' and a 'nursing diagnosis' (Kolcaba 1992a). Some nursing theorists, such as Roy (1981), Orlando (1961), Patterson and Zderad (1976) link the concept of comfort with attention to client needs (which in turn tallies with the directives of Nightingale). Kolcaba (1991) extends this idea (slightly) and argues that comfort is concerned not only with client needs but, importantly, with having one's basic human needs met. Importantly, Kolcaba (1991) does not limit these needs to one particular dimension of the person.

Perhaps not surprisingly, comfort has been contrasted with discomfort (Flaherty & Fitzpatrick 1978). It has been described as existing on a comfort–discomfort continuum (Patterson & Zderad 1976). **More contemporary writing on comfort has moved the conceptualization along, so that it is now accepted that comfort does not mean the complete absence of discomfort; in other words, people can be comfortable with a certain degree of discomfort.** It is more a matter of having one's discomfort eased, soothed, relieved; achieving an acceptable level or degree of comfort (see Kolcaba & Kolcaba 1991, Cameron 1993, Morse et al 1994, McIlveen & Morse 1995). Other nursing theorists, in attempting to explore and add to our understanding of the notion, view the concept from both a positivistic as well as a metaphysical stance. Jimenez and Sherry (1996) offer several assertions:

- That the relief of pain may not necessarily be synonymous with comfort
- That changing views on pain (incorporation of not only corporeal discomfort but also of psychic/spiritual distress) added to the debate concerning the nature of comfort
- That suffering and comfort are at opposite ends of a continuum.

Whereas, in their excellent paper on the phenomenology of comfort, Jan Morse and colleagues (1994) refer to comfort as a state of embodiment that is beyond awareness; they add that comfort is best recognized when the patient first leaves the state of discomfort. (In the opinion of the editors, such phenomenological writing and analysis of concepts essential to nursing is much underutilized as an approach to analysing concepts.) In Morse's (1992) earlier work on comfort, she referred to comfort as a state; a specific state of 'well-being' (irrespective of where the individual patient is on the illness–health continuum) that is brought about by purposeful, therapeutic nursing actions on behalf of a patient. Cameron (1993) constructed similar arguments, purporting that comfort is concerned with the nurses' individualized actions, which are geared towards health and healing (in the patient).

It is from these and other related descriptions (see, for example, McIlveen & Morse 1995) that the 'active' sense, or idea of 'comfort as process', becomes apparent. The literature also indicates that comfort is a temporary state (Morse et al 1994); just how long this temporary state lasts is unclear, as is how long a person needs to be in the state of comfort before he/she can claim to be in a 'lasting' state of comfort.

Malinowski and Stamler (2002) draw on the work of Ferrell and Ferrell (1990), and state that health professionals should cease to view comfort principally from a physiological stance and need to start considering the other dimensions of holism. However, examination of the substantive literature indicates that, within the study of the concept, work has focused on the physical subcomponents of the concept such as fatigue, nausea, vomiting and pain (Malinowski & Stamler 2002). Lastly in this section, we will not belabour the obvious point that, within the historical and current literature focusing on comfort, the definitions and uses of the term are far from consistent.

KEY ATTRIBUTES IDENTIFIED WITH COMFORT

While the precise mechanisms for identifying the key attributes remain a contested matter, two linked processes appear to be used commonly. The person undertaking the analysis needs, firstly, to interrogate the literature and identify linked 'attributes/characteristics' and, secondly, to note the attributes/characteristics that appear time and time again. Producing such a theoretically robust set of attributes that are synonymous with the concept of comfort is no easy task. Examination of the existing literature on comfort indicates that a great deal of conceptual 'speculation' has occurred and that this has resulted in a range of attributes that have been posited as part of the definition (composition) of comfort. Siefert's (2002) paper, for example, acknowledges that over 50 attributes have been identified. Such width and diversity (and the sheer number) of attributes suggests, at the very least, that additional refinement (and examination) of the concept is required; the concept appears to lack maturity. Moreover, some of these attributes appear more often than others; it is these that we will posit as key attributes.

Furthermore, identifying the attributes of comfort appears to be prefaced by an earlier conceptual decision – whether the process of comforting is an intra-and/or interpersonal process. Which of these two positions one adopts will ultimately influence the conceptualization of key attributes. As this chapter is concerned with understanding comfort within the context of nursing, one might be forgiven for immediately assuming that comfort(ing) must be an interpersonal process (given the interpersonal nature of nursing (Peplau 1952)). However, it is worth broadening our understanding by not excluding the possibility that patients (people) can provide comfort for themselves. If one accepts the argument, and thus comforting can be an intrapersonal process (which can be considered to be akin to Watson's theory of human caring), then the key attributes may look like this.

- *Cultural resonance*: Rosenbaum's (1991) work defined one aspect of comfort as congruence within one's own cultural state. Similarly, drawing on Leininger's (1981) theory of culture care, it becomes evident that a measure of personal comfort can be obtained by self-identification or assignation. In other words, one can draw personal comfort from the 'sense of belonging', identification or association/recognition with one's culture group.
- *Spiritual sourcing*: A number of pieces of literature have purported that self-comfort is obtained through connectedness to one's higher power and certain spiritual states and activities (e.g. having a personal 'peace of mind', prayer, meditation). Additionally, Letvak (1997) proposes that engaging in religiosity but not always through a specific religious affiliation is another (generic) activity that people use to provide self-comfort.
- *Drawing on one's intrapersonal resources*: Some authors have highlighted the comfort that people can gain from drawing on their intrapersonal resources (Morse 1983, Fleming et al 1987, Hamilton 1989, Arruda et al 1992, Kolcaba 1992b, 1993, Morse et al 1994). These personal resources (or characteristics) take many forms but include the following:
    - having enough strength and endurance
    - feeling self-confident and brave
    - having sufficient competence (in whatever domain they deem important)
    - feeling independent
    - being at peace or at ease with oneself
    - having a sense of being valued and/or useful.

If one subscribes to the position that providing comfort is an interpersonal process, then the key attributes may look like these.

- *Interpersonal communication*: A number of studies have identified aspects of interpersonal communication as attributes of 'providing' comfort. Morse's historical (1983, 1992) and more recent research in this area (2000) is consistent in identifying both verbal (talking) and non-verbal (supportive physical touch) as attributes of providing comfort. This position is supported the study undertaken by Fleming et al (1987); these authors found that interpersonal interactions such as active listening and talking skills provided some measure of comfort. In other research around this time, Larson (1987) found that groups of patients identified both listening and talking as crucial parts of comfort. Additional more recent research (though still research with something of a vintage) also indicated that oncology nurses regarded communication as fundamental to providing comfort.

- *Holistic interventions to soothe noxious stimuli*: Not surprisingly, there is substantial reference within the associated literature to interventions that the nurse can use to relieve the holistic discomfort or, more specifically, the noxious stimuli that cause a sense of discomfort. The historical association between pain and discomfort and the ways nurses can promote comfort by relieving pain are well documented (Fleming et al 1987, Kolcaba 1991, 1992a, b, 1993, 2001, McIlveen & Morse 1995). Similarly, attempts to relieve a patient's fatigue and promote sleep (Hamilton 1989, Gropper 1992, McIlveen & Morse 1995) have also been identified as ways to promote a patient's *physical* comfort. A growing, yet still emerging literature highlights how patients report an increased sense of discomfort when they experience anxiety, stress, suffering and uncertainty. Accordingly, interventions to reduce anxiety and help patients feel more relaxed, decrease stress and help patients feel more calm and less concerned (e.g. the interpersonal communication interventions highlighted above, the use of therapeutic humour, facilitating the exploration of choices and options) are associated with decreasing a patient's sense of psychological discomfort (Larson 1987, McIlveen & Morse 1995.) Within this range are also nursing interventions to increase the patient's sense of safety and security. Without wishing to restate the obvious, many of the interpersonal communication interventions highlighted above will increase patients' sense of trust (and thus safety and security) in their nurse(s). (This literature and process is explored in much detail in Chapter 20) In addition to these interventions, there are additional ways to promote comfort by attending to the physical environment (Arruda et al 1992, Morse et al 1994).
- *Family involvement*: Direct proximity or relative nearness to one's family as a contributor to a person's sense of comfort has been asserted by Fleming et al (1987), Hamilton (1989), Arruda et al (1992), Gropper (1992), and Siefert (2002). However, not all the research undertaken in this area has produced this finding. In a phenomenological study, Letvak's (1997) findings challenged this assertion. In addition, the author contested the idea that the absence of a family member does not necessarily obviate the nurse's ability to provide some measure of comfort. Clearly, while there is a limited consensus on this issue, there are significant implications arising from this; none more so than the inference that a person without family might not be able to be offered interpersonal comfort. The authors cited here also draw attention to the comfort than can be drawn from the familiar; not only familiar people (family, friends) but familiar objects too (e.g. a child's comfort blanket.)

While we have attempted to separate these key attributes into the two somewhat arbitrary groups, we wish to point out that some of these attributes could 'fit' comfortably with either view, i.e. they can be both intrapersonal and interpersonal processes. For example, individual patients can arrange their own physical environment to improve their sense of comfort, just as a nurse could do this for them.

ANTECEDENTS AND CONSEQUENCES

ANTECEDENTS

According to the Online Encarta Dictionary, an antecedent is 'something that comes before, and is often considered to lead to the development of, another person or thing'.

In their 1994 publication, Morse et al identified nine states or themes of discomfort reflecting the phenomenological concept of corporeality used to identify the way in which the client achieves comfort. They postulate that our limited awareness of our physical selves well prepares us for when our total health is compromised. In order to compartmentalize the varying approaches to illness and concomitant discomfiture, Morse and her colleagues separate the effects of illness into the effects upon the holistic dimensions of the entity. In reflecting on the nine themes we are able to identify a range of particular antecedents to comfort, depending on which form of discomfort is experienced.

For what Morse et al (1994) term 'the dis-eased body', the antecedents to comfort appear to be the knowledge derived from learning one's diagnosis, giving over or relinquishing some personal responsibility (for one's care of the diseased body) to caregivers and trusting in their competence and ability to provide the necessary comfort. Further, receiving the required 'treatments', interventions and/or supports necessary in order to behave 'normally' despite the influence of the diseased body are also antecedents to comfort.

For what Morse et al (1994) term 'the disobedient body', the antecedents to comfort appear to be an acceptance of the changes forced upon one by one's disobedient body, finding ways to compensate and/or control the symptoms and discovering ways that one can feel a sense of being in control; being normal. For what Morse et al (1994) term 'the vulnerable body', the antecedents to comfort appear to be increased vigilance and hypersensitivity to one's body. Also, as with the dis-eased body, trusting in the competence and ability of the caregivers to provide the necessary interventions that would minimize any sense of vulnerability appears to be an antecedent to comfort.

For what Morse et al (1994, p. 192) term 'the violated body', the antecedents to comfort appear to be the practice of 'temporarily detaching and distancing themselves from the body during violations associated with diagnostic or treatment procedures, in order to protect the self'. For what Morse et al (1994) term 'the enduring body', the antecedents to comfort appear to be a refocusing of the patient's attention in a way that gives them strength, increases hope and helps them endure in the 'here and now'.

For what Morse et al (1994) term 'the resigned body', the antecedents to comfort appear to be the patient's resignation that they must surrender the image (and function) of the former self. Comfort in these cases is prefaced by acceptance. Further, there is a particular cognitive antecedent process of 'rationalizing' that occurs. Patients are able to increase their sense of comfort, despite the changes to their bodies, by drawing comparisons with other less fortunate individuals and thinking 'Things could be much worse; just look at her'.

For what Morse et al (1994) term 'the deceiving body', the antecedents to comfort appear to be a range of patient activities centred on seeking and gaining reassurance. This most often takes the form of having investigations, annual health checks, diagnostic tests, engaging in some form of screening. For what Morse et al (1994) term 'the betraying body', the antecedents to comfort appear to be seeing and recognizing the subtle signs of stress of the betraying body and, importantly, that these subtle signs can be interpreted and given the appropriate meaning; the warning signs are recognized accurately for what they are and for the message(s) they communicate. For what Morse et al (1994) term 'the betraying mind', the antecedents to comfort appear to be accepting the support of others – be they family, friends or care givers.

Perhaps the most commonly identified additional antecedent, and one that is used by many theorists and researchers, is unmet needs; unmet needs that have inevitably led to suffering, distress and/or discomfort, followed by the appropriate intervention to reduce this discomfort. Coupled with this is a raised awareness of such changes in one's state and the patient therefore becomes acutely cognisant of the newly acquired state of comfort (Orlando 1961, Fleming et al 1987). Some nurse theorists assert that a 'rising above' or, to use Siefert's term, transcendence of the experience of discomfort is necessary in order to experience the state of comfort.

CONSEQUENCES

The majority of the consequences (or outcomes) of comfort identified in the literature are predicated upon 'the absence of symptoms, or the lack of the characteristics of discomfort' (Siefert 2002, p. 21).

This view is simplistic, given that there is no agreement regarding whether comfort is the fulcrum of nursing actions (Malinowski & Stamler 2002) or one possible intervention subsumed under the broader act of caring. There appears to be a firm consensus that the consequences of comfort are holistic (multidimensional) in nature; this is entirely intuitive given the holistic nature of comfort itself.

There also appears to be some consensus that additional work needs to be undertaken to create more 'comfort-specific' instruments and outcome measures, although some instruments do exist, such as the General Comfort Questionnaire (Kolcaba 1992a). In the main, the majority of literature refers to being 'symptom-free' (e.g. absence of pain, degree of fatigue) or a measure of the patient experiencing the absence of discomforts. In addition, the important domain of measuring whether or not a patient has their needs met also features with conspicuous regularity. A summary of some of the consequences or outcomes of comfort is provided in Table 4.1. Importantly, these authors' views of the envisioned consequences of comfort should only be considered within their own conceptual frameworks of nursing care; further, as Cameron (1993, p. 426) states, these views are 'highly subjective, context specific and extremely variable'.

Case study

Julia T. was a 38-year-old married mother of two young daughters. Julia had been diagnosed with primary carcinoma of the lower left lung 3 years previously. Following surgery and rigorous chemotherapy her prognosis was hopeful. However, after $2\frac{1}{2}$ years of remission (symptom-free) Julia developed lower abdominal pain and exploratory surgery revealed stage IV ovarian carcinoma. Further radical surgery and extensive chemotherapy proved to be of no avail as the cancer had proliferated to involve most of Julia's major organs. Her energy was dwindling rapidly and she was unable to move around in bed, too weak to sit up and requiring total assistance to maintain a reasonable degree of comfort. She was, however, lucid and aware of her diagnosis.

Julia required total nursing care, consisting of bathing, pressure area care, oral care, positioning, bowel and bladder care, hydration, an appropriate medication regimen and continuous oxygen therapy. Nursing care was negotiated with Julia to address and/or provide relief for each of these needs. Julia was able to control her pain using a patient-controlled analgesia system and this helped her rest and remain relatively free from fatigue. In each instance of these physical interventions Julia was asked what (and when) she preferred as a means of enhancing her sense of personal control. Julia knew she was dying and stated that she wanted total honesty from the team about her prognosis, however grim this was. This open communication between healthcare workers and Julia provided some measure of comfort and control for her, as she was able to prepare herself and her family for her eventual passing. Further, Julia was able to draw on her own intrapersonal 'beliefs' and 'resources' and it gave her comfort to feel that she was able to endure this experience. As she had not moved from the northern city where she born, she was able to have visits from her family and friends on a regular (and informal basis), which gave her great comfort. Julia was a devout Catholic and was also visited by her parish priest, who frequently heard her confession and gave her communion. Sometimes her husband and family joined her for the services.

Caring for Julia was not particularly problematic, even though there were constant reminders that she was dying. Being open and honest about the future provided some freedom and latitude on both sides. Julia was able to verbalize her fears, hopes and dreams for her children. Julia was encouraged to participate in this communal preparation and was very much involved in these activities. The honesty provided a forum for safe expression from carers and Julia. The nursing team were able to care for her with equal openness. In the end, Julia managed to say goodbye to her family members. Some of the nursing team were present when she said goodbye to her family and had the honour to be present when she died.

Table 4.1
Consequences of comfort cited in the literature

Author	Consequence
Kolcaba 1991, McIlveen and Morse 1995	Absence of discomfort
Morse 1983, Larson 1987, Kolcaba 1991, Arruda et al 1992	Met (satisfied) patient needs
Fagerhaugh and Strauss 1987	Increased sense of control
Tutton and Seers 2004	Relief from noxious stimuli
Leininger 1981	Increased sense of cultural integrity
Cameron 1993	Integrative balancing, increased sense of equilibrium
Larson 1987	Increased sense of being cared for and cared about
Fleming et al 1987	Reduction in the patient's sense of suffering

CONCLUSION

The literature examined for this analysis indicates that comfort is a key concept of and for nursing. Conceptual disagreement exists regarding whether comfort is a state, a condition, an intervention, an outcome/goal, a process or a continuum. However, there is a firm consensus that comfort is a holistic, multidimensional concept; having said that, the historical emphasis has been on the physiological aspects of comfort (and providing comfort). The literature also shows the lack of a universally accepted concise, 'tight' definition, although this may not be entirely surprisingly given the conceptual disagreement and the change of the concept through use (Rodgers 1989).

This chapter has also pointed out how understandings of comfort are prefaced by the question of whether it is an intrapersonal and/or interpersonal concept. Subsequent conceptual questions (and resultant answers) will be influenced by this initial choice (e.g. the nature of the key attributes). Consensus as to whether the notion of comfort can find its home as an outcome measure or an existential state of being is not forthcoming in the near future. What can be stated with reasonable confidence is that seeking to provide comfort for/with our clients remains a top priority.

REFERENCES

Arruda EN, Larson PJ, Meleis AI 1992 Comfort: immigrant Hispanic cancer patients' views. Cancer Nursing 15: 387–394

Blackstock F 1996 Comfort care: dramatic changes in a never changing nursing role. Pelican News 52(3) pp. 1–4

Cameron BL 1993 The nature of comfort to hospitalised medical-surgical patients. Journal of Advanced Nursing 18: 424–436

Collins Concise Dictionary 1988 Collins Concise (English) Dictionary. Collins, London

Crowley JE 2001 The invention of comfort: sensibilities and design in early modern Britain and early America. Johns Hopkins University Press, Baltimore, MD

Fagerhaugh, SY, Strauss A 1987 How to manage your patient's pain … and how not to. Nursing 10

Ferrell BR, Ferrell BA 1990 Comfort. In: Corr DM, Corr CA (ed) Nursing care in an aging society. Springer, New York, pp. 67–91

Flaherty GG, Fitzpatrick JJ 1978 Relaxation techniques to increase comfort level of post-operative patients: a preliminary study. Nursing Research 27: 352–355

Fleming C, Scanlon C, D'Agostino NS 1987 A study of the comfort needs of patients with advanced cancer. Cancer Nursing 10: 237–243

Gropper EI 1992 Promoting health by promoting comfort. Nursing Forum 27: 5–8

Hamilton J 1989 Comfort and the hospitalised chronically ill. Journal of Gerontological Nursing 15: 28–33

Jimenez H, Sherry LM 1996 Pain and comfort: establishing a common vocabulary for exploring issues of pain and comfort. Journal of Perinatal Education 5: 53–60

Kolcaba KY 1991 A taxonomic structure for the concept of comfort IMAGE: the Journal of Nursing Scholarship 23: 237–240

Kolcaba KY 1992a Gerontological nursing: the concept of comfort in an environmental framework. Journal of Gerontological Nursing 18: 33–38

Kolcaba KY 1992b Holistic comfort: operationalising the construct as a nurse-sensitive outcome. Advances in Nursing Science 15: 1–10

Kolcaba KY 1993 A theory of holistic comfort for nursing. Journal of Advanced Nursing 19: 1178–1184

Kolcaba KY 2001 Evolution of a mid range theory of comfort for outcomes in research. Nursing Outlook 49: 86–92

Kolcaba KY, Kolcaba RJ 1991 An analysis of the concept of comfort. Journal of Advanced Nursing 16: 1301–1310

Larson PJ 1987 Comparison of cancer patients' and professional nurses' perceptions of important nurse caring behaviours. Heart and Lung 16: 187–193

Leininger MM 1981 The phenomenon of caring: importance, research questions and theoretical considerations. In: Leininger MM (ed) Caring, an essential human need. Charles B Slack, Thorofare, NJ, pp. 3–15

Letvak S 1997 Relational experiences of elderly women living alone in rural communities: a phenomenologic inquiry. Journal of the New York State Nurses Association 28

McIlveen KH, Morse JM 1995 The role of comfort in nursing care 1900–1980. Clinical Nursing Research 4: 127–148

Malinowski A, Stamler LL 2002 Comfort: exploration of the concept in nursing. Journal of Advanced Nursing 39: 599–606

Morse JM 1983 An ethnoscientific analysis of comfort: a preliminary investigation. Nursing Papers 15: 6–19

Morse JM 1992 Comfort: the re-focusing of nursing care. Clinical Nursing Research 1: 91–106

Morse JM 2000 On comfort and comforting. American Journal of Nursing 100: 34–38

Morse JM, Bottoroff JL, Hutchinson S 1994 The phenomenology of comfort. Journal of Advanced Nursing 20: 189–195

Nightingale F 1860 Notes on nursing: what it is, and what it is not. New York

Orlando I 1961 The dynamic nurse-patient relationship: function, process and principles. Putnam New York

Patterson JG, Zderad LT 1976 Humanistic nursing. John Wiley, New York

Peplau HE 1952 Interpersonal relations in nursing. Macmillan, Basingstoke

Rodgers B 1989 Concepts, analysis and the development of nursing knowledge: the evolutionary cycle. Journal of Advanced Nursing 14: 330–335

Rosenbaum JN 1991 A cultural assessment guide: learning cultural sensitivity. Canadian Nurse 87: 32

Roy C 1981 Cited in: George JB (ed) 1985 Nursing theories, the base for professional nursing practice. Prentice Hall, Englewood Cliffs, NJ

Siefert ML 2002 A concept analysis of comfort. Nursing Forum 37: 16–23

Tutton E, Seers K 2004 Comfort on a ward for older people. Journal of Advanced Nursing 46: 380–389

Wittgenstein L 1968 Philosophical investigations 3rd edn (trans GEM Anscombe). Macmillan, New York

Wurbach ME 1996 Comfort and nurses' moral choices. Journal of Advanced Nursing 24: 260–264

A concept analysis of coping

Catherine Black

EDITORIAL

Whether it is encountered explicitly or implicitly, the concept of coping is relevant to nurses. Each day we are engaged in providing care, each time we manage a situation or learning experience, we aim to cope with whatever stressors arise. The lived experiences of patients tell us that the same intra and interpersonal dynamics, albeit prompted by different stressors, are similarly present for them. Catherine's chapter prompts us to re-examine our own attitudes towards what it is to cope and, inversely, what it is to not cope. Catherine's chapter posits a hitherto unexplored, yet immensely thought provoking view; namely, that whether or not a person is seen to be coping can be a construct of a particular social setting. The same behaviours, *vis-à-vis* the degree of coping, can be interpreted in very different ways depending on the cultural nuances and the values and beliefs of the people within the particular setting. As a result it is incumbent upon all of us to have this awareness when we attempt to determine whether or not a patient/client is coping. Furthermore, we are reminded that perhaps it is only by communicating with the person and undertaking a co-joint assessment that a credible sense of the degree of coping can be determined.

As clinicians, both the authors have worked with bereaved people and the notion of social and cultural interpretations of coping and not coping resonated with our clinical experiences. The huge variation in reactions to a bereavement and the multitude of different ways that individuals found to cope served as a poignant aide-memoire of why it is vital for practitioners not to judge another's actions (and reaction to stressors) according to our own values and beliefs; why it is crucial to help patients find their own ways rather than forcing them to fit into our own 'models' of coping.

INTRODUCTION

Coping is a word that is often used in nursing literature. Nurses have much to cope with in their professional lives, including becoming nurses (Lo 2002), suffering, loss and death among the patients they care for (Rasmussen et al 1997, Rittman et al 1997, Payne et al 1998, Richardson & Poole 2001). They also have to cope with other stressors that exist in their lives outside work. Within a healthcare setting, nurses are not the only people who need to cope. Patients, for example, have to cope with hospitalization, chronic illness, pain, bad news and terminal diagnoses (Bliss & Johnson 1995, Davis et al 1996, Pakenham 2001, Richardson & Poole 2001). It is perhaps not surprising, then, that the nursing literature makes frequent references to coping. However, it should be noted that, although the concept of coping with a specific issue is often examined, the meaning of what it is to cope is itself is rarely analysed within the nursing literature. These more capacious discussions exist mainly within psychology texts (Jones & Bright 2001).

Despite the frequency with which nurses use the term 'coping', both in literature and in their daily practice lives, there is no consensus of understanding as to what constitutes coping. This chapter will initially examine definitions of coping and compare the 'everyday' general use of the word with more 'academic' definitions. It will then go on to look at how various nursing authors have addressed ways of coping in a variety of situations and so identify the defining attributes of the concept of coping as used by nurses.

MODEL OF CONCEPT ANALYSIS

The model of concept analysis used is that outlined by McKenna (1997). The key attributes of coping will be identified and discussed. There will then be a review of the antecedents and consequences of coping. The context for this concept analysis is that of nursing in developed countries, and clinical examples of coping (and non-coping) will be used throughout. These examples are based on 'real' situations and use the perspectives of both patients and nurses as they attempt to cope with their varied stressors. In the interests of confidentiality, all names and details have been changed.

DEFINITIONS

The *New Shorter Oxford English Dictionary* (1993) defines coping as 'to contend successfully with (an opponent, difficulty, situation, etc.); deal competently with one's life or situation.' This lay definition differs from an academic definition such as that of Lazarus and Folkman (1984, p. 221) who define coping as 'constantly changing cognitive and behavioural efforts to manage specific external and/or internal demands that are appraised as taxing or exceeding the resources of the person'. These contrasting definitions show that, while coping is used both as a lay term and as an academic term, the interpretation of the concept differs significantly (Lazarus & Folkman 1984, Richardson & Poole 2001). The academic concept is based in psychology theory and draws upon physiological theory, where stress is seen to involve the person and the environment and how they react and relate and respond to one another (Folkman et al 1986). Where the demands of the environment, either internal or external, exceed the ability of the individual to manage them, they are seen as needing to use coping strategies in order to prevent themselves from becoming stressed. The cogency of this point of view notwithstanding, this may not be the interpretation of the concept that is used by nurses in daily conversation, in their practice or in their reflection on themselves or the patients.

DEFINING ATTRIBUTES

COPING AS A HOLISTIC PHENOMENON

Coping can be seen as having cognitive and behavioural aspects (Lazarus & Folkman 1984) as well as effects on motivation (Zimbardo et al 1995). Other authors posit coping as a holistic phenomenon involving physical, psychological/emotional and social perspectives and, possibly, a combination of all of these at any time (Bartlett 1998). Physical aspects of coping can be seen as unconscious physiological responses to a perceived stressor. Once a stressor has been identified, the hypothalamus in the limbic system of the brain controls the stress response. The systems involved are the sympathetic adrenal medullary response system and the hypothalamic–pituitary–adrenal axis (Jones & Bright 2001). Together these control the cardiovascular and immune systems and prepare the body for rapid physical action – fight or flight.

This physiological stress response is an ancient human response, may not always be appropriate in modern life and can have negative effects on the person. An example of this would be someone going to an appointment with a doctor to receive some test results following a biopsy. The doctor tells the patient that the results indicate the positive presence of cancer cells. The autonomic response to the stress begins and the patient's pulse and blood pressure increase. The patient begins to cope with the situation by subconsciously preparing to leave the room (flight) and is unable to comprehend or retain the further information being given. The doctor goes on to explain that the cancer is well-localized and low-grade, and that total surgical resection and cure are possible. Because of the subconscious coping reaction that is taking place the patient is unable to listen to the doctor fully and leaves the consultation aware only that he has cancer.

It can be seen from this example that the physiological stress response is not always facilitative, helpful or enabling. It could be argued that the patient's response in this scenario does not compare very closely with either of the definitions identified earlier. The patient is subconsciously attempting self-protection by leaving a situation perceived as threatening, and this is not an uncommon reaction to bad news. Healthcare professionals have learned to acknowledge this effect and might attempt to mediate situations to negate the effects of such a response. In the situation described, the doctor could have started the consultation by highlighting that the results were good news in that they showed that a complete cure was possible. The consultation could then have examined the test results in more detail, but the patient's stress response would have been lessened by the information regarding cure. The patient would have been in a position to listen to the doctor and take in more of the information being given, and so cope with the situation.

Coping strategies to help manage the physiological stress reaction have been developed. These include relaxation and visualization techniques, and what is more, these can be learned (Bottomley 1996). An example of this is the work of Bredin et al (1999). They undertook a randomized-controlled trial where patients with lung cancer either received best supportive care or attended a nurse-led clinic. Those attending the nurse-led clinic were taught a range of strategies to help them cope with their dyspnoea (breathlessness). These included breathing control, pacing of activities, relaxation techniques and psychosocial support. The study showed that, while relaxation and visualization assisted individuals' coping by helping to control breathing and heart rate, they also gave the individual a sense of control, which is a vital psychological aspect of coping (Rittman et al 1997, Bottomley 1996).

Psychological aspects and processes are often discussed in nursing literature and are also posited as the main coping 'focus' by Lazarus and Folkman (1984). They argue that there are two fundamental types of coping: problem-focused and emotion-focused. Both are psychological processes, with problem-focused coping concentrating on finding ways of solving the problem and emotion-focused coping referring to finding ways of dealing with the unpleasant emotions aroused by the event. These reactions are seen as fundamental in allowing an individual to cope effectively with any situation, and flexibility of approach is required for coping to be successful (Lo 2002).

Several authors (Bliss & Johnson 1995, Bottomley 1996, Dein & Stygall 1997, Rittman et al 1997, Payne et al 1998, Baldacchino & Draper 2001, Pakenham 2001) discuss the importance of psychological adaptation and adjustment as an aspect of coping. Rittman et al (1997) discuss how nurses limit their relationships with patients at different levels in order to protect themselves from excessive emotional demands. Additional work exists (see, for example, Payne et al 1998) that supports this argument; for example, in this study it was found that nurses choose to distance themselves from those in their care and avoid potential stressors. Instead, they focus on physical needs and are thus protected from the patient's emotions and their subsequent reaction to them. This distancing occurs over time and is a method of self-protection for the nurses, and has been studied in clinical settings that are seen as particularly stressful, such as hospices and emergency rooms (Rasmussen et al 1997, Rittman et al 1997, Payne et al 1998, Payne 2001). It is argued that without making such adjustments nurses would be unable to cope with working in such environments and would suffer from burnout (Payne 2001). **It is often said that nurses who work is settings such as hospices are 'special' to be able to tolerate the perceived stressors. It may be the case that they are indeed special, but only in that they are able to psychologically adjust to such a situation in such a way as to ensure self-protection.**

Patients are also seen as needing to make mental adjustments to life-changing situations (Bliss & Johnson 1995, Bottomley 1996, Dein & Stygall 1997). Such adjustments can be to situations such as a shortened lifespan or a change in physical ability. Individuals who are seen as not making such adjustments and adaptations are seen as 'in denial' and therefore 'not coping'. However, this depends on the individual's success or otherwise at achieving their goals, as can be seen in the following examples:

Case study 5.1
Example of coping?

Mr A. has been diagnosed with terminal cancer and told that his life expectancy is 3–4 months. He runs his own successful business and continues to go to work every day. His wife supports him and helps when asked. As his condition deteriorates, Mr A. requires a wheelchair, but his wife takes him to work every day, even if only for a few hours. Once he can no longer go to work, he has paperwork brought to his house every day. He is working on a new business deal the day before he dies.

At his funeral Mr A. is praised as being a 'fighter who never let his illness get in the way of his life'.

Case study 5.2
Example of not coping?

Mr B. has had a cerebrovascular accident and is confined to a wheelchair with extensive right-sided weakness. After rehabilitation he is discharged to a nursing home, but states that this is 'just until he can walk again'. Mr B. falls from his wheelchair most days as he attempts to maintain his independence. He refuses to let the staff use lifting equipment and one nurse injures her back trying to help him into bed. After he dies, the staff reflect that Mr B's refusal to acknowledge his condition was difficult for them to manage. They saw him as non-compliant and unpopular.

In these two examples it can be seen that the judgement concerning the appropriateness or otherwise of a lack of mental adjustment is not made by patients themselves but by those observing them. In both cases the patient was trying to maintain his independence for as long as possible, but only in the case of Mr A. was this seen as a coping well. Mr B. was seen as not coping but had the same response to his illness as did Mr A. The difference is that Mr A. was supported in his aims and his social group saw them as appropriate. **In Mr B's social situation (a nursing home) he was expected to conform to differ norms (i.e. submit to the nursing support) and only when he failed to meet expected social values did his method of coping become seen as unacceptable.**

One of the main social aspects of coping in that there is an expectation that people will cope with personal and professional stressors (Bliss & Johnson 1995, Bottomley 1996, Davis et al 1996, Rittman et al 1997, Payne et al 1998, Baldacchino & Draper 2001). Some studies (see, for example, Rittman et al 1997, Payne et al 1998) illustrate that nurses are 'expected' to be able to cope with the various emotional demands of their work – both by themselves and by others. Furthermore, nurses may judge their ability to cope by comparison with their colleagues (Rasmussen et al 1997) and if these comparisons are unfavourable this may further reduce their ability to cope. Payne et al (1998) go on to discuss that some ways of coping, for example consuming excessive alcohol, taking 'sick' days off work, may be seen as socially unacceptable. **So while there is a social expectation for individuals to cope, this is tempered by the view that not all coping responses are acceptable.**

The view that society limits the mechanisms which individuals can use in order to cope contrasts with the work of Krishnasamy (1996) who demonstrates that, although social support is complex it can provide one of the strongest resources to help individuals to cope. Long and Johnson's (2001) study found that the social isolation created by excessive infantile crying reduced the coping abilities of the parents. Where contact and support from friends and family was available it allowed the parents to have a brief respite and increased their ability to cope.

Bliss and Johnson (1995) demonstrated the complexity of social support after a diagnosis of cancer. The participants in their study discussed how, after initial cancer treatment, they wished to be seen as 'normal' and so rejected support from their social group that they perceived as being excessive. However, they did require assistance to help them manage disabling side effects of treatment and the burden of judging the appropriateness of offers of help fell on those making them. Supporters were required to ensure that the patient felt in control but also to be able to clearly identify when help was required.

This ability to identify when help is required, while maintaining the individual's sense of control, is important to nurses. The nurse–patient relationship is an addition to the patient's existing social network and should be supportive of it (Panzarine 1985). Nurses must be aware of the social support their relationship offers the patient, as well as the effect that this relationship may have on the patient's existing social networks.

COPING AS A CONSCIOUS RESPONSE TO STRESS

Within the nursing literature, the relationship between stress and coping is complex. Coping is seen as a response to a perceived stressor or stress (Folkman et al 1986, Zimbardo et al 1995, Rasmussen et al 1997, Payne et al 1998, Long & Johnson 2001, Richardson & Poole 2001) and, indeed, the terms 'stressor' and 'stress' are used interchangeably. However, psychology literature discusses that a stressor is a demand made on a person whereas stress is the outcome if the person is unable to cope with that demand (Lazarus & Folkman 1984, Jones & Bright 2001). Lazarus and Folkman (1984) describe coping and stress as inextricably linked.

In the clinical setting, when coping is discussed it is indeed always in relation to a stressor such as a life-threatening diagnosis, pain following surgery or the death of a loved one. In the professional setting, we reflect upon how our colleagues cope with difficult situations such as breaking bad news, angry or aggressive patients and emergency admissions. In these ways we do see coping as an active response to a stressor. Such a view creates a situation where coping can only be said to exist in response to a stressor and, if taken to its logical conclusion, that a person without stressors is a person who is not required to cope.

Lazarus and Folkman (1984, p. 222) address this issue in their definition of coping. They deliberately see coping as only being required when the situation is appraised as exceeding the individual's resources; hence they exclude 'automatized behaviours and thoughts that do not require effort'. This allows for coping to be seen as a highly individualized experience (see next defining attribute), but does not allow for the concept to exist without a perceived stressor. While this could be seen as existing in the case of patients, who by definition will always have illness as a stressor, can it follow for nurses in their day-to-day care?

Clinical experience shows that a working day can be completed without any conscious appraisal of events as exceeding personal resources. The day can be assessed as being successful, with all outcomes achieved to set standards and time frames. From one perspective, it could be posited that coping skills and strategies were successfully used throughout the day. Lazarus and Folkman (1984, p. 220) argue that where situations do not exceed the individual's resources the response is 'automatized adaptive behaviour' and not coping.

This highlights one of the differences between the academic and lay definitions of coping and the appropriateness of the use of the concept by nurses. A person who has successfully completed a task may not be seen as having had to cope if they do not demonstrate having any difficulties with it. Another person undertaking the same task but having problems will, on completion, be seen as having used coping strategies successfully. The relationship between stress and coping is a negative one, where it is only the lack of coping that leads to the development of stress, and so whether coping and stress are inextricably linked may be questioned. Perhaps one could offer an alternative view that posits that the inextricable relationship is between lack of coping and stress.

COPING AS AN INDIVIDUAL RESPONSE

Coping skills are not innate but are developed by individuals throughout their lives in response to different stressors and experiences (Lazarus & Folkman 1984, Zimbardo et al 1995, Bottomley 1996, Bartlett 1998, Long & Johnson 2001, Pakenham 2001, Lo 2002). Individuals may develop particular coping styles (Lazarus & Folkman 1984, Lo 2002), either problem-focused or emotion-focused, that they find successful. However, it is important that they maintain the ability to learn and use new strategies as necessary. Being reliant on one method of coping can increase stress levels if a situation is met where this particular strategy is inappropriate (Lo 2002). For example, emotion-focused coping, where the individual deals with the unpleasant emotions created by a stressor, may not be an effective strategy when coping with a flat tyre. In such a situation problem-focused skills (finding ways of solving the problem) may be more effective.

In their study Long and Johnson (2001, p. 229) describe 'peaks and troughs' of coping. Although specific triggers for changes were difficult to identify, generally small successes improved levels of coping and accumulations of perceived setbacks decreased coping levels. It is important for health professionals to acknowledge changes in the individual's ability to cope, which will depend on factors other than the immediate stressor itself. A patient in hospital will have stressors other than their illness. These could include sharing a room, lack of sleep, financial worries and family concerns. When assisting someone to cope it may be that addressing minor stressors may enable the individual to focus on the major stressor and successfully employ coping strategies. It should also be considered that, as coping skills can be developed and learned, they can also be taught and supported (Bottomley 1996, Krishnasamy 1996, Bredin et al 1999, Long & Johnson 2001). Preoperative education and advice can allow individuals to begin to develop the strategies that they may need postoperatively, although it is best if the skills being taught are congruent with the individual's existing coping style (Panzarine 1985).

MODEL CASE

Case study 5.3
A model case of coping

> I met Mr C., his wife and son an hour after Mr C. had been admitted to the hospice and several minutes after they had been told that his prognosis was that he only had days to live. I gave him some oral morphine for his pain and breathlessness and rearranged his pillows until he was comfortable. I explained that his symptoms should begin to improve and the other options we had for helping him. I asked what else I could do for him. Mr C. took my hand and looked into my eyes. There was a pause while he caught his breath to speak. 'It's OK, you know. I know you'll be here. I know you'll help.' He smiled and squeezed my hand again. I squeezed back. I looked around the room. His family were holding each other, smiling and nodding. There was a sense of calm.

ANTECEDENTS TO COPING

In order to utilize coping an individual must be in a situation where there are potential stressors. If one accepts Lazarus and Folkman's arguments then such individuals must be able to identify these stressors and appraise them in light of other stressors they are experiencing and resources that they have available. The individual needs to have some prior experience of stressors in order to identify them as potentially threatening and to have developed some coping techniques that can be used. Only once stressors have been identified and strategies developed to manage them can subconscious coping be employed.

Arguably, all patients can be seen as having their illness experience or condition as one of their potential stressors. However, without knowledge of their illness and its potential consequences they cannot appraise the nature of the threat, and so may employ inappropriate coping strategies. An individual having been given a diagnosis of cancer may decide to ask for a second opinion from a respected consultant. This process takes several weeks and consequently the cancer spreads and becomes more difficult to treat, which reduces the chances of the individual being cured. In such a case the coping strategies of gaining control and gathering information may actually harm the individual. However, they did not have knowledge and understanding of this when they made their initial decision.

CONSEQUENCES OF COPING

An individual who is successfully coping is seen as being calm, in control and making rational decisions. Nurses often espouse their intention to give increased control to patients and involve them in the decision-making process. Individuals who do not take up this option and instead ask others to make their decisions can sometimes be described as being 'in denial' or 'withdrawn' and seen as 'not coping'. Individuals who perceive themselves as 'copers' can have increased self-confidence inspired by this knowledge (Zimbardo et al 1995). The belief that they have the ability to cope with any situation means that they do not spend time deciding on the best approach to use. This creates the impression of knowledge and control of the situation, and so others then believe that the individual can cope. This confidence can be inspiring to others, so that they can also cope with the situation.

Such a situation can be seen in a clinical setting when an experienced and confident nurse is in charge when there is an emergency admission. The nurse in charge can make rapid decisions and reorganize the use of resources appropriately. Staff will be informed of the problem (emergency admission) and solution (reallocation of resources) at the same time. This prevents any chaotic response when people are wondering what to do (Zimbardo et al 1995) and so supports people in coping with the situation. A less confident and experienced person might instead ask several colleagues for advice regarding the decision. This would create uncertainty and anxiety among the team, increase stress levels and decrease coping.

EMPIRICAL INDICATORS

The literature and other sources of information accessed for this concept analysis have been unable to identify clear empirical indicators for the existence of coping. There are degrees of coping and each coping response is specific to both the individual and the stressor. The examples of Mr A. and Mr B. demonstrated that the success or otherwise of coping is not always judged by those undertaking it. Both of these men saw themselves as successfully coping with their situations but their social groups assessed them differently.

However, common empirical indicators might perhaps include the degree to which the person's behaviour is socially accepted. Coping is socially expected (Bliss & Johnson 1995, Bottomley 1996, Davis et al 1996, Rittman et al 1997, Payne et al 1998, Baldacchino & Draper 2001) and successful coping creates calmness, control and rationality. An individual displaying such traits can be seen as being an easier patient to care for, and makes the nurses' role easier. Consequently, one can assert with a degree of confidence that the opposite position might also have credibility. Therefore not coping is not often socially acceptable and unsuccessful coping (or not coping) will be followed by the absence of calmness, a lack of control and indications of irrationality. Thus, individuals displaying such traits can be seen as being less easy patients to care for as they make the nurse's role more difficult.

Nurses need to consider whether their requirement for patients to cope with difficult stressors such as hospitalization, chronic illness, pain, bad news and terminal diagnoses (Bliss & Johnson 1995, Davis et al 1996, Pakenham 2001, Richardson & Poole 2001) is because it is beneficial for the patient themselves or instead beneficial for the nurses, in that it reduces their stressors. It should also be considered that coping is the effort to manage the stressor and that, when assessing if an individual is coping or not, we should not confuse this with the outcome (Lazarus & Folkman 1984). This is especially important when individuals are using coping techniques, such as drinking excessive alcohol, that may be seen as socially unacceptable and unsuccessful coping but may actually be enabling that person to manage the stressors they are facing. Successful coping for one individual may be a psychological breakdown for another. Only the individual can be aware of all of the stressors affecting them at any given time, and only they are aware of the coping resources they have available. Being able to present a calm and rational exterior may not always be a true indicator of coping.

CONCLUSION

Coping is a concept used extensively throughout nursing literature in relation to both nurses and patients coping with a variety of situations. However, there is little discussion of what it actually means to cope. Undertaking a concept analysis using the approach described by McKenna (1997) allowed three defining attributes to be identified:

- Coping is a holistic phenomenon involving physiological, psychological and social elements; the social (cultural) element being particularly important in determining whether a person is coping/not-coping
- Coping is a conscious response to stress that produces visible behaviours in the person, namely the 'consequences' of the concept (see below)
- Coping is an individual response and, while different people may have different innate abilities to cope, the behaviours and skills associated with coping can be learned and refined.

The antecedent to coping appears to be the identification of a stressor or stressors and the consequences are that the person who is coping presents as being calm, in control and able to make rational decisions. Currently within health care, the success or degree of coping is most often judged by the outcome of the action taken, rather than whether or not the particular coping strategies used were enabling for the individual. Therefore, when nurses are assessing a person's degree of coping, for future practice it is crucial that nurses look at the *effects* or *outcomes* of the coping strategy rather than focusing on the *strategies*; particularly since such strategies are almost inevitably going to be grounded in the cultural background of the individual. Coping remains a difficult concept to measure and quantify and further work is needed to better understand it within a range of healthcare settings and cultural contexts.

REFERENCES

Baldacchino D, Draper P 2001 Spiritual coping strategies: a review of the nursing research literature. Journal of Advanced Nursing 34: 833–841

Bartlett D 1998 Stress: perspectives and processes. Open University Press, Buckingham

Bliss J, Johnson B 1995 After diagnosis of cancer: the patient's view of life. International Journal of Palliative Nursing 1: 126–133

Bottomley A 1996 Group cognitive behavioural therapy: an intervention for cancer patients. International Journal of Palliative Nursing 2: 131–137

Bredin M, Corner J, Krishnasamy M et al 1999 Multicentre randomised controlled trail of nursing intervention for breathlessness in patients with lung cancer. British Medical Journal 318: 901–904

Davis B, Cowley S, Ryland R 1996 The effects of terminal illness on patients and their carers. Journal of Advanced Nursing 23: 512–520

Dein S, Stygall J 1997 Does being religious help or hinder coping with chronic illness? A critical literature review. Palliative Medicine 11: 291–298

Folkman S, Lazarus RS, Gruen RJ et al 1986 Appraisal, coping, health status and psychological symptoms. Journal of Personality and Social Psychology 50: 571–579

Jones F, Bright J 2001 Stress: myth, theory and research. Prentice Hall, London

Krishnasamy M 1996 Social support and the patient with cancer: a consideration of the literature. Journal of Advanced Nursing 23: 757–762

Lazarus RS, Folkman S 1984 Stress, appraisal and coping. Springer, New York

Lo R 2002 A longitudinal study of perceived level of stress, coping and self-esteem of undergraduate nursing students: an Australian case study. Journal of Advanced Nursing 39: 119–126

Long T, Johnson M 2001 Living and coping with excessive infantile crying. Journal of Advanced Nursing 34: 155–162

McKenna HP 1997 Nursing theories and models. Routledge, London

Pakenham K 2001 Application of a stress and coping model to care giving in multiple sclerosis. Psychology, Health and Medicine 6: 13–27

Panzarine S 1985 Coping: conceptual and methodological issues. Advances in Nursing Science 7: 49–57

Payne N 2001 Occupational stressors and coping as determinants of burnout in female hospice nurses. Journal of Advanced Nursing 33: 396–405

Payne S, Dean S, Kalus C 1998 A comparative study of death anxiety in hospice and emergency nurses. Journal of Advanced Nursing 28: 700–706

Rasmussen B, Sandman P, Norberg A 1997 Stories of being a hospice nurse: a journey towards finding one's footing. Cancer Nursing 20: 330–341

Richardson C, Poole H 2001 Chronic pain and coping: a proposed role for nurses and nursing models. Journal of Advanced Nursing 34: 659–667

Rittman M, Paige P, Rivera J et al 1997 Phenomenological study of nurses caring for dying patients. Cancer Nursing 20: 115–119

Zimbardo P, McDermott M, Jansz J et al 1995 Psychology. A European text. Harper Collins, London

A concept analysis of dignity

Jerome Marley

EDITORIAL

Few credible nurses would deny that dignity is something they are very much aware of. Whether this is manifest as an intervention in a patient's care plan, a specific care goal or as an issue to be considered and addressed at a Research Ethics Committee meeting, dignity is encountered with predictable regularity. Yet Jerome's chapter reminds us that, despite this sense of ubiquity and nurses' experiences with dignity, it remains very difficult to encapsulate dignity in a straightforward definition. Dignity thus shares a similarity with some of the other concepts in this book, in that, while we cannot provide a succinct and universally accepted definition, we probably know it when we see it. Indeed, it might be more accurate to suggest that we recognize it more when it is missing.

What is clear is that patients are very much aware of their own dignity and are similarly aware of indignity and/or feeling dignified. While for some nurses the allure of highly technological interventions may be difficult to resist, the importance and value of maintaining a person's dignity, often through what appear to be 'simple' or 'basic' practices, should not be downplayed. Even though the technologically advanced nurse may be able to carry out the procedure quickly and proficiently, if this occurs at the expense of the person's dignity or ignores the person's need for dignity, then is this an example of good nursing care? The maintenance and preservation of dignity then, like many 'low visibility' nursing skills, is so fundamental, so basic, so unobtrusive, that it can be rejected by some in favour of the more 'overt', high tech., 'exciting' interventions and practices. This is despite the empirical evidence (such as it is) that continues to demonstrate how important dignity is to patients and despite the fact that the psychological processes of how nurses maintain and preserve dignity are not well understood.

INTRODUCTION

Even the most cursory of investigations would reveal that the concept of dignity is seen as central to the way we interact with those for whom we care. Indeed, so ingrained is this notion that it might well prove a challenge to identify what is meant by the concept. Thus, one is left with a question: if dignity is so central to what nurses do then just what is meant by the term?

The notion of structured conceptual analysis involving the adherence to investigative steps resulting in a well illuminated and fully defined concept is cautioned against in the literature (McKenna 1997). However, many of the concepts in nursing might be categorized as nebulous and developmentally immature (Morse et al 1996). Dignity is an example of such a concept. Repeatedly, the literature comments that, while the concept of dignity is a universal reference point in professional health care, and while copious research studies on dignity in clinical settings have been carried out, its components remain ill-defined (Statman 2000, Chochinov 2002, Chochinov et al 2002, Sandman 2002, Walsh & Kowanko 2002). Allied to this, it has been argued that seeking a deeper understanding of the words we use in health care is a vital goal and that using words that convey intended meanings about ideas facilitates understanding.

> Understandings arise as ideas are integrated with personal knowledge and beliefs; thus, it is always important to convey accurately and clearly what is intended. Accuracy and clarity are essential to the conveyance of meanings and are fostered by using words as they are defined in a dictionary or defined within a discipline-specific theoretical perspective.
>
> Parse 2002, p. 3

This chapter seeks to continue the process of the clarification of the concept of dignity and sets itself alongside the conceptual analysis work already done by others (Meleis 1991, Mairis 1994, Haddock 1996). This is important, as it responds to calls within the literature to specify ways in which the concept of dignity is significant for nursing theory and practice (Meleis 1991, McKenna 1997). To assist continuity with previous work the author has chosen to broadly mirror the concept analysis process described by Chinn and Kramer (1991, 1999). Following a similar path to previous authors respects the process of uncovering what has been termed 'dimensions of meaning' (van Manen 2002).

DIGNITY IN A NURSING CONTEXT

The notion of understanding dignity as an element of the collective unconscious of people, and the argument that practical attention to dignity in health care is passed on professionally and socially from generation to generation, are significant. It might be further argued that dignity is understood in broadly similar terms by health professionals and patients alike, so socially pervasive is the concept. A phenomenological study of nurses' and patients' perception of dignity echoes this point: themes identified by nurses and patients showed similarity in important elements (Walsh & Kowanko 2002). When expressions of dignity are sought in music, literature and art it is also the case that the same key components are repeatedly referred to, reinforcing the idea of an archetypal understanding.

The notion of an archetypal understanding of the concept of dignity has significance in relation to the metaparadigms that inform nursing theory and actions. It has been claimed that a paradigm provides a road map to assist in the accumulation of knowledge about selected phenomena of concern to a discipline (Conway 1992), with nursing epistemologists subscribing to a four-component metaparadigm: 'nursing', 'health', 'person' and 'environment' (McKenna 1997). Some authors point to middle-range concepts that are intimately related to the global concepts but remain abstractions from them (Moody 1990). While it may not be explicitly identified as a global component of nursing's paradigms, relegation of dignity simply to a practically grounded middle-range concept appears ill-conceived. This is because of the notion of an archetypal understanding and the claim of the universal experience of dignity as a fundamental pillar upon which professional care rests. It has been suggested that there are nine pillars of human dignity: sufficient food, potable water, shelter, sanitation, health services, healthy environment, education, employment and personal security (Diczfalusy 1997a). Accordingly, it might be said of dignity that it is at once an inherent part of being human and intertwined with what living is all about (Bournes 2000). Although currently ill-defined, when perceived as absent, dignity reminds us of how essential it is for nurses and the practice of nursing.

DEFINITIONS, CRITICAL ATTRIBUTES AND DATA SOURCES

DICTIONARIES

The *Oxford English Dictionary* (OED) (1989) notes that the word 'dignity' emerges from the trunk of the English word *digne* which in turn comes from the Latin word *dignus*, meaning 'worthy'. The OED details eight meanings of the word dignity. The first notes that dignity is a quality of being worthy or honourable and incorporates the notions of worthiness, worth, nobleness and excellence. Among the remaining meanings of the word, dignity is noted to be an honourable or high estate and a rank or title. In defining the eighth meaning of dignity, the OED echoes the idea of archetypal understanding (Danneels 2003), when it notes that, in an erroneous or fantastic rendering of the word in scientific history, dignity has been used to refer to the notion of a first principle or axiom. Webster's *Third New International Dictionary* (1971) displays an understanding of dignity that fits very easily with literature explanations of the concept. Webster's dictionary further suggests that dignity incorporates the notion of investing with dignity or honour, making illustrious and giving distinction to someone or something. This definition makes explicit the notion that dignity has at least two components. It incorporates not only the idea of intrinsic worth present in a person, situation or object but, additionally, the action of investing with the concept someone or something that may be lacking it to a degree. This notion will be returned to later.

PROFESSIONAL LITERATURE

When considering dignity it is important to make a distinction between human dignity and what has been termed contingent dignity (Sandman 2002). Human dignity refers to the fact that humans possess and retain dignity all through life by virtue of the fact that they are human. Such dignity rests upon premises of ethics and the principal of equality among humans. This view is commensurate with the Universal Declaration of Human Rights adopted and proclaimed by the General Assembly of the United Nations (UN) in 1948. The preamble states: 'Whereas recognition of the inherent dignity and of equal and inalienable rights of all members of the human family is the foundation of freedom, justice and peace in the world …' (United Nations 2003). This UN declaration clearly implies that there is a reciprocal obligation in the way in which humans should act and behave towards others, a point also found in the literature (Sandman 2002).

In addition, it has been claimed that humans also possess contingent dignity, understood as those expressions of dignity that might distinguish us from other humans. Expressions of contingent dignity might be found in certain 'deep-going' features that individuals might possess, such as being very autonomous or rational. Other expressions of contingent dignity might be found in certain personality traits such as shyness and gregariousness, or in those indefinable qualities that make us consider others as awe-inspiring or requiring of our respect (Sandman 2002).

The notions of innate and contingent dignity are visible within the literature, with repeated references not only to those standards that might reasonably be demanded by and for all, but also to those qualities of dignity suggested by individuals as being essential for them in understanding their lives.

The distinguished British zoologist and physician, Thomas Henry Huxley, stated that 'the great end of life is not knowledge but action' (Diczfalusy 1997b). Such a view offers an understanding of dignity by way of examining its antecedents in action rather than solely via theoretical exploration. The literature contains studies that outline elements that are suggested as key to an understanding of dignity (see, for example, Mairis 1994, Haddock 1996, Statman 2000, Sandman 2002, Jacelon 2003, Widang & Fridlund 2003), with the caution, however, that dignity is often talked about but rarely examined (Jacelon 2003).

Widang and Fridlund (2003) have argued that dignity comprises the conceptions of being seen as a whole person, being respected and being seen as trustworthy. Study respondents described complex physical, psychological, social and existential needs; being seen as an individual was a key way of feeling dignified and uniquely human. It has been further reported that when people were treated in their wholeness (and by extension had their uniqueness affirmed) there was a greater chance that they reported feeling a sense of well-being and feeling that they had been treated as a unique person, not as a number or a case. The ways in which respect was demonstrated included gestures such as: knocking on a room door before entering, not exposing the patient's body for longer than was absolutely necessary and not talking over the patient's head or in an offensive or patronizing manner. Patients also described how having their explanations of disease experiences accepted as true, without the dismissive gesture of requiring all explanations to be confirmed by means of a medical examination, enhanced their sense of dignity.

Other sources argue that an injury to dignity, such as not knocking on a room door or exposing a patient's body unnecessarily, are usually expressed by the patient in figurative language. Such expressions amount to the humiliation of the patient and phrases such as 'robbed of one's dignity', 'stripped of one's dignity', or simply having one's dignity 'lost' are all commonplace (Statman 2000). It might be argued that patients inherently know what for them are adequate expressions of dignity and that, since some healthcare processes contain elements of depersonalization, the patient has to surrender some degree of dignity in order to access the healthcare services (Mairis 1994). However, while a degree of depersonalization and temporary loss of dignity may be inevitable in health care, it is suggested that the patient still has three very fundamental needs:

- the need to maintain self-respect
- the need to maintain self-esteem
- the need to have their individual standards appreciated (Mairis 1994).

These views, written over a decade ago, are echoed in more recent work. For example, it is interesting to note that in Walsh and Kowanko's (2002) phenomenological study in Australia, themes similar to the points listed above were evident. In this study themes inducted from patient data showed remarkable similarity to those suggested by staff. The themes identified were:

- being exposed
- having time
- being rushed
- having time to decide
- being seen as a person
- the body as object
- being acknowledged with consideration
- discretion (Walsh & Kowanko 2002).

The contention that the degree to which a context matches a person's own dignity expectation is important and echoed by other authors, as typified by the following quotation from a study of hospitalized elders: 'A person's current dignity reflects the amount of congruence between his or her internal definition of dignity, behaviour, and the meanings he or she ascribes to the behaviour of others towards him- or herself. The greater the congruence the stronger the elder's sense of dignity' (Jacelon 2003, p. 546).

Fagermoen's (1997) study provides relevant data concerning what nurses consider to be the professional values embedded in meaningful practice. These results reveal a mirror image of the views expressed by patients when asked about dignity that are described above. Fagermoen's study of 767 randomly selected Norwegian nurses suggests that the nurses described meaningful values that related to themselves as individual professionals and values that related to the 'other' whom they were treating (Table 6.1). It is interesting to note from this study that the nurses

Table 6.1

Important values of dignity for 'self' and for 'the other'

OTHER-ORIENTED VALUES	
Process	**Outcome**
Upholding humaneness	
Upholding other's rights	Rights preserved
Fostering trust	Trust fostered
Attending to needs for help	Help recognized
Attending to needs for protection	Protection assured
SELF-ORIENTED VALUES	
Intrinsic	**Extrinsic**
Independence	Colleagues
Intellectual stimulation	Leadership
Personal stimulation	Reward structure
Creativity	Nursing as profession
Achievement	

appear to abhor treating patients as a number or case just as much as patients wish not to be treated as such.

HUMAN SOURCES

Chinn and Kramer (1991, 1999) suggest that other people can provide valuable information about the meaning of a concept, as this acts as a heuristic. Accordingly, the views of 10 people from nursing and non-nursing backgrounds were canvassed. The opinions obtained about dignity are grouped and presented in Figure 6.1.

To facilitate comparison of this new material with existing literature, it was decided to follow the same broad domains as are described in Haddock's (1996) concept analysis of dignity. Noticeably, while some similar attributes were identified, differences and additional items were also illuminated.

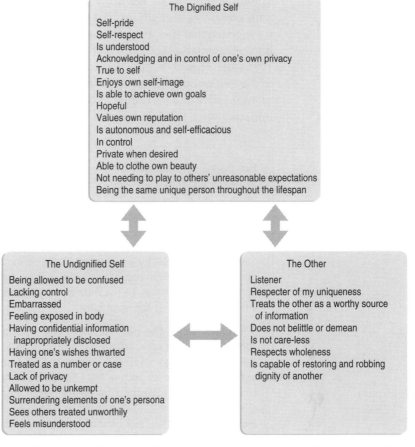

Figure 6.1 Values indicative of the presence and absence of dignity in 'self' and in 'the other'

For those consulted, dignity was seen very much as involving having pride and respect for oneself. These attributes were suggested as being evidenced within a person when they took control of their life, achieved their own goals, moved into and out of privacy and intimacy as they chose and expressed the uniqueness of their person in the way they dressed and presented themselves. Dignity was evident in human beings when they could be as much of a unique person in senior years as they were in early life. It was suggested by another source that, while an inevitable degree of depersonalization is likely in healthcare services and systems, it does not have to reach the point where patients resort to fulfilling the expectation they believe the health system has of them. In addition, it was further suggested that it is less than dignified when patients also expect the healthcare professional to fulfil the role that the patient has for them.

It is interesting to note that the notion of dignity as something that can be given to and removed from a patient by a health professional – an extension of the point made via the Webster's dictionary definition of dignity – was made repeatedly by sources. In detailing the items required of 'the other', the sources were determined to outline that dignity was a quality that existed both in and for people; that it is both possession and gift. As part of the process of creating conceptual meaning it is suggested that the multiple meanings created early in the process can be refined into representations or cases that display the concept in context (Chinn & Kramer 1999). It is argued that the case below is selected because it represents the concept to the best of our present understanding. This caution reflects the ongoing nature of progressive understanding of concepts and how they might both impact and be impacted upon through use.

Case study 6.1
An example case of dignity

Mrs Docherty had been diagnosed as having a calculus ('kidney stone') in her left kidney that was suitable for treatment with lithotripsy (disintegration of the stone by using sound/shock waves). A treatment date was arranged for the lithotripsy to be carried out as a day procedure in her local hospital. Mrs Docherty was sent notification of the appointment by post along with a small information leaflet explaining the treatment. The leaflet had been approved by a government department that specializes in analysing documents for their use of plain language. Among other things, the leaflet contained a listing of the standards of care that Mrs Docherty should expect when she attended for treatment.

On admission to the unit Mrs Docherty was greeted warmly by a nurse and shown to her bed area, which had well fitting curtains, prior to a pretreatment assessment being completed. During the assessment Mrs Docherty was encouraged by the nurse to outline her knowledge of her condition and to understand that she should expect to be treated with respect at all times, have all her questions answered to her satisfaction and opt for a different treatment method should she find lithotripsy unacceptable. In addition to the normal matters, the consent form for lithotripsy incorporated these additional elements in its attempt to ensure that Mrs Docherty fully understood her rights.

Case study 6.1
An example case of
dignity—*cont'd*

Immediately prior to treatment Mrs Docherty dressed in a gown. The gown had been specially designed by staff in consultation with patients to overlap at the side and be easily closed with a drawstring. It did not split up the back like traditional examination gowns. Once on the treatment table Mrs Docherty was covered with a sheet and only then was the area to be treated exposed. The treatment room had one of its two entrances blocked with a sign prohibiting entrance when treatment was in progress. Entry via the remaining door was strictly controlled by staff. At the beginning of treatment it was explained to Mrs Docherty that she should indicate if she was uncomfortable during treatment and the problem would be addressed. During treatment Mrs Docherty chatted with staff, who regularly determined if everything was satisfactory for her.

On completion of treatment Mrs Docherty was given instructions concerning how to care for herself. She posed a number of questions and these were answered by staff to her satisfaction. Before going home, Mrs Docherty was given the details of a 24-hour urology helpline and encouraged to call if she experienced any problems that concerned her. Mrs Docherty was asked which day suited her for a follow-up appointment and after this was booked written confirmation was given to her. Mrs Docherty was also given a questionnaire asking for her comments on the service she had received. The questionnaire audited the same standards that had been communicated to Mrs Docherty in print and by staff as normal for her to expect. On her discharge, Mrs Docherty thanked staff for their caring attitude and said she would be very happy to come back again if that was needed, comments she echoed in her returned questionnaire.

The above scenario is presented as an exemplar as it touches on many of the key attributes of the concept identified in the various sources. Staff had considered the fact that, as Mrs Docherty had not received the treatment previously she might be unsure of what was entailed. This influenced their preparation of materials that were sent to her. The materials had been examined for plain use of language as a further attempt to increase their understanding. The warm greeting reflects the fact that staff behaviour and attitude are often described as important in the maintenance of dignity (Seedhouse & Gallagher 2002). The care taken with the environment echoes the need for privacy to be respected and for unnecessary exposure to be avoided. The acknowledgement of the individual's story of his/her illness is reported as an important act by patients (Widang & Fridlund 2003). Given that patients perceive unnecessary exposure as depersonalizing, deliberate attempts were made to preserve dignity via avoidance of unnecessary exposure (Mairis 1994). The discreet way in which Mrs Docherty's body was exposed (Walsh & Kowanko 2002), being encouraged to express her level of satisfaction (Jacelon 2003) and the deliberate attempts made by staff to expose and hold up the patient's rights (Fagermoen 1997) all underscore the exemplar nature of this encounter. As an entire episode, the staff treating Mrs Docherty tried to make the experience something that was worthy of her and so the individual acts had the effect of giving her distinction (Webster 1971).

Case study 6.2
Dignity: a contrary case

Mr Hughes was a 65-year-old man who was admitted to hospital one evening at 22:45 hours with acute urinary retention. He was brought directly to a ward and was allocated a bed in a bay with three other men. The ward staff were busy as they were required to prepare patients for and receive them from theatre. Mr Hughes stated that he was in considerable discomfort due to his bladder being distended. Nursing staff told him they were very busy and would be along to see him when they had a spare minute. Mr Hughes felt confused and vulnerable. After 20 minutes a doctor arrived to begin the process of medical assessment, at the end of which a decision was made to insert a urinary catheter. Normally, experienced nursing staff carried out this procedure. After a further 30 minutes had elapsed a nurse wheeling a trolley prepared for a catheter insertion came to Mr Hughes and told him she would insert the catheter.

Although uncomfortable because of bladder distension, Mr Hughes was concerned about the procedure for inserting the catheter and told the nurse so. Standing by the sink, where she was washing her hands, the nurse responded that it was a necessary procedure and anyway he was not to worry as many men had catheters and had no problems. The nurse returned to the bedside and drew the curtains around the bed. Mr Hughes was asked to remove his trousers and underwear in preparation for the procedure. No further explanation of the need for the procedure was given. Mr Hughes was lying on the bed with his genitals exposed in preparation for the catheter insertion. The nurse quietly busied herself opening the packs she needed. Mr Hughes looked anxious but decided that it was futile to ask any further questions.

The nurse told Mr Hughes she had to clean 'the area' and began to apply a solution to his penis. At this point the nurse's name was called by a colleague and she answered, giving her whereabouts. A few seconds later the curtains opened and a nurse came into the bed area asking for a set of keys. Neither nurse acknowledged Mr Hughes's presence, although the second nurse did smile as she came in. The nurse left with the keys but a small gap remained in the curtains through which Mr Hughes could make out other people in the ward. He was unsure if they could see him.

Following the insertion of the catheter and the connection of a leg bag drainage system, the nurse told Mr Hughes he could put his pyjamas on and she would come by later to show him how to empty the drainage bag. The nurse tidied her trolley and left, closing the curtains behind her.

In contrast to the experience of the patient portrayed in the exemplar case, Mr Hughes's experience is characterized by indignity. It is argued that, because nursing is often described as a profession where dignity is promoted by the deliberate actions of the nurse (Australian Nursing Council 1995, International Council of Nurses 2000, Nursing and Midwifery Council 2002, Seedhouse & Gallagher 2002), it is justifiable to use the active term 'indignity' rather than the passive 'undignified'. Consequently, it might be further concluded that an encounter where the nurse fails to act in a manner that bestows dignity is not only an encounter where dignity is absent but one where indignity is actively present.

It was suggested in Table 6.1 that some of the outcomes of dignity involved the preservation of issues such as trust, protection and having one's rights respected and upheld. The contrary case as detailed demonstrates a negation of these issues. Despite his pain and discomfort, Mr Hughes was greeted with little in the way of understanding of his experience. There is no doubt that in a busy clinical environment there are times when competing patient needs can force staff to prioritize in favour of one patient over another. This situation was, however, not adequately explained to Mr Hughes, thus exacerbating his feelings of vulnerability. When unsure about the procedure of catheterization Mr Hughes' questions were not treated properly by the nurse. Instead of addressing Mr Hughes directly, his concerns were dismissed as not real by the nurse as she washed her hands.

Exposing genitals for a legitimate invasive examination or procedure is a regular requirement for some patients. Repeatedly, however, this issue is reported as one of the most embarrassing and potentially undignified patient experiences. Patients often realize that procedures can result in a reduction of their dignity, even though the purpose of such procedures may be to preserve or restore a central feature of dignity, such as removal of pain and restoration of bodily function (Chinn & Kramer 1999). In this scenario the reduction in dignity, however, was compounded by the intrusion of a second nurse without Mr Hughes' permission and the lack of care that left a partially naked Mr Hughes exposed to the gaze of others through badly closed curtains.

Case study 6.3
Dignity: a borderline case

> The lyrics of the song entitled 'Dignity' by Scottish singer Ricky Ross might be described as an example of a borderline case of the concept of dignity. The song tells the story of a man who for 20 years has worked in Glasgow (Scotland), clearing litter from the gutter, an unglamorous job no matter how socially necessary. Through the song the man displays sentiments that indicate that his daily experience has led him to feel somewhat belittled and devoid of respect and dignity both for what he does and for who he is. Children call him names and the reaction of some people to what he does has hardened his attitude. As a reaction to those attributes of dignity that he senses are lacking from his life, the man harbours a secret – he will buy a boat and sail along the Scottish west coast. The name of the boat will be *Dignity*.

The song clearly illustrates that the naming of the boat is not an arbitrary act. Rather it is a naming that calls into counterpoint the exemplar and contrary cases of the concept. By acquiring his dream and by naming the boat after those attributes he was robbed of in his working life, the man has refused to be completely and unavoidably influenced by his surroundings (Frankl 1963). Like the concentration camp inmates described by Viktor Frankl (1963), the street cleaner never fully allows himself to be moulded into the form of a beaten man robbed of dreams or the living of a dignified life.

EXPLORING CONTEXTS AND VALUES

Exploring the social contexts within which experience and values occur can provide important cultural meanings that influence mental representations of the experience (Chinn & Kramer 1999). With reference to nursing and dignity, understanding the concept from the position of either the patient or the nurse produces little if any divergence. Creating contexts or vantage points from which to view the expressions of dignity does little more that emphasize the key components, and only serves to illustrate these components in how they might expect to be met or in how they are planned to be met. While the ways in which dignity is experienced and valued by different social groups throughout the world may differ quite markedly, it could be argued that, no matter what actions are valued as being essential to maintain dignity, it is always the same basic concept that is being appealed to – worthiness and its maintenance. It could be argued further that a range of problems, from patient–nurse misunderstanding to global conflict, might all have a common root – a lack of congruence has been created between the understanding and expectation of dignity of one party and the understanding and provision of dignity of the other.

CRITERIA AND AN OPERATIONAL DEFINITION FOR THE CONCEPT

The exemplar case used in concept analysis is itself a full expression of conceptual meaning (Chinn & Kramer 1999). However, in the conclusion of this chapter it is appropriate to further synthesize an understanding of the concept of dignity as it is currently understood by the author and to outline some empirical indicators that can reasonably be identified from the literature. In so doing it is acknowledged that no concept analysis succeeds in capturing all that is relevant, nor can it ever provide completely definitive descriptions of concepts and the criteria or indicators by which they are recognized and developed.

Dignity is an inalienable human possession. Within each person it creates an understanding of how one should be perceived and respected and produces both common and unique understandings and expectations. Dignity is a shared concept within social groups and results in archetypical understandings of normal behaviours and the ability to identify attitudes and actions that are offensive to the individual and the group. It is possible that, while everything can be taken from a person and despite the dignity-withholding actions of others, the last of the human freedoms, the freedom to choose one's attitude, remains and can result in a complete and unaltered possession of dignity within the person (Frankl 1963).

Values and indicators of dignity expressed within nursing cluster around the acceptance and permitting of people to be who they are and not who the context or institution determines they ought to be. Understanding dignity within oneself suggests the existence of self-oriented values and possessions including independence, acceptance, creativity, hope, respect and protection. The actions that might offend the dignity of another are at once universally understood and uniquely defined. Frequently the literature refers to issues such as being embarrassed, being exposed, having oneself inappropriately spoken about, being denied privacy, being misunderstood and being treated by another as one would perceive the other to find unacceptable, as all being part of the complex concept of dignity.

CONCLUSION

This chapter does not claim to be a meta-analysis of all current literature surrounding dignity, nor all the contexts where dignity expresses itself. Rather, what is presented here draws from current knowledge and seeks to marry understandings gained and thus present another understanding of the concept of dignity. **Our human experience clearly suggests that dignity matters and if it matters then it is important to explain its components, educate professionals in its dimensions and provide resources to ensure that humans are cared for with respect to their unique and universal dignity.** Better understanding the concept of dignity may mean that nurses can both consolidate those practices that bestow dignity and identify those where dignity is challenged. To be engaged in both these activities is inherently honest nursing practice and only through honest practice can we be confident that the meeting of patient's needs and expectations can be truly facilitated.

This honesty does, however, force us to acknowledge that, despite the assertion that dignity is a concept tangibly understood by all, caution should be exercised in assuming that what we understand personally is always applicable interpersonally. In addition, as a discipline, nursing is strongly cautioned as to the need for further research and concept clarification in order that we can confidently be assured of the place of dignity in professional practice. Unless we strengthen our understandings of concepts such as dignity then, as has been suggested by other authors, we may well run the risk of blurring rather than enhancing our understanding of what good nursing care is (Sandman 2002).

REFERENCES

Australian Nursing Council 1995 Code of professional conduct for nurses in Australia. Australian Nursing Council, Canberra

Bournes DA 2000 Concept inventing: a process for creating a unitary definition of having courage. Nursing Science Quarterly 13: 143–149

Chinn PL, Kramer MK 1991 Theory and nursing: a systematic approach, 3rd edn. Mosby/Year Book, St Louis, MO

Chinn PL, Kramer MK 1999 Theory and nursing – integrated knowledge development. 5th edn. Mosby/Year Book, St Louis, MO

Chochinov HM 2002 Dignity-conserving care – a new model for palliative care. Helping the patient feel valued. Journal of the American Medical Association 287: 2253–2260

Chochinov HM, Hack T, McClement S et al 2002 Dignity in the terminally ill: a developing empirical model. Social Science and Medicine 54: 433–443

Concise Oxford English Dictionary 1995 Concise Oxford dictionary of current English, 9th edn. Clarendon Press, Oxford

Conway ME 1992 Towards greater specificity in defining nursing's metaparadigm. In: Nicoll LH (ed) Perspectives on nursing theory, 2nd edn. JB Lippincott, Philadelphia, PA

Danneels G 2003 Liturgy forty years after the Second Vatican Council: high point or recession? In: Pecklers K (ed) Liturgy in a postmodern world. Continuum, London

Diczfalusy E 1997a In search of human dignity: gender equity, reproductive health and healthy aging. International Journal of Gynaecology and Obstetrics 59: 195–206

Diczfalusy E 1997b In search of human dignity: reproductive health and healthy aging. European Journal of Obstetrics, Gynecology, and Reproductive Biology 71: 123–133

Fagermoen FG 1997 Professional identity: values embedded in meaningful nursing practice. Journal of Advanced Nursing 25: 434–441

Frankl VE 1963 Man's search for meaning. Washington Square Press, New York

Haddock J 1996 Towards further clarification of the concept 'dignity'. Journal of Advanced Nursing 24: 924–931

International Council of Nurses 2000 International code of ethics for nurses. ICN, Geneva

Jacelon CS 2003 The dignity of elders in an acute care hospital. Qualitative Health Research 13: 543–556

McKenna H 1997 Nursing theories and models. Routledge, London

Mairis ED 1994 Concept clarification in professional practice – dignity. Journal of Advanced Nursing 19: 947–953

Meleis AI 1991 Theoretical nursing: development and progress, 2nd edn. JB Lippincott, Philadelphia, PA

Moody LE 1990 Advancing nursing science through research, vol 1. Sage Publications, Newbury Park, CA

Morse JM, Mitcham C, Hupcey JE et al 1996 Criteria for concept evaluation. Journal of Advanced Nursing 24: 385–390

Nursing and Midwifery Council 2002 Code of professional conduct. NMC, London

Oxford English Dictionary 1989 Oxford English dictionary, 2nd edn. Clarendon Press, Oxford

Parse RR 2002 Words, words, words: meanings, meanings, meanings! Editorial. Nursing Science Quarterly 15(3) pp 1–2

Sandman L 2002 What's the use of human dignity within palliative care? Nursing Philosophy 3: 177–181

Seedhouse D, Gallagher A 2002 Undignifying institutions. Journal of Medical Ethics 28: 368–372

Statman D 2000 Humiliation, dignity and self respect. Philosophical Psychology 13: 523–540

United Nations 2003 Universal declaration of human rights. Available online at: http://www.un.org/Overview/rights.html

Van Manen M 2002 Care-as-worry, or 'don't worry, be happy'. Qualitative Health Research 12: 264–280

Walsh K, Kowanko I 2002 Nurses' and patients' perceptions of dignity. International Journal of Nursing Practice 8: 143–151

Webster's Dictionary 1971 Webster's third new international dictionary of the English language. G & C Merriam, Springfield, MA

Widang I, Fridlund B 2003 Self respect, dignity and confidence: conceptions of integrity among male patients. Journal of Advanced Nursing 42: 47–56

The concept of empathy

William Reynolds

EDITORIAL

Both the editors of this book are members of a minority subgroup of nurses – those who are doubly registered, sometimes euphemistically referred to as 'dual-qualified'. In essence, this means that we have undertaken one preregistration nurse education programme and then followed this up with another in a different clinical specialty. One experience that was common throughout each of these programmes was the attention given to the concept of empathy. Empathy, as Bill's chapter reminds us, has been the focus of debate, empirical and clinical work for many years. Further, while the understanding of empathy has deepened during this time, some of the debates associated with empathy are far from resolved.

Selecting one of these debates to focus on in our editorial is no easy task. However, perhaps the argument around the centrality of empathy to helping relationships is so pivotal that it cannot be ignored. Bill's chapter reminds us that Roger's seminal work on the necessary and sufficient conditions of helping relationships posits empathy at the core, at the very centre of interpersonal work. Irrespective of the cogency of Roger's position, it is difficult to imagine nurse education programmes containing no reference to empathy. The editors would add their support to Roger's position but would also add a caveat.

While we totally agree that nurses, whatever their clinical focus and specialty, need both the personal quality and individual skill base to help patients feel empathized with, there may well be times and certain clinical scenarios where being empathic may not be the most helpful response from the nurse. There is a time for consciousness-raising, which is facilitated by empathic responses, and there is a time for leaving well alone. Denial, if you will forgive the pun, is not just a river in Africa. At times denial serves as a healthy defence mechanism and practitioners need to be judicious in their decisions about when to challenge and/or confront denial. What this demonstrates is that, even when considering and using a concept so inextricably linked to compassion and care as empathy, nurses should not practice in an unthinking, ritualistic or automatic way.

INTRODUCTION

The term 'empathy' has been variously conceptualized as a behaviour, a personality dimension and an experienced emotion (McKay et al 1990). Several writers (e.g. Davis 1983, Williams 1990, Morse et al 1992, Bennett 1995, Reynolds 2000) have suggested that, as a result of the complexity of empathy, confusion exists about the meaning and components of empathy. These writers propose that empathy is a multidimensional, multiphase construct that is often considered in a narrow way as a unitary construct. This is a problem because there is a widely held view that empathy is critical to all forms of helping relationship (Reynolds 2000). In this chapter, the historical and theoretical background to empathy will be discussed. Different definitions of empathy will be presented and a construct of empathy that is relevant to clinical nursing will be considered. It will show that the relationship among the different components of empathy is still not clear.

THE COMPONENTS OF EMPATHY

Following an extensive review of the literature, Morse et al (1992) identified four components of empathy: moral, emotive, cognitive and behavioural empathy (Table 7.1). Similarly, Williams (1990) informed us that the most widely recognized components of empathy are emotional empathy, cognitive empathy, communicative empathy and relational empathy. The additional component of relational empathy was defined as patient-perceived empathy. Williams's conclusion, which did not involve moral empathy, was broadly similar to Patterson's earlier definition of empathy. Patterson (1974) described empathy as involving four concepts or stages. First, the helper must be receptive to another's communication: the emotional component. Second, the helper must understand the communication by putting him/herself in the other's place: the cognitive component. Next, the helper must communicate his/her understanding to the patient: the behavioural or

Table 7.1
Components of empathy

Component	Definition
Emotive component	The ability to subjectively experience and share in another's psychological state or intrinsic feelings
Moral component	An internal altruistic force that motivates the practice of empathy
Cognitive component	The helper's intellectual ability to identify and understand another person's feelings and perspective from an objective stance
Behavioural component	Communicative response to convey understanding of another's perspective

communicative component. Finally, Patterson suggested that empathy allowed for the possibility of the patient validating the helper's perception of the patient's world: a relational component.

The additional component of relational empathy offers the patient an opportunity to validate the accuracy of the helper's perceptions and to experience being understood. The patient's actual awareness of the helper's communication allows him/her to say, 'Yes that is how I see things' and, 'Yes that is what I would like to happen'. This assumption is consistent with Barrett-Lennard's (1981) model of empathy, where he suggested a model of the empathy cycle (Box 7.1). When the process continues, phase 1 is again the core feature, and 2 and 3 follow in cyclical mode. The total interactive sequence within which these phases occur begins with the other person being self-expressive in the presence of an empathically attending other, and this characteristically leads to further expression and feedback to the empathizing partner.

Davis (1983) suggested that one advantage of viewing empathy as a multidimensional phenomenon is that, by clearly defining the different types of reaction to others that can be called empathic, it is possible to explore systematic similarities and differences between these types of empathy, and their implications for other behaviour. The different components of empathy identified by Morse et al (1992) may all contribute to empathy but the extent to which they are all interrelated appears to be a source of disagreement among theorists. This seems particularly so in respect of the extent to which all components are necessary, or contribute to behaviours that build therapeutic, problem-solving relationships.

Box 7.1
Barrett-Lennard's
empathy cycle

Phase 1: The inner process of empathic listening to another who is personally expressive in some way, reasoning and understanding.
Phase 2: An attempt to convey empathic understanding of the other person's experiences.
Phase 3: The patient's actual awareness of the helper's communication.

In the rest of this chapter the extent to which all components are necessary, or interrelated to other components of empathy, is considered.

MORAL EMPATHY

Morse et al (1992) describe moral empathy as being an empathic disposition or trait. However, they concluded that a relationship between morality and the cognitive–behavioural components of empathy is unproven. These writers point out that such a relationship has been questioned in sociology, philosophy, nursing and developmental psychology by those attempting to understand what motivates an individual to engage in helping behaviour (Buber 1973, Hogan 1975, Gladstein 1983, Olsen 1991, Baillie 1995, Reynolds et al 2000).

The relationship of moral empathy to helping

The notion that empathy involves a social or universal morality is rooted in the philosophical belief that human beings share common needs and that they all experience the same human conditions (Hoffman 1981, Arnett & Nakagawa 1983). Inherent in this assumption is the belief that within every person is a natural willingness, or compelling desire, to reach out and help other people who are distressed or need assistance. However, several studies report a lack of correlation between trait empathy, as measured on the Hogan Empathy Scale (Hogan 1969) and measures of cognitive–behavioural empathy (Conklin & Hunt 1975, Forsyth 1979, Reynolds 1986). This suggests that cognitive–behavioural empathy is not necessarily dependent upon trait or moral empathy.

Hogan (1969) described trait empathy as the ability to take the moral point of view; to consider the implications of one's behaviour for the welfare of others. Like Morse et al (1992), he also called this tendency empathic disposition and suggested that this trait heightens one's sensitivity to the expectations of others.

Commenting upon the reported lack of correlation between his empathy scale and measures of cognitive–behavioural empathy, Hogan (1975) suggested that individuals might sometimes display relatively high levels of cognitive–behavioural empathy even though they might be low in trait empathy, or empathic disposition. He further claimed that whether a helper is empathic or not in a moral sense is irrelevant. What matters most is whether the patient perceives the helper as caring about their welfare. His assumption was supported by the findings from Reynolds's (1986) study of student nurses' empathy in Scotland. Hogan (1975) also claimed that too much helper reliance on trait empathy might foster a tendency to overidentify with the patient's problems, leading to a loss of objectivity. This suggests that there may be a relatively limited amount of trait empathy necessary in a helping relationship. This view was endorsed by Morse et al (1992), who identified cognitive–behavioural empathy as being the therapeutic component. That conclusion is consistently reported by many researchers concerned with the measurement, teaching and therapeutic effects of empathy (Truax & Carkhuff 1967, Gazda et al 1982, McKay et al 1990, Reynolds 2000).

The correlation between moral empathy and cognitive–behavioural empathy

Hogan's conclusions are unproven; however, a number of studies demonstrating a lack of correlation between his measure of trait empathy and measures of cognitive–behavioural empathy lend support to his assumptions about the relevance of trait empathy to helping. Generally, studies investigating the validity of the Hogan scale have reported a correlation between scores on the scale and likeability (Hogan & Manikin 1976), non–aggressive behaviour (Gray 1978), mature reasoning (Daurio 1978) and low anxiety (Kendall et al 1978, Reynolds 1986), all qualities that seem related to an attractive interpersonal style. An alternative explanation for the lack of correlation between Hogan's scale and other measures of empathy may be the different conditions under which the scales were administered. Trait empathy is always self-reported while patients have been used in many studies to rate cognitive–behavioural empathy.

Forsyth (1979) used the Hogan Empathy Scale (trait empathy) and the Barrett-Lennard Relationship Inventory (cognitive–behavioural empathy) to measure registered nurses' empathy. Results revealed that only 50% of nurses perceived themselves as being high in trait empathy, while 98% of the subjects were rated high in cognitive–behavioural empathy. Forsyth concluded that patients might perceive nurses as being empathic whether they are or not. An alternative explanation was offered by Barrett-Lennard (1974), who suggested that relating to another person empathically involves certain distinct phases and that different scales 'tap' the process at different points. **In spite of Forsyth's concern about the possible limitations of patient ratings, Kurtz and Gruman (1972) and Reynolds (1986) reported evidence that patient-perceived empathy is a better predictor of therapeutic outcomes than any form of self-rated empathy.**

Similarly, Reynolds (1986) reported that basic nursing students scored lower than other professional groups on trait empathy (as measured by the Hogan Empathy Scale) and higher than other professional groups on cognitive–behavioural empathy (as measured by the Empathy Construct Rating Scale (ECRS; LaMonica 1981). Furthermore, as patient ratings of students on the ECRS increased among measures, their anecdotal descriptions of their relationship with their nursing student suggested that they perceived the student to be more empathic in a cognitive–behavioural sense. Typical examples of patient comments included: 'She seems to listen because after a pause she continues to focus on and investigate what I had been saying previously.'

It is possible that the dependent and passive nature of the hospitalized patients' role accounts for their perceptions. However, the specific and detailed nature of patients' comments in Reynolds' (1986) study indicates that they were being truthful. These data suggest that cognitive–behavioural empathy might be relatively independent of moral empathy.

EMOTIVE EMPATHY

Mehrabian and Epstein (1972) described emotional empathy as being a vicarious emotional response to the perceived emotional experiences of others. This affective state has been variously referred to as empathic concern or empathic emotion (Morse et al 1992, Reynolds 2003). Stotland (1969) argued that there is a critical difference between cognitive empathy and empathic emotional responsiveness. Whereas the former is recognition of another's feelings, the later also includes the sharing or communication of those feelings. According to Gladstein (1977), a person's emotional distress is 'contagious'. By that it is meant that an empathic response is aroused in an individual when the emotional distress of another is perceived. Empathy then takes on the characteristic of a feeling state that is characterized by feelings of warmth, compassion and concern for others (Davis 1983).

Bateson et al (1983) make a distinction between personal distress in a helper aroused by the distress of another, which leads to egoistic motivation, and empathy, which leads to altruistic motivation. In other words, Bateson et al are arguing that emotional empathy does not always result in helping behaviours but that sometimes it can motivate people to behave in a truly altruistic way. Bateson et al (1983), who conceptualized empathy as an experienced emotion, sometimes referred to it as sympathy. They stated that research has not made it clear what evokes such a reaction and Reynolds (2003) suggests that this is still the case 20 years later. Adler (1989) informs us that Bateson et al have suggested that trying to see the world from another person's point of view helps to facilitate emotional empathy. A further possible explanation is that listening, identification and understanding of the other person' s feelings might result in emotional empathy.

The relationship of emotive empathy to helping

The relationship of empathic emotion and helping has been investigated in terms of its association with non-aggressive behaviour (Buss 1961, Fesbach 1964, Milgram 1965, Mehrabian & Epstein 1972). Findings indicate that emotional empathy was associated with low levels of aggression. However, the extent to which emotional empathy results in helping distressed individuals to problem-solve remains unresolved. Mehrabian and Epstein (1972) tested the hypothesis that a person who has a high level of emotional empathy is less likely to engage in aggressive behaviour and more likely to engage in helping behaviour, particularly when the stress from the other person is immediate. Results indicated that subjects who scored highly on a measure of emotional empathy were more likely to engage in non-aggressive behaviours than low scorers. Helping behaviours were defined as sociability, concern over acceptance and 'succorance', with Mehrabian et al defining 'succorance' as an approval-seeking tendency.

These data suggest that those perceived to be high in emotional empathy are emotionally responsive to the other person's needs. While approval-seeking behaviour may contribute to sociability, several studies have found a negative relationship between helping and social attractiveness (Krebs 1970). Sensitivity to rejection sounds similar to egoistic motivation, which may hinder the ability to view the world from another person's viewpoint. At best it seems reasonable to assume that, since these behaviours are non-aggressive, they might signal a commitment to care, or concern for the other person. **That point is roughly analogous to Rogers' (1957) concept of warmth, which, he suggests, contributes towards the empathic** process by encouraging patients to be personally expressive to a person who appears to be committed to listening to them.

The relationship of emotive empathy to sympathy

A further issue relating to emotive empathy is the extent to which it is similar to sympathy or pity, which are alternative terms used by Bateson et al (1983) for empathy. Everyone does not necessarily accept the distinction between empathy and sympathy and there is ambiguity in the use of terms. For example, Szalita (1976) proposed that empathy involves, 'placing oneself in the "shoes" of another in order to permit sympathetic understanding of the other's mental life' (p. 145). However, empathy in this case means 'understanding' rather than 'siding with'. Travelbee (1966) viewed sympathy as genuine concern for the patient, coupled with a desire to help the patient to alleviate stress. Her description of sympathy as warmth, kindness, a transient type of compassion, a caring quality experienced on a feeling level and communicated to another, shows it to be somewhat similar to empathy as conceptualized by others.

In contrast to Travelbee (1966), Kalish (1971) emphasized that with empathy the helper remains separate and objective. According to Kalish, with sympathy the helper experiences the patient's feelings as if they were his/her own. Similarly, Rogers (1975) is careful to keep empathy in the realm of perceiving the other as if we were the other, but remembering this 'as if' condition. Gazda et al (1975, p56) expressed the difference between empathy and sympathy quite clearly: 'Empathy and sympathy are different. Sympathy means that the helper experiences the same emotions as the helpee. Fortunately it is not necessary to experience the helpee's feelings to be helpful. You can understand how the other person feels and that is what is meant by empathy'.

Johnstone et al (1983) proposed that pure sympathy is self-defeating in the therapeutic relationship because merely experiencing another person's negative feelings can immobilize a helper. That view is reflected by Peplau's (1987) conclusion about the efficacy of the counselling relationship. She suggested that when a helper feels bad they could become overwhelmed by the distress of the other person. Peplau suggested that the language of the helper should be investigative and designed to assist the patient to control negative feelings, such as anxiety, not colliding with the stress of the patient. That is not to say that emotional empathy is non-therapeutic, but the possibility remains that there may be a fixed degree of emotional empathy necessary in a helping relationship.

COGNITIVE EMPATHY

Irrespective of different theoretical orientation, the concept of empathy, originating from the German word *Einfühlung* as used by Lipps (1903) (which means literally 'feeling within'), refers to the ability of the other person to 'know' experientially what another person is feeling at any given moment, seeing through the other person's eyes. That description is compatible with the cognitive components of empathy cited by Williams (1990) and Morse et al (1992). 'Feeling within' could also be related to emotional empathy, but knowing what another person is feeling, seeing through the other person's eyes, seems dependent on an ability to identify another person's feelings and perspectives from an objective stance.

Lipps' (1903) contribution to our understanding of empathy might explain why a review of the psychology and nursing literature reveals a persistent tendency to refer to empathy as a perceptual rather than a communicative skill. Empathy has regularly been referred to as a kind of attitude, or way of perceiving, that the helper assumes, not something that he says or does. References to empathy as a human quality or perceptual skill indicate that a necessary condition of empathy is that the observer understands in some sense the affective state of another (Smither 1977). Thus Shafer (1959, p. 343) wrote: 'Empathy may be defined as the inner experience of sharing and comprehending the momentary psychological state of another person.' And Kalish (1973, p. 1548):

> *Empathy is the ability to enter into the life of another person, to accurately perceive his current feelings and their meanings. In empathy the helper borrows his patient's feelings in order to fully understand them, but he is always aware of his own separateness and realizes that the feelings of the patient are not his own.*

References to comprehending the psychological state of another and accurately perceiving current feelings and their meanings are examples of cognitive function such as perceiving, imagining, analysing, judging and reasoning. The reference by Kalish (1973) to borrowing the patient's feelings in order to understand, implies that she makes a distinction between emotional empathy, or sympathy, and cognitive empathy. This view is compatible with Rogers' (1951) suggestion that empathy is not an emotional identification. Rogers pointed out that the helper perceives the patient's hopes and fears, but does not experience them.

The relationship of cognitive empathy to behavioural empathy

An issue relating to cognitive empathy is the extent to which it is related to behavioural empathy. Rogers (1951) referred to an earlier paper that he had presented (in 1940), in which he recognized the interaction between cognitive empathy and the verbal skills of the helping person. In his paper he outlined the principles and techniques of a new approach to psychotherapy, which became known as non-directive counselling. Rogers drew attention to the counsellor's clarification and acceptance of the patient's feelings and perceptions. Reporting on a comparison of directive and non-directive (recorded) counselling interviews, Rogers reported that non-directive counsellors were more likely to respond in a manner that indicated recognition of their patients' feelings and attitudes. Subsequently, Rogers (1957) concluded that the techniques of counselling are less important than what he described as the necessary and sufficient conditions of therapeutic change. These necessary conditions were, he argued, operative in all effective types of helping relationships. The necessary and sufficient conditions for change that have received the greatest amount of attention all relate to the helper's attitude, cognition and behaviour. Rogers suggested that a patient learns to change when the helper is warm (committed to the patient), genuine (non-defensive) and empathic (successful in communicating understanding of the patient's current feelings).

In spite of Rogers's (1975) later reluctance to describe empathy as a communication skill, it seems logical to conclude that the necessary conditions for therapeutic change can be observed in the helper's behaviour. For example, Truax and Carkhuff (1967) pointed out that the helper's ability to know what another person means is dependent on a verbal ability to clarify and accept the patient's feelings, as well as a cognitive ability to perceive, judge and reason. According to Truax and Carkhuff, an empathic response is determined by how well we communicate understanding of a person's feelings and the meaning attached to those feelings. Failure to communicate understanding means that either we give a hurtful response, such as a put down, or a neutral response, such as unsolicited advice. These low-level responses prevent a therapeutic relationship from developing (Truax & Carkhuff 1967).

COGNITIVE–BEHAVIOURAL EMPATHY

In spite of frequent references to empathy as a human quality emphasizing moral, emotive and cognitive qualities, alternative views can be found in the literature. Several theorists have conceptualized empathy in a manner that emphasizes its cognitive–behavioural components. Thus Truax (1961, p. 2) wrote:

> Accurate empathy involves more than just an ability of the therapist to sense the patient's 'private world' as if it were his own. It also involves more than just the ability of the therapist to know what the patient means, Accurate empathy involves the sensitivity to current feeling and the verbal ability to communicate this understanding in a language attuned to the patient's feelings.

The Truax definition has shifted the emphasis from a way of perceiving to a way of communicating, from a trait or human quality to a form of interaction.

The interpersonal nature of the concept of empathy

Following the Truax definition of empathy, there has been an increasing tendency among theorists (e.g. Zoske et al 1983) to argue that empathy is an interpersonal concept comprising a specific set of interpersonal or communication skills, rather than being an instinctive quality possessed by certain persons. Empathy has been increasingly been viewed in a cognitive–behavioural way and described as a skill and an ability (Morse et al 1994, Jaffrey 1995, Reynolds 2000, Mercer & Reynolds 2002). For example, Aspey and Roebuck (1975, p. 11) see empathy as: 'the ability to communicate your understanding of the other person's feelings'. Similarly, Valle (1981, p. 784) stated that: 'Empathy is the ability to respond to the feelings and reasons for the feelings the patient is experiencing in a manner that communicates an understanding of the patient'.

Even authors who tend to emphasize empathy from the perspective of the person who is receiving help (relational empathy) stress the communicative aspect of the empathic process. Barrett-Lennard's (1962) definition has been cited frequently: 'The degree of empathic understanding is conceived as the extent to which the other person is conscious of the immediate awareness of another'(p. 3). In more recent times Reynolds (2000, p. 11) stated that: 'Empathy involves communicating understanding of the patients' experience in order that this can be validated by the patient'.

The increasing tendency to conceptualize empathy as a type of interpersonal relationship has encouraged a view that empathy skills are teachable and measurable. Nevertheless, the teaching and measurement of empathy poses a problem given the absence of an agreed theoretical framework and operational definition. Reynolds (1998, 2000) argued that a major problem faced by nurses is knowing when they are showing empathy. He suggested that there was a need for a construct of empathy that reflected what patients wanted from their relationships with nurses. Reynolds (1987) identified conceptual disagreement among a sample of nurse educators. That study revealed that teachers who viewed empathy in a cognitive–behavioural way tended to be more certain that it could be taught and measured than teachers who viewed empathy as a moral attitude or cognitive attribute possessed by a few. The latter group regarded empathy as an art, or an innate quality, suggesting that the concept defied measurement. This conceptual confusion is unsurprising in view of the fact that some theorists are inconsistent in their approach.

EMPATHY AS AN ATTITUDE

Carl Rogers (1957) described empathy as a way of being with another person. By this he meant an approach one assumes in relationship with the other person. That view suggests that empathy is an attitude rather than a skill, or, as Barrett-Lennard suggested, an interpersonal process. However, it is likely to be an interpersonal process that is dependent on and facilitated by a range of cognitive–behavioural skills that can be observed. This seems logical, since Forchuk and Reynolds (2001) reported that, during their relationships with nurses, patients in both Canada and Scotland were able to describe a range of attributes that separated the high empathizer from the low empathizer.

The view that empathy is dependent upon a range of helper attributes was also expressed by de la Mothe (1987, p. 7), who wrote: 'I have no doubt that the empathic process depends on a range of skills for fulfilment, but it is not itself a skill'. The conclusion reached by de la Mothe resulted from his extensive review of the frequent publications of Carl Rogers and Rogerian theorists. These publications reinforced his assumption that high empathizers possess certain attitudes, cognitive abilities and behaviours that facilitate a helping relationship.

Rogers (1951) proposed that a crucial characteristic of an empathic relationship is that it is free of defensiveness. **Commenting on this point, Truax (1975) suggested that a high empathizer is able to provide a non-threatening, safe, trusting or secure relationship. He also said that the basic philosophy of the helper is represented by an attitude of neutrality towards the other person, respect for the individual's capacity and right to self-direction, and for the worth and significance of each other**. Additionally, the high empathizer is able to understand, be with and grasp the meaning of the other person's communication on a moment-to-moment basis. Truax, like Rogers, implies that empathy is an interpersonal process or relationship that is dependent on the attitude of the helper. His description of empathy sounds similar to the moral and cognitive components of empathy that were described by Morse et al (1992) and does not specifically refer to behavioural empathy. This definition is inconsistent with Truax's (1961) earlier suggestion that empathy included a verbal ability, not just a willingness to know what the other person meant.

EMPATHY AS A SKILL

In the earlier definition provided by Truax (1961), empathy is more than a way of being with a person, it is more than an attitude or cognitive ability. His conceptualization of empathy at that time included the verbal ability needed to communicate to the other person the helper's understanding of what they meant. Egan (1986, p. 99) suggested: 'It's the helper's way of saying I'm with you, I've been listening carefully to what you've been saying and expressing, and I'm checking if my understanding is accurate.'

In spite of Rogers' (1975) reluctance to comment on how the empathic relationship might be implemented behaviourally, he does concede that empathy is a process that can be observed through the behaviour of the helping person. He points out that this is indicated by the wide use of measurement scales developed to infer the ability of professionals to offer empathy to others (e.g. Barrett-Lennard 1962, Truax 1967, Wilt et al 1995). In more recent times Forchuk and Reynolds (2001) pointed out that, since patients can clearly describe empathic skills, empathy does have a behavioural component that can be observed by patients and measured by professionals.

Rogers' (1975) concern about how professionals were conceptualizing empathy was related to his view that warmth and genuineness are just as important as the form of words that the helper uses. He regards these conditions as being part of empathy, in the sense that a patient is unlikely to make self-disclosures unless the helper is perceived as being warm and genuine. Equally, Rogers made it clear that merely reflecting feelings or focusing on the patient's last words indicates an absence of cognitive empathy.

In spite of his reluctance to focus on the helper's responses, Rogers continued in subsequent productions to imply that the attitudes and cognitive ability of the helper are conveyed through the communication of the helper. He stated that:

> *While I am experiencing an attitude of annoyance toward another person, but unaware of it, then my communication contains contradictory messages. My words are giving out a message, but I am also in subtle ways communicating the annoyance I feel and this confuses the other person and makes him distrustful, though he may be unaware of what is causing the difficulty.*
>
> *Rogers 1990, p. 51*

SUMMARY OF VIEWS IN THE LITERATURE ABOUT THE MEANING OF EMPATHY

The views expressed in the literature points to a general tendency to define empathy at two levels. First, there is a conceptual definition of empathy as an attitude, which Rogers (1975) describes as a way of being with another person. Second, there is an operational level of empathy as a communication skill. These two levels incorporate the multidimensional levels of empathy identified in the literature. The first level includes Rogers' (1957) conditions of warmth, genuineness and empathic listening. Warmth and genuineness might be similar to, or influenced by, the moral and emotive components of empathy. Rogers's frequent descriptions of empathic listening are compatible with cognitive empathy, involving imagination, reasoning and perception. The second level includes the helper's ability to communicate warmth and genuineness, as well as their cognitive awareness of the other person's world.

Several writers have combined the two levels of empathy to make Rogers' (1957) facilitative conditions into observable behaviours. For example Egan (1986, p. 95) wrote: 'Empathy is the ability to enter into and understand the world of the other person and communicate this understanding to him or her'. This two-level definition describes empathy as an attitude and, when operationalized, it is a cognitive–behavioural skill.

Truax and Carkhuff (1967) also combined the two levels of empathy. This conceptualization underpinned the development of two cognitive–behavioural measures of empathy, the Truax Accurate Empathy Scale, and the Carkhuff Scale for Empathic Understanding. Bachrach et al (1974) stated that the Carkhuff and Truax scales changed Rogers's idea of empathy from a way of being that the helper assumes into something the helper does. Similarly, Reynolds (2000, p. 7) argued strongly for the two levels of empathy when he stated that: 'Empathy is a form of interaction involving communication of the helper's attitudes and an understanding of the patient's world'.

These views influenced several attempts to teach cognitive–behavioural empathy. Examples include training programmes for educators (Gazda et al 1984), criminal justice personnel (Sissons et al 1981) and nurses (LaMonica et al 1986, Hughes et al 1990, Reynolds 2000).

CONCLUSION

Clearly there is much to learn about the nature of empathy. However, it has been shown that there is a need for a construct of empathy that reflects what patients want from their relationships with nurses and other clinicians. Recent literature (Reynolds & Scott 1999, 2000, Reynolds et al 2000, Mercer & Reynolds 2002) reveals that patients want clinicians to communicate understanding of their feelings and their attached meanings. Unless nurses and others are able to achieve that, it is unlikely that they will be able to understand the patient's responses to health problems, or to achieve outcomes desired by the patient. In such circumstances, patients are in danger of receiving less than appropriate care, both from the moral and the professional perspective.

REFERENCES

Adler C 1989 Altruism may be a powerful motive. Science Monitor p. 11

Arnett R, Nakagawa GG 1983 The assumptive roots of empathic listening: a critique. Communication Education 32: 368–378

Aspey D, Roebuck F 1975 A discussion of the relationship between selected student variables and the teacher's use of interchangeable responses Human Education 1: 3–10

Bachrach H, Luborsky L, Mechanick P 1974 The correspondence between judgments of empathy from brief samples of psychotherapy; supervisors judgments, and sensitivity tests. British Journal of Medical Psychology 47: 337–340

Baillie L 1995 Empathy in the nurse patient relationship. Nursing Standard 9(20): 29–30

Barrett-Lennard G 1962 Dimensions of therapist response as causal factors in therapeutic change. Psychological Monographs: General and Applied 76: 1–36

Barrett-Lennard G 1974 Empathy in human relationships: significance, nature and measurement. Unpublished paper presented at the Annual Conference of the Australian Psychological Society, Perth

Barrett-Lennard G 1981 The empathy cycle: refinement of a nuclear concept. Journal of Counseling Psychology 28: 91–100

Bateson CO, Quinn B, Fultz J et al 1983 Influences of self-reported distress and empathy on egoistic versus altruistic motivation to help. Journal of Personality and Social Psychology 45: 706–718

Bennett J 1995 Methodological notes on empathy: further considerations. Advanced Nursing Science 18: 36–50

Buber M 1973 Elements of the interhuman. In: Stewart J (ed) Bridges not walls. Addison-Wesley, Menlo Park, CA

Buss A 1961 The psychology of aggression. John Wiley, New York

Conklin R, Hunt A 1975 An investigation of the validity of empathy measures. Counselor Education and Supervision 15: 119–127

Daurio S 1978 The development of socio-political intelligence. Unpublished doctoral thesis, Johns Hopkins University, Baltimore, MD

Davis M 1983 The effects of dispositional empathy on emotional reactions and helping: a multidimensional approach. Journal of Personality 51: 167–184

De la Mothe M 1987 Empathy revisited. Unpublished PhD thesis, Open University, Milton Keynes

Egan G 1986 The skilled helper. Brooks-Cole, New York

Fesbach S 1964 The function of aggression and the regulation of aggressive drive. Psychological Review 71: 257–272

Forchuk C, Reynolds W 2001 Clients' reflections on relationships with nurses: comparisons from Canada and Scotland. Journal of Psychiatric and Mental Health Nursing 8: 45–51

Forsyth G 1979 Exploration of empathy in nurse–client interaction. Advanced Nursing Science 1: 53–61

Gazda G, Walters R, Childers W 1975 Human relations development: a manual for health sciences. Albyn & Bacon, Boston, MA

Gazda G, Childers W, Walters R 1982 Interpersonal communication: a handbook for health professionals. Aspen, Rockville, MD

Gazda G, Ashbury F, Balzer F et al 1984 Human relations development: a manual for educators, 3rd edn. Albyn & Bacon, Boston, MA

Gladstein G 1977 Empathy and counselling outcome: an empirical and conceptual review. The Counseling Psychologist 6: 70–79

Gladstein G 1983 Understanding empathy: integrating counselling developments and social psychology perspectives. Journal of Counseling Psychology 30: 467–482

Gray C 1978 Empathy and stress as mediators in child abuse: theory, research and practice implications. Unpublished doctoral dissertation, University of Maryland, College Park, MD

Hoffman M 1981 The development of empathy. In: Rushton J, Sorrentino RR (eds) Altruism and helping behaviour. Lawrence Erlbaum, Hillsdale, NJ

Hogan R 1969 Development of an empathy scale. Journal of Consulting and Clinical Psychology 33: 307–316

Hogan R 1975 Empathy: a conceptual and psychometric analysis. The Counseling Psychologist 5: 14–18

Hogan R, Maniken A 1976 Determinants of interpersonal attraction: a clarification. Psychological Reports 26: 235–238

Hughes J, Carver E, Mackay R 1990 Learning to use empathy. In: Mackay R, Hughes J, Carver E (eds) Empathy in the helping relationship. Springer, New York

Jaffrey L 1995 Patient care: from nurse to patient and back again. Nursing Standard 9: 50–51

Johnstone J, Cheek J, Smither R 1983 The structure of empathy. Journal of Personality and Social Psychology 43: 1299–1312

Kalish B 1971 An experiment in the development of empathy in nursing students. Nursing Research 20: 202–211

Kalish B 1973 What is empathy? American Journal of Nursing 73: 548–1552

Kendall P, Finch A, Montgomery L 1978 Vicarious anxiety: a systematic evaluation of a vicarious threat to self-esteem. Journal of Counselling and Clinical Psychology 46: 997–1008

Krebs D 1970 Altruism: an examination of the concept and a review of the literature. Psychological Bulletin 73: 258–302

Kurtz R, Gruman D 1972 Different approaches to the measurement of therapist empathy and their relationship to therapy outcomes. Journal of Counseling and Clinical Psychology 39: 106–105

LaMonica E 1981 Construct validity of an empathy instrument. Research in Nursing and Health 4: 389–400

LaMonica E, Oberst M, Madea A, Wolk R 1986 Development of a patient satisfaction scale. Research in Nursing and Health 9: 43–50

Lipps T 1903 Einfühlung, innere Nachahmung, und Organenempfindungen. Archiv für die gesamte Psychologie 1: 185–204

McKay R, Hughes J, Carver E 1990 Empathy in the helping relationship. Springer, New York

Mehrabian A, Epstein N 1972 A measure of emotional empathy. Journal of Personality 40: 525–543

Mercer S, Reynolds W 2002 Empathy and quality of care. British Journal of General Practice 52(Suppl): S9–S12

Milgram S 1965 Some conditions of obedience and disobedience to authority. In: Steiner ID, Fishbein M (eds) Current studies in social psychology. Holt, Rinehart & Winston, New York

Morse J, Anderson G, Botter J et al 1992 Exploring empathy: a conceptual fit for nursing practice? IMAGE: Journal of Nursing Scholarship 24: 273–280

Morse J, Miles M, Clarke D, Doberneck B 1994 Sensing patient needs: exploring concepts of nursing insight and receptivity used in nursing assessment. Scholarly Inquiry for Nursing Practice 8: 233–260

Olsen D 1991 Empathy as an ethical and philosophical basis for nursing. Advanced Nursing Science 14: 62–75

Patterson C 1974 Relationship counseling and psychotherapy. Harper & Row, New York

Peplau H 1987 Interpersonal constructs for nursing practice. Nurse Education Today 7: 201–208

Reynolds W 1986 A study of empathy in student nurses. MPhil thesis, Dundee College of Technology, Dundee

Reynolds W 1987 Empathy: we know what we mean, but what do we teach? Nurse Education Today 7: 265–269

Reynolds W 1998 A study of the effects of an empathy education programme on registered nurses' empathy. PhD thesis, Open University, Milton Keynes

Reynolds W 2000 The development and measurement of empathy in nursing. Ashgate, Aldershot

Reynolds W 2003 Developing empathy. In: Barker P (ed) Psychiatric and mental health nursing: the craft of caring. Edward Arnold, London

Reynolds W, Scott B 1999 Empathy: a crucial component of the helping relationship. Journal of Psychiatric and Mental Health Nursing 6: 363–370

Reynolds W, Scott B 2000 Do nurses and other professional helpers normally display much empathy? Journal of Advanced Nursing 31: 226–234

Reynolds W, Scott A, Austin W 2000 Nursing, empathy and perception of the moral. Journal of Advanced Nursing 32: 235–242

Rogers C 1951 Client-centred therapy. Houghton Mifflin, New York

Rogers C 1957 The necessary and sufficient conditions of therapeutic personality change. Journal of Consulting Psychology 21: 95–103

Rogers C 1975 Empathic: an unappreciated way of being. The Counseling Psychologist 5: 2–10

Rogers C 1990 A way of being. Houghton Mifflin, Boston, MA

Shafer R 1959 Generative empathy in the treatment situation. Psycho-Analysis Quarterly 38: 342–373

Sissons A, Arthur D, Gazda G 1981 Cited in Mackay R, Hughes J, Carver E (eds) Empathy in the helping relationship. Springer New York

Smither S 1977 A reconsideration of the developmental study of empathy. Human Development 20: 253–276

Stotland E 1969 Exploratory investigations of empathy. In: Berkowitz L (ed) Advances in experimental psychology 14. Academic Press, New York

Szalita A 1976 Some thoughts on empathy. Psychiatry 39: 142–152

Travelbee J 1966 Interpersonal aspects of nursing, FA Davis, Philadelphia, PA

Truax C 1961 A scale for the measurement of accurate empathy. Discussion paper 20. Wisconsin Psychiatric Institute, Madison, WI

Truax C 1967 A scale for rating accurate empathy. In: Rogers C, Gendelin E, Kiesler D, Truax C (eds) The therapeutic relationship and its impact: a study of psychotherapy with schizophrenia. University of Wisconsin Press, Madison, WI

Truax C 1975 The meaning and reliability of accurate empathy ratings: a rejoinder. Psychological Bulletin 77: 397–399

Truax C, Carkhuff R 1967 Toward effective counseling and psychotherapy: training and practice. Aldine Press, Chicago, IL

Valle S 1981 Interpersonal functioning of alcoholism counsellors and treatment outcome. Journal of Studies on Alcohol 42: 783–790

Williams C 1990 Biopsychological elements of empathy: a multidimensional model. Issues in Mental Health Nursing 11: 15–26

Wilt D, Evans C, Muenchen R, Guegold G 1995 Teaching with entertainment films: an empathetic focus. Journal of Psychosocial Nursing 33: 5–14

Zoske J, Pietrocarlo D 1983 Dialysis training exercises for improved staff awareness. American Association of Nephrology and Technicians Journal 19–39

A critical examination of the concept of empowerment

James Dooher and Richard Byrt

EDITORIAL

Those who study the modern history of nursing will be aware of a feature of our culture – the phenomenon of how nurses embrace the latest 'hot' concept so that certain ideas and practices become 'in vogue'. During the 1970s, within the UK, the latest 'hot' concept was the nursing process. In the 1980s it was the idea of Project 2000 and the movement of nurse education into higher education. Coupled with that was the in-vogue idea of community care. In the 1990s clinical supervision and 'reflective practitioners' could be described as being 'in vogue'. In the first decade of the new millennium, and not without a distinct sense of irony that is not lost on the editors, the 'hot concept' in the UK is the notion of re-kindling past values and re-introducing phased-out practices as a means to bolster falling standards of care (e.g. the re-introduction of 'Matrons').

A further concept that was very much in vogue in the 1990s was empowerment. Whether this was linked to the growing service user movement or the increased political lobby of health service consumer groups, or was a bona fide paradigmatic shift in nurses' thinking is undear. Nevertheless, in order to be regarded as avant garde one had to be

niliar with the idea and concept of empowerment. Yet Jim and Richard's
apter reminds us of the ambiguity surrounding the concept and, more
rryingly, the micro- and macro-level implications of genuine attempts to
power health service users. While few nurses (and other healthcare
ctitioners) would openly deny that they believe empowerment is a good
g, the evidence of major shifts in power within healthcare
ider–consumer relations suggests that little has changed, despite the
oric about empowerment.

It is within this context that the time-honoured attempts of some
nurses to attain professional status make the least sense. While we have
neither the space nor the scope within this book for a thorough debate
about whether or not nursing is a profession (and the associated
debate about whether or not nurses should aspire to professional status),
it is very difficult to reconcile the perpetual drive to be seen as a
profession with the inherent power imbalance this propagates and with
nurses' claims that they wish to empower patients. It is difficult to
envisage how the great strength of nurses (their ability to form close,
therapeutic, interpersonal relationships with patients) would not be
further eroded by the construction of additional professional obstructions
(e.g. professional distance, professionals as experts, professionals as
holders of the power).

INTRODUCTION

The concept of empowerment is one that many nurses are no doubt familiar with,
yet it remains a difficult concept to define. Even though attention to the conceptual
clarity of empowerment is a relatively recent addition to the nursing literature, several publications have identified problems with obtaining a clear and concise definition (e.g. Byrt & Dooher 2002, Chevannes 2002). While this literature includes
many definitions of empowerment, the concept is often used vaguely; with
assumptions that it is necessarily a good thing (Kendall 1998, Byrt & Dooher 2002,
Houston & Cowley 2002). The vagueness and lack of clear definitions indicate that
clarity of conceptualization is an essential precursor to the effective implementation of empowerment and participation strategies. Further, assumptions about the
value of empowerment are often made uncritically without examining the evidence for the advantages and disadvantages. Accordingly, in this chapter the definitions of the concept of empowerment will be explored, followed by an
examination of the key attributes and dimensions of the concept that have been
described in the relevant theoretical and empirical literature. Following this, the
inextricable link between empowerment and power will be explored. While the
chapter does not adhere strictly to an established approach to concept analysis, it

adopts a critical and systematic review of the literature as a means of enhancing understanding of the concept.

DEFINITIONS AND MEANINGS OF EMPOWERMENT

Several authors (Kendall 1998, Dooher & Byrt 2002, 2003) have commented that *some* writing on empowerment is largely rhetorical as it does not consider methods of implementation in order to benefit health service users and their carers. Indeed, according to Simpson (2003, p. 136) 'Much time is spent in extolling the virtues of empowering service users… but little practical guidance is given on how this is to be achieved.'

Criticisms of empowerment, as both a concept and a reality in everyday nursing practice, are far-reaching. Many practitioners express their dislike of the term 'empowerment', suggesting that it is an 'in vogue' expression that has become so tired and overused that it no longer has meaning in health terms. Such doubts have been echoed in critiques that suggest that 'the term can be interpreted in so many ways that it is not clear what purpose it serves' (Brown & Piper 1995, p. 641).

Another problem is that definitions and models often appear to be based on the perspectives of academics, managers or professionals rather than on those of service users and carers. Within the extant literature there is often evidence of limited understanding of the complexity and multifaceted nature of empowerment (Byrt & Dooher 2002). This often results in definitions in the literature that refer only to a limited number of aspects or dimensions of empowerment (see, for example, Malin & Teasdale 1991, Ellis-Stoll & Popkess-Vawter 1998, Skinner & Cradock 2000). In addition, definitions and the scope of studies on empowerment often reflect the discipline (such as nursing, social work, psychology, sociology) of particular authors (see, for example, Melluish 1998, Morrall 1998, Oliver & Barnes 1998, Tones & Green 2002, Westwood 2002, Godfrey 2003, McHugh 2003). Empowerment has been criticised for being a culture-bound concept (Mok 2001). The assumption that empowerment is a good thing, leading to health improvement and to patients being healthier, has been challenged by Chevannes (2002), supported by Reece and White (2002, p. 115) who stated that empowerment has 'become so value laden that it appears to have lost credibility'.

Recently, empowerment appears to have become almost a cliché; a word that has become virtually obligatory in writing on both local and national health services. **Confusion about the meaning of empowerment may relate to the endless conceptualization of the term and the lack of translation into meaningful outcomes that underpin real change.** While we do not wish to appear premature, our review of the literature has enabled us to distil the key attributes and dimensions of empowerment and this has led to our tentative definition of empowerment.

> *Empowerment involves increases or transfers in power involving four dimensions. These include individual or psychological empowerment, in which the individual experiences increased power or control. Other dimensions relate to service-initiated empowerment, where professionals or managers enable service users or carers to increase their power. Empowerment also includes the achievement of actual change (in health services and/or wider society) and social inclusion. Achieving the latter involves gaining greater power within society, with the availability of increased life opportunities, and the reduction of discrimination.*
>
> *Byrt & Dooher 2003, p 1f).*

KEY ATTRIBUTES OF EMPOWERMENT

Several authors examine the links between psychological (individual) and social change dimensions of empowerment (Falk-Rafael 2001, Ritchie 2001, Houston & Cowley 2002). Empowerment often involves participation: 'the involvement of service users/carers in responsibility and/or decision making, which has an intended impact [given outcome] on services and/or policies which affect the individual participant and/or other service users/carers' (Byrt & Dooher 2002, p. 2). In relation to participation, empowerment is a state whereby an individual is afforded and/or, more importantly, affords himself/herself, the opportunity to contribute to a given outcome, in relation to the individual and/or other service users/carers. Empowerment requires interdependence between the individual and the community in which they live. This is in contrast to the often celebrated state of independence, which may produce isolation and, consequently, limited opportunities to participate.

Empowerment has cognitive, affective (or emotional) and behavioural (or action) components. For example, an individual with cerebral palsy might be empowered in the following ways.

- *Cognitive*: Recognition and realization that the way they have been treated in wider society is stigmatizing and discriminatory. A growth in understanding of the injustice and inappropriateness of other people's negative attitudes, and of discrimination in job opportunities. Increased awareness and questioning of the lack of access to certain buildings for people with physical disabilities.
- *Affective (emotional)*: Development of increased self-esteem, self-confidence and anger at discrimination. They might also experience a feeling of pride about their efforts to challenge stigmatization, discrimination and social exclusion. They might also experience a sense of solidarity with other individuals experiencing the social effects of disability (Oliver & Barnes 1998).

- *Behavioural (action)*: They could experience empowerment through their participation in efforts to change stigmatization, discrimination and social exclusion. This could include action as an individual, e.g. campaigning or running workshops to enable health professionals to develop services to meet the needs of individuals with disabilities. The behavioural (action) component could also involve collaboration for change with other people, e.g. through membership of the voluntary organization 'Scope' or participation in a Department of Health advisory group concerned with enabling the social inclusion of individuals with disabilities.

Some individuals may experience satisfaction from the cognitive and/or affective components of empowerment alone. However, within health services, many service users and carers may find empowerment meaningless unless they are able to participate in actions that result in desired changes, either in services or in wider society (Dooher & Byrt 2002, 2003). Within nursing, if empowerment remains as a theoretical construct, its utility is diminished if not thwarted. It becomes more useful when it shifts from a cognitive/emotional or abstract state to become tangible through behaviour and action. **Indeed, empowerment is of little use to the activity of nursing unless it can be effectively implemented in busy healthcare settings and, most importantly, result in positive benefits to service users and their informal carers.**

The effective implementation of care to empower the patient results in positive outcomes. These include psychological gains, such as increased self-esteem, satisfaction with care and feeling in control, in relation to having influence on the care and treatment given. In contrast to empowerment, helplessness is a response to an individual's absence of control over a given circumstance, which may, according to Seligman (1975) and Atkinson et al (2003) produce depression and other emotional distress. Such an inverse relationship led Tones and Green (2002) to suggest that the helpless person is in a diametrically opposed position to the empowered individual. This leads us to think of a continuum of empowerment, which is illustrated in Figure 8.1. In contrast to the individual who experiences helplessness,

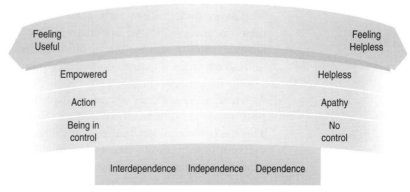

Figure 8.1 The empowerment paradigm

an empowered person is more likely to be able to achieve their goals, acknowledge personal expectations and recognize the value that their goals will have upon their life.

Atkinson et al's (2003) research suggests that outcomes that are independent of responses are quickly learned: in other words, if the person has no control, they quickly give up (Atkinson et al 2003). In contrast, when a person has been in partial control, they are much more determined to keep trying to regain that control. Outcome-sensitive or instrumental behaviours (i.e. behaviours dependent on the achievement of goals) reinforce successful action but equally confirm failure. For this reason, empowerment may be seen as a dangerous thing for vulnerable people, as it may increase the risk of failure and perhaps reconfirm feelings of loss of control and helplessness.

Most definitions of empowerment refer to increases in the power of individual(s), sometimes involving transfers of power from one individual or group to another (Byrt & Dooher 2002). Importantly, a distinction should be drawn between empowerment as an individual, gaining control in relation to their specific health problems, and as a response to wider social inequalities. The notion of one individual exerting 'power over' another, with resultant inequalities of power (Breeze 2002) can be contrasted with the more complex notion of 'power with' or power-sharing. The latter involves a social process of enhancement, together with a transfer of power and a package of rights that has been achieved through concordance (Ghaye 2000).

Psychological empowerment, sometimes referred to as self-empowerment, has a direct link to health, in particular mental health. Its components, listed in Figure 8.2, include: self-confidence and increased self-efficacy. Psychological empowerment also involves a heightened internal locus of control, leading to health outcomes that are directly related to the individual's belief that they are able to influence their health and attain particular goals. Perceptions about self-determination and control are at the heart of self-empowerment and, associated with well-being; contribute greatly to self-esteem, self-confidence, self-respect, self-worth and self-reliance. In turn, this produces a sense of coherence in relation to one's environment and enables the person to function at their optimum potential (Tones & Green 2002).

These aspirations cannot be achieved in isolation (see Fig. 8.1), as it is the inter-relationships in which we are involved that underpin our sense of worth, competence, capability and feeling of authenticity. It becomes harder to increase low self-esteem when one finds oneself in a minority or isolated through social exclusion or discrimination.

These adverse effects of and on the 'self', on one's self-esteem, self-efficacy and positive self-identity, are often decreased through a process of consciousness-raising. This has been considered in relation to the psychological empowerment of individuals of minority ethnic groups, older people, women and individuals who are transgendered, lesbian or gay (Dooher & Byrt 2002, 2003). For example, women-only groups may help women to gain confidence and self-respect, enabling them to progress towards recovery or a more empowered position (Ifill 2003). Professionally

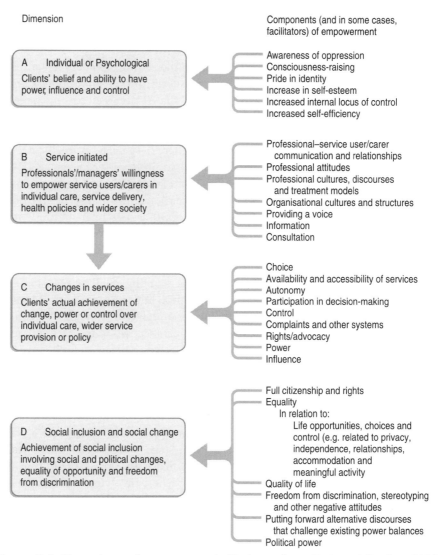

Figure 8.2 Dimensions of empowerment (Redrawn from Byrt and Dooher 2002, p. 24, with permission of Quay Books, Mark Allen Publishing Ltd, Salisbury)

initiated empowerment and participation is a dimension that is particularly important to the successful redistribution of power and frequently it is the influence of professionals in either facilitating or hindering the process that determines the outcome.

As a result of acknowledging the limitations of existing definitions and through consideration of the extant literature on empowerment, Byrt and Dooher (2002) argued that empowerment could be effectively and more completely defined and conceptualized as consisting of four dimensions rather than a single dimension. They distinguish between: individual or psychological; service-initiated; service change; and social inclusion and social change (see Fig. 8.2).

POWER AND OPPRESSION

Having highlighted the relationship between empowerment and power, it is necessary to examine issues of power (and oppression) in more detail. This is undertaken in the belief that this enhanced understanding should provide additional meaning for the concept of empowerment.

Issues of power and oppression are increasingly becoming agenda items for service planners. There have been noticeable developments in increased empowerment and participation of service users and 'survivors' within some consultation processes. Some authorities, including conflict theorists, have argued that meaningful participation and empowerment cannot occur unless there is a redistribution of power. Others, again including consensus theorists, consider that disempowered individuals or groups can increase their power without subsequent loss of power for others (Morgan 1999). It has been argued by conflict theorists that, without redistribution of power, services will merely preserve the status quo, perhaps enabling small increases in empowerment but retaining oligarchic elements that undermine equity. Morgan (1999, p. 138) has defined oligarchy as: 'power and decision-making … concentrated in the hands of a few'. According to this perspective, empowerment involves service users taking, or being given, more power and, by default, this takes away at least some power from providers.

This notion assumes that power is quantifiable and that its distribution can be measured. However, considering that power, at its simplest, needs to be viewed in cognitive, emotional, behavioural and economic terms, measuring it is methodologically problematic. This difficulty poses a problem for those relinquishing a proportion of their stake as well as for those who are receiving it. Often, recipients feel more satisfied with any redistribution if it has been achieved through oppositional approaches, involving the raising of consciousness and reducing oppression through direct challenges to people in positions of power (Byrt & Dooher 2002).

Consensus theorists argue that increases in the power of service users or carers do not necessarily result in diminished power for professionals and others. Barnes and Bowl (2001) state that some empowerment is concerned with:

> *… notions of partnership, [in which] shared decision making, or negotiation may be a more appropriate way of conceptualizing the nature of the relationship being sought. A model of partnership practice which enables the knowledge and insights of both user and professional to be drawn on in developing problem-solving strategies, not only has the potential to produce better outcomes for the user, it can also provide learning opportunities for professional actors to develop better practice.*

Both oppositional and collaborative approaches can initiate psychological empowerment in the individual, as well as initiating collective action to bring about social change. Sometimes, the latter has involved challenging and attempting to address inequalities in the provision of particular services, or in access to life opportunities or social inclusion, including the elimination of discriminatory attitudes. However, some aspects of power imbalance and inequality appear difficult to change because of the considerable vested financial and other interests of dominant groups such as pharmaceutical companies (Reznick 1997, Hogg 1999, Baggott 2000).

Godfrey (2003, p. 175) described the effects of discourses in wider society, including powerful familial, legal and institutional structures, that influence discriminatory attitudes. She concluded: 'it is more realistic to think of empowering patients, not from the premise of them as powerless, but as individuals with views and understanding about their illnesses and social life which deserve to be heard by nurses and other health professionals'.

Those who are marginalized by professionals and have not been afforded any power are more likely to feel like pawns in a strategic power game over which they have no control. However, the evidence does not suggest a damning indictment of authoritarianism in health care. Gloomy, perhaps, but there are many examples of increasing empowerment and/or participation, sometimes with redistributions of power, which have apparently successfully enabled participation in care and treatment decisions, and where users have found a voice to express their experience of problems and oppression (Dooher & Byrt 2002). The success of attempts to increase service user and carer empowerment and participation depends, in part, on the extent to which the application of these concepts is either intrinsic to all organizational goals or considered important, compared with other goals. The latter may complement or conflict with empowerment. For example, there may be a 'conflict of individual right to autonomy versus duty of care' (Breeze 2002, p. 109).

The motivation of managers and professional leaders and their interest in increasing empowerment or participation is also important. To devolve power may not be an instinctive action, particularly when leadership through power has often been the norm. Managers who operate from a power through leadership stance may be more willing to devolve appropriate elements of their role. The motivation to devolve or share power may be subdivided into the valance, or value, the manager places upon it and their expectations in terms of outcome. In many cases, mental health service users are empowered solely on terms dictated by professionals, and if either valence or expectation is low for those professionals, empowerment is less likely to happen.

SPECIFIC ORGANIZATIONAL AND INDIVIDUAL-PRACTITIONER-LEVEL PRACTICES LINKED WITH EMPOWERMENT

The extant literature identifies a number of practices that are linked with empowerment. While not exhaustive, the following list describes specific ways that can be used to empower service users.

- *Value the individual*: This has been emphasized, for example, in services for older people with Alzheimer's disease and related conditions. In these services, respect for personhood, the unique and individual identity of the person, has been stressed by a number of authors (e.g. Innes & Capstick 2001, Martin & Younger 2001, Simpson 2003).

- *Use clear, accessible information, language and explanations with the avoidance of jargon* (Brooks 2001, Dooher & Byrt 2003).

- *Encourage service users to 'find their voice'*: Several authors have outlined ways in which individuals from oppressed groups have 'found a voice', expressed their views, perspectives and feelings, e.g. from the use of the arts in health projects (Dooher & Byrt 2003).

- *Wherever possible, provide a choice – the possibility of deciding between two or more options* (Hogg 1999): However, 'the extent to which individuals have sufficient power to make *genuine* free choices will depend on the nature of their social, economic, cultural and material circumstances' (Tones & Green 2002, p. 101).

- *Wherever possible, offer the service user control – the capacity to have influence or power over decisions about health care, treatment and service* (Hogg 1999): For example, Miers (1999) and McHugh (2003) consider issues of male professional control over services for women with breast cancer and maternity services, respectively.

- *Wherever possible, respect the service user's autonomy*: Uphold service users' capacity to make informed choices for themselves, involving 'not just a sense of self, but also awareness of options and knowledge of the implications and consequences of choosing a particular course of action'(Hendrick 2000, p. 30).

- *Consider and address issues of accessibility*: Provide easily available information about services, complaints systems and life opportunities (Evans & Byrt 2000) Ensure there is adequate availability of staff and managers to service users and carers (Hogg 1999).

- *Respect service users' and carers' rights and make advocacy services available* (Sang 2003, Teasdale 1998).

- *Practise with a continued sense of equality*: This includes respecting the diversity and common humanity of all health service participants; providing opportunities for partnership with health service and managers in decision-making and other aspects of participation (Byrt & Dooher 2003, Florin & Coulter 2001, Hogg 1999).

- *Establish an organizational culture that enables empowerment through offering the components listed above* (Byrt 2001, Whyte & Carton 2002).

CONSUMERISM AND PROFESSIONALISM

It can be argued that consumerist participation is influenced, in part, by paternalism and professional fears that genuine empowerment may reduce professional autonomy and directly challenge the notion of expertise. We assert that professionals are generally reluctant to hand over their hard-earned expertise, as they may have studied for years, if not decades, to establish their position. It could even be said that the education process itself socializes trainees to protect 'their' discipline despite the fact that service users and their carers are often more knowledgeable (Saks 2002). Professional acknowledgement of the expertise of service users and carers can be seen as a first step in the shift of professional power in their favour (Fisher & Gilbert 2001, Florin & Coulter 2001). Such a shift would also reflect and demonstrate changes in attitude towards service users and carers (Kohner & Hill 2000).

There is a considerable literature on the power bases of health service professionals, particularly that of doctors (Rogers & Pilgrim 2003, Saks 2002). The power of the doctors' 'dominant medical culture' and the consumerist approach to health care possibly reinforce the 'current dominant medical discourse' as well as minimizing service users' influence (Ward 2000). Smith and Forster (2000) argued that some medical practitioners need to be more prepared to admit to and apologize for mistakes and to make it clear to the public, service users and carers what, as doctors, they are realistically able to achieve.

Professionals can go some way to redressing power imbalances by considering how and what they communicate. Professional discourses, with the use of specialist language, psychobabble and jargon, can be disempowering (Dooher & Byrt 2003). Participatory communication and decision-making is partly determined by professionals' perceptions of service users' class, social status and ability to articulate their views (or make a complaint against them (Evans & Byrt 2002)). If users and carers do not feel empowered by their interactions, their service user status is likely to be perpetuated. It is, therefore, crucial to the prevention and resolution of situations that professionals 'talk the language' of the people they serve, thus promoting the professional–client relationship (Florin & Coulter 2001).

How informed and assertive patients are, together with clinicians' 'readiness' to communicate and take their views seriously, has a direct impact on the instigation of empowerment/participatory dialogue (Paterson 2001). Moreover, the promotion of clinical governance and public participation in National Health Service and primary care trusts and in strategic health authority decision-making have increased the pressure to change (Evans & Byrt 2002). Even relatively simple initiatives, such as involving patients in the design and refurbishment of waiting rooms, may convey the message that patients are valued partners.

BENEFITS AND DRAWBACKS OF EMPOWERMENT

As we stated earlier in this chapter, the common conception of empowerment among nurses is that it is a good thing (Byrt & Dooher 2002). Yet such simplistic ideas do not give full acknowledgement to the potential drawbacks of a healthcare service that is genuinely driven by attempts to empower service users. We have summarized these benefits and potential drawbacks in Table 8.1.

Table 8.1   Benefits and drawbacks of empowerment

Benefits	Drawbacks
May result in increases in psychological empowerment, eg: raised self-efficacy, self-esteem, self-confidence, self-worth and pride in identity	May lead to decreases in psychological empowerment, particularly if strategies to increase participation fail to take account of individuals' wishes to be involved and their specific aptitudes, self-beliefs and skills
Has the potential to value the individual service user/carer and his/her views	Service users/carers likely to feel devalued if their views are not taken seriously or acted on, or if there is tokenism or pseudoparticipation
Service users/carers benefit from opportunities for their perspectives to be voiced and appreciated. This also enables professionals and managers to provide services that meet the expressed needs of service users/carers	If there is a clash of perspective, professionals and managers may be likely to dictate the extent and nature of empowerment and participation
Reported benefits from involvement in decision-making and responsibility	Individuals can be disempowered if there is a mismatch between their wish for empowerment/participation and the expectations of others
Information, explanation and consultation may be valued by some service/users carers, whether or not their power is increased or participation at higher levels is involved	According to some authors, genuine empowerment and participation cannot occur unless there are changes in the distribution of power
Mutual giving and receiving support in some participatory mechanisms, eg, self-help groups	Not all individuals feel able, or wish, to be involved in this way. The giving of support may be left to a few participants
Participation of service users/carers, including expression of their views and choices helps to ensure that the services meet their needs	The views, choices and other participation of service users/carers may: a) conflict with other organizational goals and priorities b) be difficult to take forward because of lack of resources
In professional–client communication and relationships based on empowerment and participation models, there is greater emphasis on quality, a partnership approach, and respect for the expertise of the service user/carer	Some service users/carers want a professional relationship and communication in which they play a passive role, with the professional as an expert
Service user/carer participation has contributed to improvements in services	Such participation has often not resulted in improvements related to: a) issues of most importance to service users/carers b) changes in wider society related to increased social inclusion and life opportunities
The skills of service users and carers benefit both other people in similar circumstances, and specific health services	Service users and carers may consider that they lack the requisite skills, or organizations may fail to recognize the skills they have. Resources may be needed to enable both service users/carers and professionals to gain skills in relation to empowerment and participation

Table 8.1 Benefits and drawbacks of empowerment—cont'd

Benefits	Drawbacks
Many empowerment and participation approaches emphasize the rights of service users and carers	Charters of rights for service users and carers in health services in the UK are not legally enforceable and may not be reflected in practice. The rights of some individuals may conflict with their responsibilities or the rights of other service users or carers, the public or professionals
Empowerment and participation in community health projects are often found to increase social cohesion and decrease isolation	Some people may not desire these goals. Other goals may be more important to them
Empowerment and participation can lead to action and successfully bringing about change	The extent of change often depends on resources and the decisions of people in positions of power
Service users and carers who actively participate are not representative of other service users and carers	Some service users and carers: prefer this representation to their own direct participation. Also, other individuals, including professionals, may not be representative of their constituencies

CONCLUSION

In our attempts to discover the meaning and practical application of empowerment in health care we have found it essential to recognize the complexity of this concept and the difficulties associated with its implementation. This complexity is, in part, explained by the multidimensional nature of empowerment. Empowerment has a dynamic, humanistic and individual essence. However, blanket policies and overuse of the term have only served to undermine honourable, well-intentioned attempts by service users, professionals and managers to empower recipients of health care and their informal carers. Empowerment is clearly very closely linked to power, and issues of power and control. It is impossible, in a meaningful way, to discuss empowerment without simultaneously considering power (and control). Accordingly, genuine attempts to empower service users (and their families), we believe, must produce change.

The complexity of empowerment is further illustrated by the fact that an individual could feel that they had power according to one dimension but experience disempowerment in relation to others. Thus, a woman might experience a high level of self-efficacy and feel that members of her multiprofessional team enabled her empowerment and participation, as an equal partner in care and in treatment decisions. However, similarly to many of the respondents in a study by Priestley (1999), she might argue that those aspects of empowerment and participation were unimportant, as they had no effect on the discrimination she faced in wider society; or on the attitudes of people who saw her, not as a girlfriend, mother, artist and a woman who enjoys clubbing but solely as someone in a wheelchair to be stereotyped, patronized or ignored.

REFERENCES

Atkinson RL, Atkinson RC, Smith EE et al (eds) 2003 Hilgard's introduction to psychology, 14th edn. Harcourt College Publishers, Fort Worth, TX

Baggott R 2000 Public health, policy and politics. Macmillan, Basingstoke

Barnes M, Bowl R 2001 Taking over the asylum. Palgrave, Basingstoke

Breeze J 2002 User participation and empowerment in community mental health nursing practice. In: Dooher J, Byrt R (eds) Empowerment and participation: power, influence and control in contemporary health care. Quay Books, Dinton, Salisbury

Brooks F 2001 Why user involvement in primary health care? In: Gillam S, Brooks F (eds) New beginnings. towards patient and public involvement in primary health care. King's Fund/University of Luton, London

Brown PA, Piper SM 1995 Empowerment or social control? Differing interpretations of psychology in health education. Health Education Journal 54: 115–123

Byrt R 2001 Power, influence and control in practice development. In: Clark A, Dooher J, Fowler J (eds) The handbook of practice development. Quay Books, Dinton, Salisbury

Byrt R, Dooher J 2002 Empowerment and participation: definitions, meanings and models. In: Dooher J, Byrt R (eds) Empowerment and participation: power, influence and control in contemporary health care. Quay Books, Dinton, Salisbury

Byrt R, Dooher J 2003 Service users and their desire for empowerment and participation. In: Dooher J, Byrt R (eds) Empowerment: and the health service user. Quay Books, Dinton, Salisbury

Chevannes M 2002 Empowerment and ethnicity. In: Dooher J, Byrt R (eds) Empowerment and participation: power, influence and control in contemporary health care. Quay Books, Dinton, Salisbury

Dooher J, Byrt R (eds) 2002 Empowerment and participation: power, influence and control in contemporary health care. Quay Books, Dinton, Salisbury

Dooher J, Byrt R 2003 Empowerment: and the health service user. Quay Books, Dinton, Salisbury

Ellis-Stoll CC, Popkess-Vawter S 1998 A concept analysis on the process of empowerment. Advances in Nursing Science 21: 62–68

Evans S, Byrt R 2002 The power to complain? In: Dooher J, Byrt R (eds) Empowerment and participation: power, influence and control in contemporary health care. Quay Books, Dinton, Salisbury

Falk-Rafael AR 2001 Empowerment as a process of evolving consciousness: a model of empowered caring. Advances in Nursing Science 24: 1–16

Fisher B, Gilbert D 2001 Patient involvement and clinical effectiveness. In: Gillam S, Brooks F (eds) New beginnings: towards patient and public involvement in primary health care. King's Fund/University of Luton, London

Florin D, Coulter A 2001 Partnership in the primary care consultation. In: Gillam S, Brooks F (eds) New beginnings: towards patient and public involvement in primary health care. King's Fund/University of Luton, London

Ghaye T 2000 Is this a case of the emperor's new clothes? In: Ghaye T, Gillespie D, Lillyman S (eds) Empowerment through reflection: the narratives of healthcare professionals. Quay Books, Dinton, Salisbury

Godfrey J 2003 The lesbian, gay man's and transgendered experience as users of healthcare services. In: Dooher J, Byrt R (eds) Empowerment and participation: power, influence and control in contemporary health care. Quay Books, Dinton, Salisbury

Hendrick J 2000 Law and ethics in nursing and health care. Stanley Thornes, Cheltenham

Hogg C 1999 Patients, power and politics: from patients to citizens. Sage, London

Houston AM, Cowley S 2002 An empowerment approach to needs assessment in health visiting. Journal of Clinical Nursing 11: 640–650

Ifill W 2003 Women's needs in a medium secure unit: a former patient's perspective. In: Dooher J, Byrt R (eds) Empowerment and participation: power, influence and control in contemporary health care. Quay Books, Dinton, Salisbury

Innes A, Capstick A 2001 Communication and personhood In: Cantley C (ed) A handbook of dementia care. Open University Press, Buckingham

Kendall S 1998 Introduction. In: Kendall S (ed) Health and empowerment: research and practice. Edward Arnold, London

Kohner N, Hill A (eds) 2000 Help! Does my patient know more than me? Kings Fund, London

McHugh N 2003 Giving birth to participation: are women empowered within the maternity services? In: Dooher J, Byrt R (eds) Empowerment: and the health service user. Quay Books, Dinton, Salisbury

Malin N, Teasdale K 1991 Caring versus empowerment: considerations for nursing practice. Journal of Advanced Nursing 16: 657–662

Martin GW, Younger D 2001 person-centred care for people with dementia: a quality audit approach. Journal of Psychiatric and Mental Health Nursing 8: 443–448

Melluish S 1998 Community psychology: a social action approach to psychological distress. In: Barker P, Davidson B (eds) Psychiatric nursing: ethical strife. Arnold, London

Miers M 1999 Involving clients in decision making: breast care nursing. In: Wilkinson G, Miers M (eds) Power and nursing practice. Macmillan, Basingstoke

Mok E 2001 Empowerment of cancer patients: from a Chinese perspective. Nursing Ethics 8: 69–75

Morgan I 1999 Power and politics. Hodder & Stoughton, London

Morrall P 1998 Clinical sociology and empowerment. In: Barker P, Davidson B (eds) Psychiatric nursing: ethical strife. Arnold, London

Oliver M, Barnes C 1998 Disabled people and social policy. Longman, Harlow

Paterson B 2001 Myth of empowerment in chronic illness. Journal of Advanced Nursing 34: 574–581

Priestley M 1999 Disability politics and community care. Jessica Kingsley, London

Reece J, White C 2002 Women's empowerment – myth or reality. In: Dooher J, Byrt R (eds) Empowerment and participation: power, influence and control in contemporary health care. Quay Books, Dinton, Salisbury

Reznick P 1997 Twenty-first century democracy. McGill–Queen's University Press, Montreal

Ritchie L 2001 Empowerment and Australian community health nurses' work with aboriginal clients: the sociopolitical context. Qualitative Health Research 11: 190–205

Rogers A, Pilgrim D 2003 Mental health and inequality. Palgrave, Basingstoke

Saks M 2002 Empowerment, participation and the rise of orthodox biomedicine. In: Dooher J, Byrt R (eds) Empowerment and participation: power, influence and control in contemporary health care. Quay Books, Dinton, Salisbury

Sang B 2003 Patient and public participation in health systems: some basic principles. In: Dooher J, Byrt R (eds) Empowerment: and the health service user. Quay Books, Dinton, Salisbury

Seligman MEP 1975 Helplessness. Freeman, San Francisco, CA

Simpson R 2003 Participation of older people and their carers in care. In: Dooher J, Byrt R (eds) Empowerment: and the health service user. Quay Books, Dinton, Salisbury

Skinner TC, Cradock S 2000 Empowerment: what about the evidence? Practical Diabetes International 17: 91–95

Smith ML, Forster HP 2000 morally managing medical mistakes. Cambridge Quarterly Heathcare Ethics 9: 38–53

Teasdale K 1998 Advocacy in health care. Blackwell Science, Oxford

Tones K, Green J 2002 The empowerment imperative in health promotion. In: Dooher J, Byrt R (eds) Empowerment and participation: power, influence and control in contemporary health care. Quay Books, Dinton, Salisbury

Ward D 2000 Totem not taboo. Groupwork as a vehicle for user participation. In: Kemshall H, Littlechild R (eds) User involvement and participation in social care. Research informing practice. Jessica Kingsley, London

Westwood S 2002 Power and the social. Routledge, London

Whyte L, Carton G 2002 Creating and maintaining strategies for empowering clients within high secure settings. In: Dooher J, Byrt R (eds) Empowerment and participation: power, influence and control in contemporary health care. Quay Books, Dinton, Salisbury

A concept analysis of facilitation

Carole McIlrath

EDITORIAL

On first consideration the reader could be forgiven for wondering, is a book on the essential concepts of nursing the correct place to include a concept analysis of facilitation? Similarly, why do nurses need to have an understanding of the composition, dynamics and processes of facilitation? The editors' view is that facilitation can be regarded as one of many concepts that nurses encounter and use in everyday practice, without perhaps being fully aware that that is what they are doing. Accordingly, if nurses do frequently encounter and use facilitation, yet lack a full awareness of this, then it is entirely understandable that they would question the inclusion of facilitation in this book.

As editors we will not belabour the obvious point that we have already made in Chapter 1, although it may warrant a quick reminder that nurses do encounter and use a whole range of concepts in everyday practice without having a full awareness of them. Interestingly, Carole's chapter reminds us that, although the concept is not commonly understood, increased attention is being given to facilitation within nursing literature, clinical practice and nurse education. Indeed, this paradigmatic or, more appropriately, pedagogical shift in nurse education can be thought of as one of the most significant developments in nurse education over the last few decades. The movement from students as passive recipients to active (and proactive) participants in a learning process can be seen to parallel the processes of shifting the way patients (and their families) are viewed. A patient as a partner in the care episode rather than being someone who is 'done unto' is not only underpinned by a significant body of evidence (see, for example, much of the literature emanating from heathcare service user groups, e.g. Mind, NSF) but simultaneously begets the need for nurses to be facilitative rather than 'doing for'.

A further issue that underpins the value of this concept analysis is that of the expanding role of the modern-day, contemporary nurse. The traditional image of the nurse as one who inevitably works in a hospital, often an acute care hospital, as one who stays by the bedside and personifies Nightingalian nursing traits is now thankfully consigned to the realm of history. Contemporary nurses can be found in many settings, many of which would not be synonymous with these traditional images (e.g. nurses offering education to secondary schoolchildren on communicable diseases and safe sex practices.) It is within many of these 'new', broader functions that the nursing role perhaps becomes one of facilitator more than perhaps a 'hands-on' clinician.

INTRODUCTION

Facilitation is a word often used by politicians, academics, the media, civil servants and 'modern' organizations, to name but a few. Concomitantly, an examination of contemporary nursing parlance will show that it is now common to encounter the term (and concept) within different nursing-related areas. For example, nurse managers, nurse teachers, clinical nurse specialists and practice development nurses often talk about facilitation. It has become fashionable to be called a 'facilitator'; however, what is meant by the concept of facilitation, and how the concept is 'used' suggest that it is not always well understood.

As mentioned in Chapter 1, concept analyses are widely recognized to be important for the development of nursing theory and practice for a range of reasons, including the following. First, according to Chinn and Kramer (1995), concepts are used in theory development in that theories are constructed from clarified concepts. Watson (1991) offered similar remarks, suggesting that concepts are the building blocks from which theories can be built. Secondly, analysis is necessary if the concept is to be operationalized, permitting researchers to specify what counts as an instantiation of the concept and perhaps to devise measuring instruments. Thirdly, concept analysis improves practice by offering nurses a clearer understanding of what certain terms mean. As McKenna (1997) argued, if a concept is unclear then any work on which it is based is similarly likely to be unclear.

Accordingly, this chapter is therefore aimed at presenting a concept analysis of facilitation using Walker and Avant's framework (1995). The chapter also aims to help define the attributes or characteristics of the concept in the hope that those nurses who practice facilitation of learning may obtain a greater understanding of the process and underlining principles involved.

SELECTION OF THE CONCEPT: WHY FACILITATION?

The importance of facilitation to an organization should not be underestimated. This importance has been recognized within the National Health Service (NHS) in recent years, when facilitation has become increasingly central to the work of health service organizations, particularly following the introduction of clinical and social care governance. Indeed, many NHS trusts in Northern Ireland have employed Nurse Facilitators over the past few years, to promote personal and professional development, clinical services and aspects of practice development.

Historically, most nurses will have learnt, or have been taught (or both) within organizational and educational systems that were largely prescriptive. Such systems had a significant number of rules (aims, behavioural objectives, lesson plans, assessment essays and examinations) that influenced and coloured nurses' expectations and governed or controlled their behaviour (Townsend 1990). It is naive to assume that, because nurses undertook training or development under the direction of a teacher, learning was being facilitated. According to Rogers (1983), in contrast to the facilitation of learning, the practice of teaching is a highly overrated function.

Prescriptive organizational systems were influenced by the 'traditional' management approach, referred to as 'theory X', which stemmed from the work of McGregor (1961). This system persisted within most NHS organizations until the early 1990s (although it should be noted that, despite many organizational developments, even today some organizations possibly continue to use this directive approach). This theory holds the views that staff are unmotivated and unreliable; they prefer to be directed rather than think for themselves; they require rules, structures and hierarchies; they lack creativity; they are only motivated by money; and they do not want to take responsibility. Such pervasive and prevailing views within the NHS undoubtedly influenced nurse education, which is hardly surprising given that, during this time, nurse education was (in the main) hospital- and not university-based. Such nurse education held the view that education/training programmes should be highly structured in order to motivate staff to learn; teachers should 'tell students how to do it' and the teacher held responsibility for ensuring that learning took place. As organizations continued to change because of increasing demands for quality of care, increased competition, increases in public expectations and technology, it became clear that this approach stifled innovation and the ability to respond quickly and effectively to change (Bee & Bee 1998).

There is a body of evidence (see, for example, Bee & Bee 1998) that suggests that most NHS organizations have moved away from the aforementioned approach over the past decade, towards what McGregor (1961) termed his 'theory Y – facilitative approach'. This theory, in contrast to the views of theory X, suggests that staff can demonstrate creativity when involved in developing/planning services; they want responsibility; they have a desire to learn and to achieve their potential to the benefit of both patients and organization. There is evidence to suggest that this 'theory Y' view has been embraced by many educationalists over the past decade, with many nurse educators advocating a move from the traditional teacher role to that of facilitator. It is also becoming more widely recognized that nurses want to take more responsibility for their learning; they are highly motivated to learn; they believe responsibility for learning should rest with the nurse and not the teacher/facilitator and that training programmes should be flexible to suit the nurses' needs (Bee & Bee 1998).

Although the activities inherent in facilitation have been referred to within education since the beginning of the 20th century, the term 'facilitation' primarily stems from the work of the humanistic psychotherapist Carl Rogers (1969). The characteristics of Rogers' (1969) client-centred counselling approach were transplanted into and applied to education. This resulted in the formulation of his student-centred approach to learning. This approach emphasized the need for student-centred learning environments, which stress the freedom for individual development as a means to enable student participation, involvement and self-evaluation. This leads students to become more adaptable and self-directed.

Rogers (1969) viewed the teacher as a facilitator of learning; a provider of resources for learning and someone who shares his/her feelings as well as his/her knowledge with the students. Rogers (1983) suggested that the only person who is educated is the person who has learned how to learn; the person who has learned how to adapt and change; the person who has realized that no knowledge is secure, that only the process of seeking knowledge gives a basis for security. However, although Rogers' (1983) approach advocated the shift from teacher to facilitator, his work fails to provide clear guidelines on how to implement the process of facilitation.

WHY IS FACILITATION IMPORTANT TO NURSING?

Following on from the UK Central Council for Nursing, Midwifery and Health Visiting statement (UKCC 1986) that in the future nurses would need to be adaptable, analytical practitioners committed to life-long learning, and have a problem-solving rather than task-centred approach to nursing, much of the nursing education literature advocated that nurse teachers should act as facilitators. From the 1980s through to the 1990s much of the literature on facilitation was based upon the work of Heron (1977), Brookfield (1986), and Townsend (1990). **Heron (1977) and Brookfield (1999) perceive facilitation as an active teaching method whereas Townsend (1990), on the other hand, views facilitation as 'a way of life'**

where the facilitator becomes a co-learner, sharing responsibility and control with the student.

Facilitation, as an activity within nursing practice as well a nursing education, should not be underestimated. Patients and their families determine the meaning of their current state of health and well-being within the context of their sociocultural environment, and should be empowered to determine their own needs and direction of therapeutic care (Dooher & Byrt 2003). The nurse, the patient and the patient's family interact within an increasingly complex healthcare environment. The knowledge and skills required for nursing practice have become progressively more diverse (Pearson 1992). Nursing specialties need practitioners who can function as expert clinicians, role models and leaders, within the context of both the specialty and the broader nursing community. Education programmes designed to prepare nurses for specialist practice need to balance the requirements and standards of the practice setting with the need for an education process that fosters the development of leadership, critical thinking and creativity (Cutcliffe 2003). To this end, educational programmes should aim to achieve a balance between the broader professional and educational needs of the individual and the needs of the practice setting. Emphasis is placed on the learning *process* (i.e. the understanding of how and why; and the broad application of principles) although, in some contexts, *outcomes* may be measured as a means of validating performance standards.

Being an effective facilitator is both a skill and an art. It is a skill in that people can learn certain techniques and can improve their ability with practice. It is an art in that some people just have more of a natural or innate ability for it than others. A good facilitator is concerned with: the outcome of the meeting or planning session; with how the people in the meeting participate and interact; and also with the process. While achieving the goals and outcomes that everyone wants is, of course, important, a facilitator also wants to make sure that the process is sound, that everyone is engaged and that the experience is the best it can be for the participants.

SELECTION OF FRAMEWORK FOR ANALYSING THE CONCEPT

The selection of a concept analysis framework should be contingent upon a variety of factors. The philosophical underpinnings of the approach, the analytical goals, the analytical steps and the practicality of the techniques for furthering understanding of areas of nursing practice all warrant consideration if the approach to be used is to be effective and of benefit to nursing enquiry (Cahill 1996). The methods of concept analysis described by Walker and Avant (1995) and Rodgers (1989) seem to be the two approaches that are most often seen in the nursing literature. Walker and Avant (1995) suggest the use of a step-by-step approach to concept analysis (Box 9.1).

Walker and Avant (1995) report that the basic purpose of their analysis is to distinguish between the defining attributes of a concept and its irrelevant attributes.

Box 9.1
Walker and Avant's
eight-step concept
analysis methodology

- Select a concept
- Aims of analysis
- Identify uses of the concept
- Determine defining attributes
- Develop model case(s)
- Construct additional cases
- Identify antecedents and consequences
- Define empirical referents

Walker & Avant 1995

Furthermore, their rigorous approach also serves the purpose of refining ambiguous concepts, developing operational definitions and clarifying overused, vague concepts that are prevalent in nursing practice. As noted in previous chapters, Walker and Avant's (1995) approach has been subject to heavy criticism because of its linear approach, positivistic nature and oversimplistic procedures (Morse 1995, Morse et al 1996). Nevertheless, given the number of concept analyses published in the nursing literature that have used this method, I have decided to undertake my analysis of facilitation using the approach advocated by Walker and Avant (1995), its limitations notwithstanding. It has been selected because of its structured, systematic approach and in the hope that additional systematic consideration might help reduce any sense of vagueness that might be associated with this particular concept.

STAGE 3: USES OF THE CONCEPT

Once the concept has been selected the process of exploring conceptual meaning can begin. This stage uses multiple sources of 'evidence' (or resources) to generate and refine criteria, which can be used to identify the concept. Walker and Avant (1995) describe how the sources of 'evidence' at this stage in the analysis are dictionary and other forms of definitions, and thesauruses. While such definitions do not give a complete sense of meaning for the concept, they can help to clarify common usage, which is helpful in identifying the scope of subsequent work (Table 9.1).

While these definitions view facilitation as a conscious process to guide and achieve some action, they do not speak to the range or type of 'problem' that facilitation may help address. Furthermore, the definitions are broad and do not specify the different forms that facilitation can take. From the definitions, however, it is clear that one purpose of facilitation is to help individuals and groups learn in order to both solve problems and simultaneously grow and develop. What the facilitator is aiming to do is trying to make individuals or group members more competent, more powerful and more in control of their own destinies. Examples of

Table 9.1
Definitions of the term facilitation from the available literature

Source	Definition
Beckett & Wall 1985	Facilitation is a process to guide another person to meet their needs
Oxford English Dictionary 1994	Facilitation is to make easy, promote, help forward through action or result
Schwarz 1994	Facilitation is to increase ease of performance of any action
Cross 1996	Facilitation is an active, positive process in which change or the movement towards a desired outcome takes place
Burrows 1997	Facilitation is a goal-orientated dynamic process, in which participants work together in an atmosphere of genuine mutual respect, in order to learn through critical reflection
Durgahee 1998	Facilitation involves providing a framework for thinking, feeling and developing insight
Kitson et al 1998	Facilitation is a technique by which one person makes things easier for others

facilitation within nursing include a team learning how each person is perceived by others to improve interpersonal relationships between group members; a training course where learning is focused on developing personal leadership skills and knowledge; and a clinical example would involve a nurse working with a patient, facilitating the patient's deeper and more comprehensive understanding of his/her drug regimen. Beyond these definitions there is little literature which defines the term facilitation. Many studies appear to concentrate more on defining facilitation styles, how to facilitate and why facilitate; see, for example, Heron (1977), King (1984), Burnard (1989) and Bentley (1993).

NURSES' USE OF FACILITATION

In addition to examining definitions to help analyse a concept, Walker and Avant (1995) also suggest that asking a group of people with experience of the concept to define it as another source. Accordingly, 10 registered nurses were asked to attend a focus group in an attempt to determine their understanding of facilitation. The nurses were all at postgraduate level from a mixture of acute, primary care and mental health settings. Seven nurses were NHS-employed practice development nurses and the other three were primary care nurses who co-facilitated the Royal College of Nursing Primary Care Leadership Programme in Northern Ireland. These nurses were selected purposely, as I felt they would have experience of the concept. Summaries of emerging themes from the focus group discussions are listed in Box 9.2.

Box 9.2
Nurses' definition of the concept 'facilitation'

Facilitation:
- is a dynamic process
- encourages critical reflection
- encourages critical thinking
- is a goal-orientated process
- requires an effective facilitator
- creates a climate for members to share their diverse knowledge and experience
- creates a climate of mutual trust, respect and acceptance
- encourages collaborative learning and mutually beneficial relationships
- does not exist to maintain or change the status quo
- is not a short-term solution to conflict
- is a process for negotiation
- is a process to establish understanding between individuals and groups
- is proactive rather than reactive

STAGE 4: DETERMINE CRITICAL ATTRIBUTES

The next step in concept analysis, according to Walker and Avant (1995) is to identify the critical attributes. Jasper (1994) observed that defining attributes are those that must be present for a pure example of the concept to exist, while Walker and Avant (1995) describe defining attributes as those characteristics of a concept that arise again and again. The purpose of identifying the defining attributes of a concept is to provide a basis for its occurrence as a phenomenon as differentiated from another similar or related one. However, it is important to realize that, because it is possible for two people to identify slightly different attributes for the same concept, all findings must be viewed tentatively (Walker & Avant 1995).

A DYNAMIC GOAL-ORIENTATED PROCESS

Focus group members identified facilitation as a proactive rather than a reactive process. This concurs with the *Oxford English Dictionary* (Allen 1994) definition of facilitation as a means of facilitating or moving forwards. Further consensus of this critical attribute is evident within the extant literature. Harvey et al (2002) for example, suggested that, where the primary purpose of facilitation is to achieve set task or goals, the role is largely concerned with providing practical help and support. However, where facilitation is focused more broadly on developing and empowering individuals and teams, there is at least an equal emphasis on the development of a helping (enabling) process or relationship. While the process of facilitation is focused on the other person and their needs and wants, it helps if a structure is used to make sure that the learning takes place.

The key features of the facilitation process include identifying a learning need, setting goals, identifying learning resources, planning and carrying out the facilitation, assessing and evaluating the learning (Townsend 1990). Bee and Bee (1998) view these features as technical processes; the tools and techniques that help the group structure and analyse the problem and formulate a solution. Personal and interpersonal processes are equally important within facilitation. For example, the effective facilitator would be mindful and watchful of how individuals are responding and dealing with a situation and how individuals within a group are reacting with each other and with the facilitator.

Facilitation involves goal investigation, questioning assumptions and thinking outside the usual framework. This includes elements of negotiation to ensure a balance between challenge and support in which individuals assume responsibility for their own learning and the facilitator's role is to question, probe, challenge, encourage, guide and mediate in an environment of mutual trust and cooperation.

GENERAL MUTUAL RESPECT

Facilitation is fundamentally about respect for participants. The *Oxford English Dictionary* (Allen 1994) describes respect as 'to feel or show esteem or regard'. Respect means being able to suspend judgement and giving individuals what Carl Rogers (1969) called unconditional positive regard. It means listening without feeling the need to advise, argue, criticize, persuade or collude; essentially, showing that one accepts individuals all of the time. Focus group members felt strongly that, if facilitation is to be effective, respect must be offered sincerely. Equally, respect must be mutual.

A facilitator must therefore be able to be sensitive and responsive to individuals but similarly to interaction between individuals and the subtleties of group dynamics. It is essential to build trust among the facilitators and the participants to challenge personal assumptions and accept challenges from others.

CRITICAL REFLECTION

A further critical attribute of facilitation is reflection. Critical reflection is often identified as a teaching and learning method that is used in nursing education (Durgahee 1998). In essence, engaging in critical reflection entails a continual questioning of assumptions and actions (Brookfield 1987); for instance Why do I react this way to this particular patient? What is it about dealing with bereavement that makes me feel uncomfortable? Burnard (1989) extended the definition and highlighted that critical reflection also involves seeing other possibilities, intelligently discriminating between choices and options, and identifying new ideas.

Critical reflection then appears to include aspects of questioning and analysing and these are behaviours that the facilitator engages in. Critical reflection, within a process of facilitation, encourages nurses to question their own and other's assumptions, thoughts and attitudes. According to Durgahee (1998), critical reflection within facilitation should enable a professional response or reasoned opinion;

it should inform appropriate judgement of value, truth, empathy; and should enhance appreciation of clinical and interpersonal techniques (Durgahee 1998). The skills of self-evaluation and critical reflection enable growth, enhance significant learning and promote self-direction.

COLLABORATIVE LEARNING

The last critical attribute I have identified for facilitation is collaborative learning. The word 'collaborate' is derived from the Latin *collaborare* which means 'to labour together'. Collaboration is frequently equated with a bond, union or partnership characterized by mutual goals and commitments (Henneman et al 1995). It is non-hierarchical in nature and assumes power based on a knowledge or expertise as opposed to power based on role or function.

Focus group members highlighted the importance of collaboration within the process of facilitation particularly during and after critical reflection sessions. They felt more supported when there was collaboration and were able to share experiences, perspectives, different ways of thinking and working, which maximized their learning. Durgahee (1998) argued that learning is maximized when it is shared, and it is more enriching to have others in the process. It enables comparison and testing of perspectives, which contribute to the process of clarification and analysis, grounding issues in different contexts, encouraging emic learning.

STAGE 5: DEVELOPMENT OF A MODEL CASE

Once the critical attributes have been defined, Walker and Avant (1995) suggest progressing to the formulation of a model case. Rodgers (1989) advocated for the use of a 'real life' example to demonstrate a model case. A model case provides evidence of what the concept definitely is and should include all the critical attributes. Accordingly, the following cases are all derived from 'real' situations and scenarios. In the interests of confidentiality, personal details have been changed.

Case study 1
A model case of facilitation

Four district nursing managers shared an interest in developing a more effective district nursing service for their patients. They felt that district nurses were like sponges, soaking up referrals and were unable to say 'no' to anyone who sent a referral to them. This resulted in high levels of sick leave, low morale and reduced time for professional development. After contacting a nurse facilitator from the Royal College of Nursing a facilitative approach was agreed to take forward this practice development initiative.

Time was spent on building a relationship based on trust, acceptance and acknowledging the value of their differing opinions. The process of facilitation

Case study 1
A model case of
facilitation—*cont'd*

was discussed and there was mutual agreement that the group would be called the referral criteria group, which would involve a collaborative partnership approach where mutual goals and commitments were agreed. The main aim of the group was meet twice a month over a 3-month period to develop referral criteria for district nursing services within their Trust.

Through a critical reflection approach the facilitator encouraged the nurse managers to question their assumptions, thoughts and attitudes. They were then forced to examine their current ways of working and think outside the usual framework, which led to the development of referral criteria and a protocol for referral to the district nursing service. Throughout the process the facilitator encouraged members to question, probe and challenge each other while ensuring that there were high levels of support within an environment of mutual trust and cooperation.

Because of the success of the group it was agreed that it would meet again in 6 months to evaluate the effectiveness of the referral criteria and protocol.

Each of the critical attributes is present in the case above. Goal orientation is established when they decide what they can achieve in the time available. By building a relationship they demonstrate genuine mutual respect for each other. Critical reflection is evident by reviewing current district nursing practice and looking at new ways of working and there is also evidence of collaboration through mutual goals and commitments.

Borderline cases contain only some of the critical attributes of the concept. They may even contain most or all of them but differ substantially in one of them. These cases are inconsistent in some way and as such they help us see why the model case is not (Walker & Avant 1995).

Case study 9.2
Facilitation: a borderline
case

Ann works as a staff nurse on a medical ward. She would like to develop her career and is interested in working as a health visitor. However, because she lacks postregistration educational qualifications and experience working in the community, she is unsure how to make this transition. She makes an appointment to see Laura, a professional nurse facilitator from the Trust she is working in.

When Ann arrives for her appointment, they decide what they will do in the time available. Laura asks Ann some probing questions that enable Ann to recognize some aspects of her career background and a career pathway that best suits her. Ann then asks Laura about some aspects of other career pathways until she is sure which one she will engage in. Time is spent on building a relationship based on trust, acceptance and acknowledging the value of their differing opinions.

Ann discusses her ambitions to become a health visitor based on the information shared with her during their meeting, but Laura does not feel that health visiting would be a suitable career for Ann and encourages her to develop as a Nurse Practitioner, as Laura feels there are more opportunities for career development in this area. Ann accepts that this other specialty of nursing would be in her best interests and agrees to follow that career pathway.

In this example most of the critical attributes of facilitation are met. Goal orientation is established when Ann and Laura decide what they can achieve in the time available and by building a relationship they demonstrate genuine mutual respect for each other. As a facilitator, however, Laura does not encourage Ann to challenge Laura's thoughts and personal assumptions that Ann does not seem suitable to work as a health visitor; therefore the attribute 'critical reflection' has not been met. Ann assumes that this is indeed the case and opts to follow another career pathway.

Walker and Avant (1995) identify that a related case is an instance of a concept that is related to the concept being studied but which, on closer examination, is found to be different.

Case study 9.3
Facilitation: a related case

> John, a senior nurse manager, decides to review the hospital policy on managing patients with aggressive behaviour. To ensure that practice staff take ownership of the policy and to ensure that it is appropriate to practice he decides to facilitate a steering group made up of ward managers. During the first meeting with the steering group John gives a presentation on the current policy and the proposed changes he feels need to be implemented. He also gives the group copies of other related policies, which he has obtained from colleagues who work in other NHS trusts. Following a brief discussion with the group around the current policy, how it links to practice and recommendations for change, John advises the group that he will draft a proposal to the Trust Executive Team outlining his recommendations for changes to the current policy.

This example is more evident of a form of prescriptive teaching or briefing, as opposed to facilitation. John educates the group on the current policy and related policies from other Trusts and informs them of the changes he feels are necessary. He also takes responsibility for drafting the proposal with his recommendations without including the views of the group.

In considering the concept of facilitation it is apparent that there are several concepts that are similar and related to, but not the same as facilitation. That is, they are not in themselves critical attributes nor do they contain all of the defining characteristics of facilitation, for example teaching. Where teaching generally involves the transmission of skills or knowledge, facilitation involves helping the participants discover for themselves.

Walker and Avant (1995) identify that a contrary case illustrates 'what the concept is not'.

Case study 9.5
Facilitation: a contrary case

> Shauna works as a community psychiatric nurse. She receives a referral from Ian's general practitioner asking for Shauna to arrange a programme of anxiety management for Ian. Shauna writes a letter to Ian advising him of her visit. When she arrives she explains that she will visit him for 1 hour each week for a period of 6 weeks during which time she will educate him on the signs and symptoms of anxiety, causes and triggering factors and develop a plan for him to follow when he feels anxious beyond this.

This clearly contains none of the attributes of facilitation; however, it is particularly useful to illustrate 'what facilitation is not'.

STAGE 6: IDENTIFY ANTECEDENTS AND CONSEQUENCES

Once the cases have been identified, the next step is to specify the characteristics present whenever the concept occurs. The identification of antecedents and consequences is an important, although sometimes ignored, step in the analysis of a concept (Unsworth 2000). According to Walker and Avant (1995), antecedents are those events or incidents that must occur prior to the occurrence of the concept, and consequences are those events or incidents that occur as a result of the occurrence of the concept. The antecedents and consequences of the concept of facilitation are listed in Table 9.2.

EMPIRICAL REFERENTS

The final step in the analysis of a concept, using Walker and Avant's (1995) framework, is to determine the empirical referents for the critical attributes. Walker and Avant (1995) declare that empirical referents provide the clinician with clear, observable phenomena with which to diagnose the concept. Empirical referents are measurable, observable or verifiable components of the concept (Goosen 1989). Walker and Avant (1995) recognize that empirical referents and critical defining attributes may be identical and therefore critical defining attributes, previously identified, must be sought in practice.

Owing to the multifactorial nature and complexity of facilitation the empirical referents are difficult to define. Suanmali (1981) and Conti (1985) offer instruments in the measurement of effective facilitation. Burrows (1997), however, has identified that on close examination these tools contain ambiguous and vague

Table 9.2
Antecedents and consequences

Antecedents	Consequences
A facilitator and one or more people	Self-discovery
Goal orientation towards learning	Evaluation of attitudinal differences
Skilled, knowledgeable and self-aware facilitator	Self-development
Open, non-threatening environment	Learning
Commitment from all participants	Enhanced decision-making
Understanding of the process from all participants	Participants more personally responsible for learning
Collaboration	Enriched quality of life
Reciprocity in the facilitator–participant relationship	

terms and it is difficult to ascertain precisely what behaviours would be looked for. Testing the extent to which facilitation occurs within nurse education would be best done by systematic observation of a sample of interactions between the facilitator and the participant. An observer could note, for example, whether an attempt was made to demonstrate genuine mutual respect and critical reflection. However, this would be a subjective measure of the presence of the concept, as it would depend on the observer's perceptions and, as such, would not be the most reliable measure. Therefore, there appears to be a need for the development of a highly reliable, effective facilitation measurement tool.

CONCLUSION

While the term 'facilitation' has been widely used within nurse education, the concept, nature and scope of facilitation remain poorly articulated. If nurse educators are going to participate in facilitation then they would benefit from some firmer conceptual 'foundations' from which to work. Much of the literature on facilitation is based upon the work of Heron (1977), Brookfield (1986) and Townsend (1990). Beyond this, the majority of studies appear to concentrate more on defining facilitation styles, how to facilitate and why facilitate.

With the introduction of clinical governance, it is likely that facilitation will become more central to the work of NHS organizations in the near future (Royal College of Nursing 1998). Therefore, it is likely that there will be additional opportunities in the future, as well as those existing at the moment, where an effective facilitator would benefit our discipline. Through careful analysis, the critical defining attributes of the concept of facilitation have been identified and explored, leading to a more thorough understanding of facilitation. Finally, with regard to the concept analysis approach employed, Walker and Avant's (1995) tool provided a useful guide for the systematic analysis of the concept and provided clear guidelines for carrying out certain stages of the analysis.

According to Walker and Avant (1995) concept synthesis is one of the most exciting ways of beginning theory building. It is based on observation, qualitative or quantitative evidence, literature or some combination of these. Therefore, if we apply this to facilitation it could be tentatively defined as:

... a dynamic, goal orientated process in which participants collaboratively learn through critical reflection within an atmosphere of genuine mutual respect.

REFERENCES

Allen RE 1994 The pocket Oxford dictionary of current English. Clarendon Press, Oxford

Beckett C, Wall M 1985 Role of the clinical facilitator. Nurse Education Today 5: 259–262

Bee F, Bee R 1998 Facilitation skills. Institute of Personnel Development, London

Bentley T 1993 Facilitation: providing opportunities for learning. McGraw-Hill, Maidenhead

Brookfield SD 1986 Understanding and facilitating adult learning. Open University Press, Milton Keynes

Brookfield SD 1987 Developing critical thinkers: challenging adults to explore alternative ways of thinking and acting. Open University Press, Milton Keynes

Brookfield SD 1999 Discussion as a way of teaching: tools and techniques for University teachers. Open University Press, Buckingham

Burnard P 1989 Teaching interpersonal skills: a handbook of experiential learning for health professionals. Chapman & Hall, London

Burrows DE 1997 Facilitation: a concept analysis. Journal of Advanced Nursing 25(2): 396–404

Cahill J 1996 Patient participation: a concept analysis. Journal of Advanced Nursing 24: 561–571

Chinn PL, Kramer MK 1995 Theory and nursing: a systematic approach, 4th edn. Mosby/Yearbook, St Louis, MO

Conti GJ 1985 Assessing teaching style in adult education: how and why. Lifelong learning: the adult years, vol 8, part 8, pp. 7–11, 28

Cross K 1996 An analysis of the concept of facilitation. Nurse Education Today 16: 158–164

Cutcliffe JR 2003 A historical overview of psychiatric/mental health nurse education in the United Kingdom: going round in circles or on the straight and narrow? Nurse Education Today 23: 338–346

Dooher J, Byrt R 2003 Empowerment: and the health service user. Quay Books, Dinton, Salisbury

Durgahee T 1998 Facilitating reflection: from a sage on stage to a guide on the side. Nurse Education Today 18: 158–164

Goosen GM 1989 Concept analysis: an approach to teaching physiologic variables. Journal of Professional Nursing 5: 31–38

Harvey G, Loftus-Hills A, Rycroft-Malone J 2002 Getting the evidence into practice: the role and function of facilitation. Journal of Advanced Nursing 37: 577–588

Henneman EA, Lee JL, Cohen JI 1995 Collaboration: a concept analysis. Journal of Advanced Nursing 21: 103–109

Heron J 1977 Dimensions of facilitator style. University of Surrey, Guildford

Jasper MA 1994 Expert: a discussion of the implications of the concept as used in nursing. Journal of Advanced Nursing 20: 769–776

King EC 1984 Affective education in nursing. A guide to teaching and assessment. Aspen Systems Corporation, Rockville, MD

Kitson A, Harvey G, McCormack B 1998 Enabling the implementation of evidence-based practice: a conceptual framework. Quality in Health Care 7: 152

McGregor H 1961 The human side of enterprise. McGraw-Hill, Maidenhead

McKenna H 1997 Theory and research: a linkage to benefit practice. International Journal of Nursing Studies 34: 431–437

Morse JM 1995 Exploring the theoretical basis of nursing using advanced techniques of concept analysis. Advances in Nursing Science 17: 31–46

Morse JM, Mitcham C, Hupcey JE et al 1996 Criteria for concept evaluation. Journal of Advanced Nursing 24: 385–390

Pearson A 1992 Knowing nursing: emerging paradigms in nursing. In: Robinson K, Vaughan B (ed) Knowledge for nursing practice. Butterworth Heinemann, London, pp. 213–226

Rodgers BL 1989 Concepts, analysis and the development of nursing knowledge: the evolutionary cycle. Journal of Advanced Nursing 14: 330–335

Rogers C 1969 Freedom to learn. Merrill Publishing, Columbus, OH

Rogers C 1983 Freedom to learn for the 80s. Bell and Howell Columbus as cited in Burrows DE 1997 Facilitation: a concept analysis. Journal of Advanced Nursing 25(2): 396–404

Royal College of Nursing 1998 Guidance for nurses on clinical governance. RCN, London

Schwarz R 1994 The skilled facilitator. Jossey-Bass, San Francisco, CA

Suanmali C 1981 The core concepts of andragogy. Unpublished doctoral dissertation, Department of Higher and Adult Education, Teachers College, Columbia University

Townsend J 1990 Teaching/learning strategies. Nursing Times 86(23): 66–68

Walker LO, Avant KC 1995 Strategies for theory construction in nursing, 3rd edn. Appleton & Lange, Norwalk, CT

Watson SJ 1991 An analysis of the concept of experience. Journal of Advanced Nursing 16: 1117–1121

United Kingdom Central Council for Nurses, Midwives and Health Visitors 1986 Project 2000: a new preparation for practice. UKCC, London

Unsworth J 2000 Practice development: a concept analysis. Journal of Nursing Management 8: 317–326

Delineating the concept of fatigue using a pragmatic utility approach

Karin Olson and Janice M. Morse

EDITORIAL

The chances are that any nurse who has ever worked repeated shifts on a busy unit will have an experiential familiarity with the concept of fatigue. Furthermore, the likelihood of having encountered a fatigued patient is high. Fatigue can be an insidious and pervasive concept and, as Karin and Jan's chapter reminds us, nurses clearly need to be vigilant for signs of fatigue developing in patients. However, within a healthcare context, it is not only patients who can suffer from fatigue.

There appears to be a high level of consensus that fatigue can be an issue for healthcare practitioners. In addition to the literature covered in this chapter, there is a well-established literature on the problems of fatigue in 'junior' doctors (perhaps more so in the UK) and an associated debate *vis-à-vis* the number of hours junior doctors should work. This literature shows how 'performance' (i.e. the practitioner's clinical performance) is, not surprisingly, affected by fatigue. Thought processes slow down, problem-solving ability is impaired and concentration is more difficult. These are just a few of the well-documented problems resulting from fatigue in practitioners. Interestingly, there is a much less substantial literature on fatigue in nurses than there is for junior doctors, and also interestingly, there is a parallel literature that argues in *favour* of longer hours and extended shifts for nurses.

Perhaps this debate is exemplified by the discussion around the issue of 8- or 12-hour shifts for nurses (and that is not to exclude alternative models such as the case for 9-hour shifts.) In simplistic terms, those in favour of 8-hour shifts appear to point to the evidence regarding the lower frequency of mistakes and higher quality of care that often results from 8-hour shifts. Those in favour of longer (12-hour) shifts point to the evidence that indicates higher levels of satisfaction in nurses and sometimes in patients. While the editors would not presume to have the answer to this debate, what we would advocate is that additional support mechanisms should be ensured for those nurses who work longer shifts. Given the well-documented evidence of the relationship between fatigue and quality of care (incidence of mistakes, etc.) thought must be given to how these nurses can avoid (or minimize) their own experiences of fatigue.

INTRODUCTION

It was a dark and stormy afternoon during the winter of 1995 in northern Alberta. My colleague, a nurse in the outpatient gastrointestinal cancer clinic, was normally an 'upbeat' person despite the challenges of her clinical work, but not today. Upon my inquiry she noted that subsets of her patients were somehow unable to manage the tremendous fatigue that accompanied their treatments and were withdrawing from protocols that had the potential to offer them increased survival with good quality of life. This was not the experience of all the patients, but she was unable to identify the factors that distinguished those who managed fatigue from those who did not. She wanted to understand fatigue better so that she could provide appropriate nursing interventions. Informal discussions with other nursing colleagues led to the realization that others had noted profound fatigue in some of their patients as well. Together, we decided to review the related research literature.

We noted a growing number of nursing studies about cancer-related fatigue (CRF). Table 10.1 shows conceptualizations that were available at that time (1996), plus several that have been published since then. The literature review became a springboard for a systematic evaluation of fatigue as a concept using the approach outlined by Morse et al (1996). This analysis showed that the existing conceptual definitions were incongruent; each one seemed to explain only part of what we saw in our clinical practice. We had patients with advanced disease and low haemoglobin levels who reported no fatigue and patients with similar disease and treatment profiles and normal haemoglobin levels who reported marked fatigue. Some patients reported profound fatigue after a single treatment while others completed their whole chemotherapy series without reporting fatigue.

While the existing definitions within the reviewed literature fit the clinical settings in which these definitions were developed, colleagues working on the concept

Table 10.1 Seven conceptual frameworks for cancer-related fatigue

Model/First author	Antecedents	Attributes	Manifestations	Consequences	Definition
Integrated Fatigue Model (Piper 1986, Piper et al 1987)	Alterations in physiological and psychological processes	Decline in cognitive and muscular functioning, alertness, and motivation	Decreased physical and mental performance, tired, need more sleep, lack vigour, feel weak, decreased energy, decreased stamina and motivation, increased irritability eyestrain, headache	Acute fatigue is protective. Chronic fatigue may lead to aversion to activity with a desire to escape	In contrast to tiredness, subjective fatigue is a whole-body tiredness, disproportionate to exertion, influenced by circadian rhythm and variable in unpleasantness, duration and intensity
Organizing Framework (Alistars 1987)	Physical and psychosocial stressors due to cancer and treatment				
Energy Analysis Model (Irvine et al 1994)	Energy deficits arising from fall in energy supplies or rise in energy demand	Decline in muscular function, increased emotional lability	Increased symptom distress and mood disturbance	Decreased weight is a consequence of disrupted energy transformation and reduced functional status	A subjective experience of weariness, tiredness or lack of energy that varies in degree, frequency, duration
Psychobiological–Entropy Model (Winningham 1996)	An imbalance between activity and rest caused by cancer, its treatment and/or related symptoms	Decline in muscular function	In contrast to weakness, individuals say they are 'unable' to do certain things (voluntary component)	Decreased activity followed by decreased functional status	A feeling state that has an impact on the individual's perception of his or her ability to engage in usual activities. May be relieved by rest (acute) or persists over time (chronic)

Continued

Table 10.1 Seven conceptual frameworks for cancer-related fatigue—cont'd

Model/First author	Antecedents	Attributes	Manifestations	Consequences	Definition
Ream and Richardson Model (Ream & Richardson 1996)	Pathological or psychological condition that can be perceived and evaluated by a cognitively aware person	Whole body unpleasant feeling including physical, cognitive, and emotional dimensions	Irritability, impaired thought processes, inability to cope, poor motivation, family conflict	Reduced quality of life	A subjective unpleasant, unrelenting symptom incorporating total body, range from tiredness to exhaustion, interferes with ability to function
Glaus Model (Glaus 1998)	Stressors associated with disease and treatment	Physical, cognitive and affective changes	Unpleasant weakness, decreased ability, increased tiredness, need for sleep and rest	Reduced quality of life	Fatigue is a stress response, complicated by the linguistic and cultural context in which it occurs
Magnusson model (Magnusson et al 1999)			Loss of energy, strength, control, condition, pace, initiative ability, coordination, well-being, sociability	Social limitations, reduced self-esteem, reduced quality of life	

evaluation project suspected that the definitions were too context-based to fit fatigue as manifested in our oncology setting. In addition, however, we suspected that efforts to add specificity regarding the nature of fatigue had inadvertently shifted the conceptual boundaries to the point that definitions now included significant elements of allied concepts such as boredom, tiredness and exhaustion (Olson et al 2002). Normally, one might expect the addition of specificity to tighten a conceptual definition but in this case, probably owing to the close proximity of the related concepts, the conceptual boundaries became less clear. To address these concerns, our concept evaluation group decided to seek a conceptual definition that was sufficiently abstract to be generalizable to instances of fatigue across both ill and non-ill contexts and thus one that would show the essential characteristics of fatigue.

Concepts are abstract but, when they are developed close to a context, it is difficult to remove the characteristics that make it particular to that context and to see the essential nature of the concept. Morse calls concepts developed close to the context 'low level' concepts (personal communication 2003). We hypothesized that, by comparing and contrasting the same concept in different contexts, the 'noise' or characteristics particular to individual contexts could be identified and removed, leaving the concept in its purest form, and that, when we recontextualized the concept, it would fit our clinical setting. However, the risk of high-level abstraction is that the concept may be so 'pure' that it seems superficial and elementary, lacking sufficient information to be of use in clinical practice (Morse et al 1996).

Morse developed an approach – pragmatic utility – that facilitates the decontextualization – recontextualization process. This approach was ideal for our analysis of fatigue because it provided an opportunity to remove concepts from the contexts in which they were initially identified (decontextualization) and identify the attributes of the fatigue that were common across contexts. We are currently conducting a series of studies using ethnoscience to track the manifestations of those attributes back into the contexts of interest (recontextualization). Decontextualization begins with a critical appraisal of the literature, tracing the development of fatigue across contexts, the ways it has been used in published studies, and the assumptions that underlie existing research. Assessment of pragmatic utility is organized around the following guiding principles: clarity regarding the purpose of the inquiry, assurance of validity, identification of analytic questions and synthesis of findings (Morse 2000). Thus theorists who take this approach are in a position to comment on the logical coherence of a concept and are in stronger position to recontextualize it. In this chapter, the principles of pragmatic utility are used to compare fatigue as a concept across five contexts.

CLARITY REGARDING PURPOSE OF THE INQUIRY

As with many concepts in nursing, the use of fatigue in both 'everyday' language and as a scientific concept contributes to confusion regarding its meaning. In order to ensure that we would capture the fullest 'everyday' meaning of fatigue, we reviewed a series of transcripts from our previous study of fatigue in individuals with advanced cancer (Olson et al 2002) and identified words and phrases used to talk about fatigue. As can be seen in Figure 10.1, the overlaps in the definition of these words and phrases are significant but not completely congruent. Thus, it was unclear whether these words and phrases were synonyms or were concepts representing distinct but related clusters of behaviours. To help us clarify this point, we used the words and phrases in Figure 10.1 as keywords in our searches of electronic databases.

ENSURING VALIDITY

Fatigue occurs in many contexts in addition to cancer. Similarly, there are many aspects to the experience of cancer that are distinct from fatigue. We reasoned that, by searching the published literature for descriptions of fatigue across populations in which it was well recognized, we could isolate the unique set of attributes that were common across these populations, but could also possibly outline variations in the manifestation of fatigue across populations. Thus, in addition to examining the 'fatigue'-related literature that emanates from the substantive area of cancer care, we also examined four other populations in which fatigue was commonly understood to be a prominent component. Chronic fatigue syndrome (CFS) and

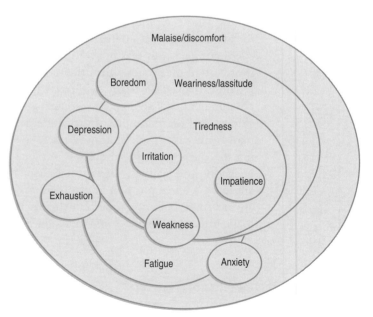

Figure 10.1 Keywords in searches of electronic databases

depression represented fatigue related to illness, shift workers were chosen to represent work-related fatigue and athletes were selected to represent fatigue related to a leisure activity.

These populations were selected because a brief examination in these substantive areas showed that there was sufficient literature available and the populations also had some unique features that would permit the development of highly informative analytic questions. CFS was selected because, although there are many theories about its antecedents, the aetiology of CFS remains unclear and the diagnostic process may take many months. Similar to the diagnostic experience of many individuals with advanced cancer, by the time a diagnosis is made the degree of disability is profound and the long-term adverse consequence on quality of life are significant. We reasoned, therefore, that the manifestation of fatigue in CFS would be similar to that of cancer patients.

Individuals diagnosed with a major depressive disorder were selected because, in the experience of my clinical colleagues, the manifestations of depression and fatigue are sufficiently similar that one is often mistaken for the other. We hypothesized that by examining the manifestations of depression more carefully, we could identify important clinical differences between depression and fatigue. Shift workers were chosen because their fatigue is primarily attributable to sleep disruption, a common antecedent of fatigue in cancer patients. We hypothesized, however, that, since shift workers are essentially healthy and therefore more able to adapt to sleep disruption, their fatigue would be manifested differently from that in cancer patients, despite common attributes. Athletes were included because their fatigue is primarily due to physical exertion, also a common antecedent of fatigue in cancer patients. We expected to find the same attributes described by cancer patients but hypothesized that, since fatigue is an element of a training program, viewed positively and 'chosen' since it is an essential precursor to improved performance, the manifestation of fatigue in athletes would be different.

The terms in Figure 10.1 were used as key words to search relevant databases for the five study populations (CINAHL, Medline, PubMed, Psych INFO, SPORT discus, and CancerLit) for 1995–2001. Abstracts were searched to identify articles that discussed the conceptual nature of fatigue in shift workers, athletes and individuals diagnosed with CFS, cancer or depression. All identified papers were reviewed and indexed using Procite bibliographic software. The reference lists of these papers were also reviewed to identify key papers and books, particularly those that may have been published prior to 1995. Six domains of fatigue – muscular changes, cognitive changes, sleep disruption, emotional changes, changes in body sensation and social disruption – were consistently identified across all five study populations. Our database currently includes over 1000 references. Table 10.2 shows authors who identified significant variations in manifestations of fatigue by population, stratified by these domains, and concludes with the attributes of fatigue common across the study populations.

Table 10.2 Domain for identifying attributes of fatigue across five populations

Domains	Shift work	Cancer	CFS	Athletes	Depression	Common Attributes
Muscular changes	Deterioration in physical performance following night work in older (34+ years) workers (de Zwardt et al 1993)	Deterioration of physical ability (Alistars 1987), weakness and muscle atrophy (Blesch et al 1991, Nail & Winningham 1993, Baracos et al 1994, Winningham et al 1994, Messias et al 1997, Ream & Richardson 1997, Berger 1998, Woo et al 1998, Stone et al 1999, Schwartz 2000), interferes with self care (Rhodes et al 1988)	Weakness (Bates et al 1994, MacDonald et al 1996, Wright & Beverley 1998, Mullis et al 1999), heavy limbs, loss of coordination (Fry & Martin 1996, Fisher 1997, Lloyd 1998, Nisembaum et al 1998, Lovell 1999)	Muscle fatigue (Costill et al 1988, Sahlin et al 1998), impaired performance/ metabolic fatigue (MacKinnon 1996, Green 1997), performance affected by changes in circadian rhythm (Manfredini et al 1998) sore and stiff muscles (Jurrell 1998), respiratory muscle fatigue (Nava et al 1992), chronic muscle strains, tendinitis, tissue fatigue (Welsh & Woodhouse 1992)	Slowness of movement (Wool 1990)	Decline in speed, coordination and strength out of proportion to energy expenditure
Cognitive changes	Deterioration in mental performance (de Zwardt et al 1993), performance lapses and errors (Wool 1990, Welsh & Woodhouse 1992), decreased alertness (Akerstedt 1995),	Decline in capacity for attention and concentration (Cimprich 1993, Winningham et al 1994, Mitler et al 1997, Berger 1998, Broeckel et al 1998, Dumont 1999, Hann et al 2000), problems with reasoning (Alistars 1987)	Difficulty with concentration, attention, memory (Berrios 1990, Ray et al 1992, Fry & Martin 1996, MacDonald et al 1996, Fisher 1997, Buchwald et al 1998, Lloyd 1998, Nisembaum et al 1998, Saltzstein et al 1998, Stone et al 1998, Lovell 1999)	Jet lag affects memory recall among athletes, thus affecting performance (Manfredini et al 1998)	Problems with thinking, reasoning (Davidson et al 1982, Shepherd & Lees 1992, Depression Guideline Panel 1994, Klein et al 1996, Vercoulen et al 1997)	Decline in thinking ability

	decreased concentration (Gillberg et al 1994)					Decline in sleep quality
Sleep disruption	Shorter-stage (Piper et al 1987) and REM sleep (Mitler et al 1997), reduced sleep quality (Sluiter et al 1999), reduced sleep length (Tepas & Carvalhais 1990)	Significant sleep disturbance (Engstrom et al 1999, Miaskowski & Lee 1999), disturbed activity and sleep patterns (Irvine et al 1994, Hoskins 1997, Berger 1998, Broeckel et al 1998, Berger & Farr 1999) poor sleep quality (Hann et al 2000)	Initial insomnia followed by hypersomnia or insomnia (Tiersky et al 1997)	Disturbed sleeping pattern (Kindermann 1986)	Initial insomnia; some individuals may become hypersomniac (Koenig et al 1993)	
Emotional changes	Emotional exhaustion, (Sluiter et al 1999), depression, anxiety (Tepas & Carvalhais 1990, Scott et al 1998, Scott 2000, Ferrell et al 1996)	Feel low, decreased self esteem, (Schwartz 2000) feel useless (Ferrell et al 1996)	Emotional lability, (Fisher 1997) depressed mood, (Koenig et al 1993) worthless, guilty, thoughts of death (Manu et al 1989)	Irritable, excitable, emotional lability, (Kuipers & Keizer 1988) mood disturbance (Morgan et al 1988, MacKinnon 1996, Naessens et al 2000)	Sense of hopelessness, helplessness (Koenig et al 1993)	Increased emotional fragility

Continued

Table 10.2 Domain for identifying attributes of fatigue across five populations—cont'd

Domains	Shift work	Cancer	CFS	Athletes	Depression	Common Attributes
Changes in bodily sensation	Cold (Akerstedt 1995), heavy eyelids, difficulty keeping eyes open (Gillberg et al 1994), sleepy at work	Weary (Irvine 1994) legs like spaghetti, run out of steam quickly (Nail & Winningham 1993), feeling drained (Ream & Richardson 1997), bone tired (Ferrell et al 1996)	Visual loss, paresthesias (Komaroff & Buchwald 1998)	Fatigue at rest (Naessens et al 2000), frequent infections (Hendrickson & Verde 1994)	Decreased energy, decreased appetite, (Buckwalter & Babich 1990) decreased stamina (Berrios 1990)	Decreased control over body processes
Social disruption	Disrupted family and social life (Walker 1985, Scott 2000)	Loss of social, family and work roles (Pearce & Richardson 1996)	Reduced interaction with others (Ray et al 1992, Fisher 1997)	Loss of desire to compete (Costill et al 1988, Kuipers & Keizer 1988)	Loss of sexual interest (Casper et al 1985), social withdrawal (Davidson et al 1982, Koenig 1993, McEnany et al 1996)	Diminished social network

IDENTIFYING SIGNIFICANT ANALYTIC QUESTIONS

The following analytical questions evolved from our reading of the literature outlined in Table 10.2 and guided our critical analysis of it:

- Are tiredness and exhaustion manifestations of fatigue or are they distinct concepts, representing clusters of behaviours that serve different purposes?
- What is the role of adaptation in tiredness, fatigue and exhaustion?
- Are there any 'early' signs that distinguish tiredness, fatigue and exhaustion?

SYNTHESIS OF RESULTS

FATIGUE IN SHIFT WORKERS AND ATHLETES

A comparison of the literature pertaining to shift workers and athletes suggests that in both populations fatigue results when individuals are not able to adapt. Shift workers must adapt to lack of sleep and decreased sleep quality (Tepas & Carvalhais 1990, Akerstedt 1995, Sluiter et al 1999). A basic principle of athletic training is that correct training facilitates adaptation toward one's maximum potential (Hoffman 2002, Bompa 1999). Adaptation follows rest in both populations. For shift workers, failure to adapt results in the inability to stay awake at work. Athletes who fail to adapt become unable to perform at the level to which they are normally capable. Table 10.2 documents the attributes of incomplete adaptation in these populations.

In both shift workers and athletes, there appear to be at least two distinct states – one associated with complete adaptation and one associated with incomplete adaptation. Bartley and Chute (1947), early investigators of work-related fatigue, argued that symptoms relieved by rest were not attributable to fatigue but to some other phenomenon – they proposed boredom. In the nursing fatigue literature, this state is called acute fatigue. In the clinical setting, patients refer to this state by saying they are tired. For the remainder of this chapter, we have labelled this state *tiredness*. Many authors have noted that the sensations associated with tiredness are protective mechanisms, similar to those associated with acute pain, intended both to serve as a signalling system that energy resources are low and to slow energy expenditure while adaptation is still relatively simple to accomplish.

The sensations associated with lack of adaptation, on the other hand, serve a different purpose: they indicate that significant energy resources have been expended, that adaptation is no longer easily attainable and that further energy expenditure must be halted to prevent complete collapse. The shift worker literature overflows with descriptions of 'trying to stay awake' and 'heavy eyelids'. Similarly, athletes 'try to keep going'. For the remainder of this chapter, we have labelled this state *fatigue*. Bartlett (1953) noted that, since the sensations associated with fatigue are the result of excessive energy expenditure, they arrive too late to be of any practical value as 'early warning signs'.

Both the shift worker literature and the athlete literature implied a third state beyond fatigue. Several authors discussed involuntary sleep while at work (Akerstedt 1995, Sluiter et al 1999) and there is a growing body of literature on athletes describing overtraining syndrome. Overtraining syndrome is associated with indicators over which the athlete has no control such as increased resting heart rate and a delayed return of the heart rate to normal levels following exercise (Kuipers & Keizer 1988). For the remainder of this chapter, we have labelled this state *exhaustion*. The primary difference between fatigue and exhaustion is related to control. Individuals who experience fatigue are able to 'keep going'; those who experience exhaustion are not.

FATIGUE IN CANCER, DEPRESSION AND CHRONIC FATIGUE SYNDROME

Individuals diagnosed with cancer, depression or CFS bring unique challenges to the adaptation process that are associated with their illnesses. Regardless of which aetiological hypothesis of cancer-related fatigue one supports, it is clear that the adaptation processes upon which individuals have relied at other challenging times are altered. In the midst of managing a life-threatening illness, one would want to access all the coping skills one had managed to acquire. The signs and symptoms associated with cancer and its treatment, however, interfere with that process. The manifestations of cancer-related fatigue shown in Table 10.2 show the magnitude of this interference. All these manifestations alter the ability of an individual with cancer to adapt.

The literature on CFS is filled with manifestations of the challenges individuals with CFS bring to the adaptation process. Given the length of time required for the diagnostic process – often at least 6 months – the severity of the manifestations increases significantly before treatments become available. The similarities between the manifestations of fatigue in cancer and CFS are striking. Although depression is often a co-morbidity for a significant group of individuals with CFS, Moss-Morris and Petrie (2001) identified unique cognitive styles characteristic of depression and CFS. This is further supported by the work of van der Linden et al (1999), who document the existence of a 'pure' fatigue that either resolved or evolved into a psychiatric disorder within 6 months. Individuals diagnosed with depression experience cognitive and sleep alterations similar to those reported by individuals with cancer or CFS, but a sense of hopelessness and helplessness distinguishes them from non-depressed individuals with cancer or CFS. The primary change in their muscular function is related to decreased speed, consistent with the expected neurovegetative characteristics of depression, rather than muscle weakness, atrophy or loss as seen in cancer and CFS.

Unlike the literature on athletes and shift workers, the literature on cancer, depression and CFS is less clear about the existence of the three distinct states previously labelled as tiredness, fatigue and exhaustion. Our group described one behavioural pattern (Gliders) that characterized individuals who reported tiredness and three behavioural patterns (Boredom, Disorganized and Over-exerters) used by individuals who reported fatigue (Olson et al 2002). In retrospect, we think that the Over-exerter pattern probably represents exhaustion, since it is character-ized by overestimating the amount of available energy. The Disorganized pattern appears to represent fatigue and the Boredom pattern represents an incomplete response to tiredness that will eventually evolve into a Disorganized pattern.

Given the similarities in the fatigue manifestations of individuals with cancer and those with CFS, the behavioural patterns for tiredness, fatigue and exhaustion developed for the cancer population may fit the CFS population as well, but this needs to be established in future studies. Berrios (1990) described three distinct states in fatigue related to depression that ranged from normal fatigue after work to feelings of decreased stamina and finally to feelings of unexplained fatigue. Our current study of individuals diagnosed with a major depressive disorder will show the extent to which all three states (tiredness, fatigue and exhaustion) are indeed present among depressed individuals.

ANALYTIC QUESTIONS

ANALYTIC QUESTION 1: ARE TIREDNESS AND EXHAUSTION MANIFESTATIONS OF FATIGUE OR ARE THEY DISTINCT CONCEPTS, REPRESENTING CLUSTERS OF BEHAVIOURS THAT SERVE DIFFERENT PURPOSES?

This analysis provides some support for the existence of tiredness and exhaustion as distinct concepts separate from but closely related to fatigue through adaptation; each serves a distinct purpose. Tiredness, fatigue and exhaustion all occur in response to stressors, are characterized by changes in sensation, decline in muscular and cog-nitive function, increased emotional lability and sleep disruption, and result in social withdrawal. **Tiredness, fatigue and exhaustion can be distinguished from each other, however, by the rate of onset and recovery and the perceived relationship to energy expenditure** (Table 10.3). Tiredness occurs gradually and, as expected, following work or exercise, and recovery takes place, as expected, following rest.

Fatigue also occurs gradually but sooner than expected, given the amount of energy expended, and recovery takes longer than expected. The unexpectedness of fatigue triggers anxiety, a distinctly different emotional response from the irritabil-ity and impatience associated with tiredness. Fatigue and exhaustion both occur sooner than expected, given the energy expended, and recovery takes longer than

Table 10.3
Distinguishing characteristics of tiredness, fatigue and exhaustion

	Tiredness	Fatigue	Exhaustion
Rate of onset and recovery	Gradual	Gradual	Sudden
Perceived relationship to energy expenditure	Consistent with energy expenditure	Out of proportion to energy expenditure	Energy expenditure not possible

expected. In contrast to fatigue, which occurs gradually, exhaustion occurs suddenly without any perceptible antecedent.

ANALYTIC QUESTION 2: WHAT IS THE ROLE OF ADAPTATION IN TIREDNESS, FATIGUE AND EXHAUSTION?

Our analysis of the literature outlined in Table 10.2 has given rise to the following proposed relationships between tiredness, fatigue and exhaustion in the context of adaptation:

- *Tiredness* is a precondition for fatigue. It occurs in proportion to the amount of energy expended and develops over time. Two outcomes of tiredness are possible – complete adaptation and non-adaptation. Individuals who adapt to tiredness return to a 'normal' state where they no longer 'feel tired'. Some authors have labelled tiredness 'acute fatigue'. Individuals who are unable to adapt to tiredness progress to fatigue.
- *Fatigue* results from the inability to adapt to tiredness. It is out of proportion to the amount of energy expended. It develops over time but is reported sooner than expected, indicating a loss of stamina. Some authors have labelled fatigue 'chronic fatigue'. Two outcomes of fatigue are possible – complete adaptation and non-adaptation. Adaptation to fatigue takes longer than adaptation to tiredness. During the adaptation process, individuals may report the manifestations of tiredness. If adaptation is complete, these individuals return to a normal state in which they no longer feel tired. If adaptation is incomplete, they may remain tired or return to fatigue. Fatigued individuals unable to adapt progress to exhaustion.
- *Exhaustion* is an undesirable outcome of fatigue. It can be distinguished from fatigue by its rapid onset and, frequently, the absence of any identifiable energy expenditure ('but I didn't do anything'). Recovery from exhaustion is slower than the recovery from fatigue. During the recovery process individuals may report manifestations of fatigue and eventually tiredness, before returning to a normal state.

Previous discussions of fatigue have not discussed adaptation in any detail nor addressed its role as a process that links tiredness, fatigue and exhaustion. The above hypotheses provide a possible explanation for our clinical observation regarding the wide variation in fatigue among patients with similar disease and treatment processes – some were able to adapt while others were not. In a previous study, we labelled individuals who experienced tiredness but who were able to adapt as 'Gliders' (Olson et al 2002). Three groups of individuals demonstrated non-adaptive patterns in that study; those in the 'Disorganized' pattern demonstrated behaviours that we now recognized as fatigue while those in the 'Overexertion' pattern demonstrated behaviours that we now have labelled exhaustion. The third non-adaptive pattern, 'Bored', is one that we believe could lead to fatigue, at least in the context of cancer.

ANALYTIC QUESTION 3: ARE THERE ANY 'EARLY' SIGNS THAT DISTINGUISH TIREDNESS, FATIGUE AND EXHAUSTION?

The manifestations of fatigue and exhaustion arrive too late to be of any value as early warning signs of an overexpenditure of energy. Teaching individuals to be more aware of the manifestations of tiredness, however, may aid in protection from fatigue and exhaustion. Thus, we are currently using ethnoscientific methods to identify the attributes of tiredness and exhaustion, to refine the attributes of fatigue and to identify the manifestations of tiredness, fatigue and exhaustion in the five populations identified above. Linking the attributes and manifestations of these three concepts will help us begin to recontextualize them. Future studies to identify physiological markers of the manifestations of tiredness, fatigue and exhaustion are being planned, further facilitating the recontexualization process. By focusing on the refinement of the manifestations of tiredness, fatigue and exhaustion and related physiological indicators, we hope to identify 'early warning signs' useful in protection from fatigue and exhaustion. Our objective is to detect fatigue potential as early as possible so that strategies supporting adaptation can be implemented.

A NEW CONCEPTUALIZATION OF FATIGUE

In this chapter, we have used the principles of pragmatic utility to further delineate the concept of fatigue. The cross-contextual analysis presented in this chapter made it possible to strip away more of the contextual 'noise', facilitating the identification of two new attributes of fatigue not previously identified – declining control over body processes and emotional fragility. Our group's current working definition of fatigue, consistent with the hypotheses outlined above in the response to Analytic Question 2, is that fatigue is a marker for incomplete adaptation to stressors. The stressors are unique to the context in which they occur. Viewed from the perspective of stress theory (Cannon 1920, Selye 1952, 1956, 1971), fatigue occurs during the resistance phase of the general adaptation syndrome. We are still some way from having an answer for our cancer nursing colleagues about the most appropriate nursing interventions for managing fatigue, but we are getting closer.

REFERENCES

Akerstedt T 1995 Work hours sleepiness and the underlying mechanisms. Journal of Sleep Research 4(Suppl. 2): 15–22

Alistars J 1987 Fatigue in the cancer patient: a conceptual approach to a clinical problem. Oncology Nursing Forum 14: 25–30

Baracos V, Urtasun R, Humen D et al 1994 Physical fitness of patients with small cell lung cancer. Clinical Journal of Sport Medicine 4: 223–227

Bartlett F 1953 Psychological criteria of fatigue. In: Floyd W, Welford A (eds) Symposium on fatigue. HK Lewis, London, pp. 1–5

Bartley S, Chute E 1947 Fatigue and impairment in man. McGraw Hill, New York

Bates D, Buchwald D, Lee J et al 1994 A comparison of case definitions of chronic fatigue syndrome. Clinical Infectious Diseases 18(Suppl 1): S11–S15

Berger A 1998 Patterns of fatigue and activity and rest during adjuvant breast cancer chemotherapy. Oncology Nursing Forum 25(1): 51–61

Berger A Farr L 1999 The influence of daytime inactivity and nighttime restlessness on cancer–related fatigue. Oncology Nursing Forum 26(10): 1663–1671

Berrios G 1990 Feelings of fatigue and psychopathology: a conceptual history. Comprehensive Psychiatry 31: 140–151

Blesch K, Paice J, Wickham R et al 1991 Correlates of fatigue in people with breast or lung cancer. Oncology Nursing Forum 18(1): 81–87

Bompa T 1999 Periodization: theory and method of training. Human Kinetics, Windsor, Ontario

Broeckel J, Jacobsen P, Horton J et al 1998 Characteristics and correlates of fatigue after adjuvant chemotherapy for breast cancer. Journal of Clinical Oncology 16: 1689–1696

Buchwald D, Pearlman T, Kith P et al 1998 Screening for psychiatric disorders in chronic fatigue and chronic fatigue syndrome. Journal of Psychosomatic Research 42: 87–94

Buckwalter K, Babich K 1990 Psychologic and physiologic aspects of depression. Nursing Clinics of North America 25: 945–954

Cannon W 1920 Bodily changes in pain, hunger, fear, and rage, 2nd edn. Harper & Row, New York

Casper R, Redmond E, Katz M et al 1985 Somatic symptoms in primary affective disorder. Archives of General Psychiatry 42: 1098–1104

Cimprich B 1993 Development of an intervention to restore attention in cancer patients. Cancer Nursing 16: 83–92

Costill D, Flynn M, Kirwan J et al 1988 Effects of repeated days of intensified training on muscle glycogen and swimming performance. Medicine and Science in Sports and Exercise 20: 249–254

Davidson J, Miller R, Turnbull C et al 1982 Atypical depression. General Hospital Psychiatry 39: 527–534

Depression Guideline Panel 1994 Depression: serious, prevalent, detectable. Patient Care 15: 30–63

De Zwardt B, Bras V, Dormolen M et al 1993 After-effects of night work on physical performance capacity and sleep quality in relation to age. International Archives of Occupational and Environmental Health 65: 259–262

Dumont M 1999 Report on the effects of night work. Unpublished report prepared for the Canadian Union of Postal Workers

Engstrom C, Strohl R, Rose L et al 1999 Sleep alterations in cancer patients. Cancer Nursing 22: 143–148

Ferrell B, Grant M, Dean G et al 1996 'Bone tired:' the experience of fatigue and its impact on Quality of Life. Oncology Nursing Forum 23: 1539–1547

Fisher G 1997 Chronic fatigue syndrome: a comprehensive guide to symptoms, treatments and solving the practical problems of CFS. Warner, New York

Fry A, Martin M 1996 Fatigue in the chronic fatigue syndrome: a cognitive phenomenon? Journal of Psychosomatic Research 41: 415–426

Gillberg M, Keckllund G, Akerstedt T 1994 Relations between performance and subjective ratings of sleepiness during a night awake. Sleep 17: 236–241

Glaus A 1998 Fatigue in patients with cancer. Springer-Verlag, Berlin

Green H 1997 Mechanisms of muscle fatigue in intense exercise. Journal of Sports Science 15: 247–256

Hann D, Denniston M, Baker F 2000 Measurement of fatigue in cancer patients: further validation of the Fatigue Symptom Inventory. Quality of Life Research 9: 847–854

Hendrickson C, Verde R 1994 Inadequate recovery from vigorous exercise. Physician and Sports Medicine 22: 56–63

Hoffman J 2002 Physiological aspects of sport training and performance. Human Kinetics, Windsor, Ontario

Hoskins C 1997 Breast cancer treatment related patterns in side effects, psychological distress, and perceived health status. Oncology Nursing Forum 24: 1575–1583

Irvine D, Vincent L, Graydon J et al 1994 The prevalence and correlates of fatigue in patients receiving treatment with chemotherapy and radiotherapy. Cancer Nursing 17: 367–378

Jurrell K 1998 Surface EMG and fatigue. Physical Medicine and Rehabilitation Clinics of North America 9: 933–947

Kindermann W 1986 Das Übertraining Ausdruck einer vegetativen Fehlsteuerung. Deutsche Zeitschrift für Sportsmedizin 37: 238–244

Klein D, Kocsis J, McCullough J et al 1996 Mood disorders: symptomatology in dysthymic and major depressive disorder. Psychiatric Clinics of North America 19: 41–53

Koenig H, Cohen H, Blazer D et al 1993 Profile of depressive symptoms in younger and older medical inpatients with major depression. Journal of the American Geriatric Society 41: 1169–1176

Komaroff A, Buchwald D 1998 Chronic fatigue syndrome: an update. Annual Review of Medicine 49: 1–13

Kuipers H, Keizer H 1988 Overtraining in elite athletes. Sports Medicine 6: 79–92

Lloyd R 1998 Chronic fatigue and chronic fatigue syndrome: shifting boundaries and attributions. American Journal of Medicine 105: 7S–10S

Lovell D 1999 Chronic fatigue syndrome among overseas development workers: a qualitative study. Journal of Travel Medicine 6: 16–23

MacDonald K, Osterholm M, LeDell K et al 1996 A case-control study to assess possible triggers and cofactors in chronic fatigue syndrome. American Journal of Medicine 100: 548–554

McEnany G, Hughes A, Lee K 1996 Depression and HIV. Nursing Clinics of North America 31: 57–80

MacKinnon L 1996 Overtraining and recovery in elite athletes: extension of a model to identify indicators of overtraining. Research report, Australian Sports Commission, Belconnen, Australian Capital Territory

Magnusson K, Moller A, Ekman T et al 1999 A qualitative study to explore the experience of fatigue in cancer patients. European Journal of Cancer Care 8: 224–232

Manfredini R, Manfredini F, Fersini C et al 1998 Circadian rhythms, athletic performance, and jet lag. British Journal of Sports Medicine 32: 101–106

Manu P, Matthews D, Lane T et al 1989 Depression among patients with a chief complaint of chronic fatigue syndrome. Journal of Affective Disorders 17: 165–172

Messias D, Yeager K, Dibble S et al 1997 Patients' perspectives of fatigue while undergoing chemotherapy. Oncology Nursing Forum 24: 43–48

Miaskowski C, Lee K 1999 Pain, fatigue, and sleep disturbances in oncology outpatients receiving radiation therapy for bone metastasis: a pilot study. Journal of Pain and Symptom Management 17: 320–332

Mitler M, Miller J, Lipsitz J et al 1997 The sleep of long-haul truck drivers. New England Journal of Medicine 337: 755–761

Morgan W, Costill D, Flynn M et al 1988 Mood disturbance following increased training in swimmers. Medicine and Science in Sports and Exercise 20: 408–414

Morse J 2000 Exploring pragmatic utility: concept analysis by critically appraising the literature. In Rodgers B, Knafl K (ed) Concept development in nursing, 2nd edn. WB Saunders, Philadelphia, PA, pp. 333–352

Morse J, Hupcey J, Mitcham C et al 1996 Criteria for concept evaluation. Journal of Advanced Nursing 24: 385–390

Moss-Morris R, Petrie K 2001 Discriminating between chronic fatigue syndrome and depression: a cognitive analysis. Psychological Medicine 31: 469–479

Mullis R, Campbell T, Wearden A et al 1999 Prediction of peak oxygen uptake in chronic fatigue syndrome. Journal of Sports Medicine 33: 352–356

Naessens G, Chandler J, Kibler W et al 2000 Clinical usefulness of nocturnal urinary noradrenaline excretion patterns in the follow-up of training processes in high-level soccer players. Journal of Strength and Conditioning Research 14: 125–131

Nail L, Winningham M 1993 Fatigue. In: Groenwald S, Frogge M, Goodman M, Yarbro C (eds) Cancer nursing: principles and practice, 3rd edn. Jones & Bartlett, Boston, MA, pp. 608–619

Nava S, Zanotti E, Rampulla C et al 1992 Respiratory muscle fatigue does not limit exercise performance during moderate endurance run. Journal of Sports Medicine and Physical Fitness 32: 39–44

Nisembaum R, Reyes M, Mauwle A et al 1998 Factor analysis of unexplained fatigue and interrelated symptoms. American Journal of Epidemiology 148: 72–77

Olson K, Tom B, Hewitt J et al 2002 Evolving routines: preventing fatigue associated with lung and colorectal cancer. Qualitative Health Research 12: 655–670

Pearce S, Richardson A 1996 Fatigue in cancer: a phenomenological perspective. European Journal of Cancer Care 5: 111–115

Piper B 1986 Fatigue. In: Carrieri-Kohlman V, Lindsay A, West C (eds) Pathophysiological phenomena in nursing: human responses to illness. WB Saunders, Philadelphia, PA, pp. 219–234

Piper B, Lindsey A, Dodd M 1987 Fatigue mechanisms in cancer patients: developing nursing theory. Oncology Nursing Forum 14: 17–23

Ray W, Cullen S, Phillips S 1992 Illness perception and symptom components in chronic fatigue syndrome. Journal of Psychosomatic Research 36: 243–256

Ream E, Richardson A 1996 Fatigue: a concept analysis. International Journal of Nursing Studies 33: 519–529

Ream E, Richardson A 1997 Fatigue in patients with cancer and chronic obstructive airway disease: a phenomenological enquiry. International Journal of Nursing Studies 34: 44–53

Rhodes V, Watson P, Hanson B 1988 Patients' descriptions of the influence of tiredness and weakness on self-care abilities. Cancer Nursing 11: 186–194

Sahlin K, Tonkonogi M, Soderlund K 1998 Energy supply and muscle fatigue in humans. Acta Physiologica Scandinavica 162: 261–266

Saltzstein B, Grace W, Hubbuch M, Perry J 1998 A naturalistic study of chronic fatigue syndrome among women in primary care. General Hospital Psychiatry 20: 307–316

Schwartz A 2000 Daily fatigue patterns and effect of exercise in women with breast cancer. Cancer Practice 8: 16–24

Scott A 2000 Shift work and health. Primary Care 27: 1057–1079

Scott A, Monk T, Brink L 1998 Shiftwork as a risk factor for depression. International Journal of Occupational and Environmental Health 3 (Suppl. 2): S2–S9

Selye H 1952 The story of the adaptation syndrome. Acta, Montreal, Quebec

Selye H 1956 The stress of life. McGraw-Hill, New York

Selye H 1971 Hormones and resistance, part 1. Springer, New York

Shepherd C, Lees H 1992 ME: is it a genuine disease? Health Visitor 65: 165–167

Sluiter J, van der Beek A, Frings-Dresen M 1999 The influence of work characteristics on the need for recovery and experienced health: a study of coach drivers. Ergonomics 42: 573–583

Stone P, Richards M, Hardy J 1998 Fatigue in patients with cancer. European Journal of Cancer 34: 1670–1676

Stone P, Hardy J, Broadly K et al 1999 Fatigue in advanced cancer: a prospective controlled cross sectional study. British Journal of Cancer 79: 1479–1486

Tepas D, Carvalhais A 1990 Sleep patterns of shiftworkers. Occupational Medicine 5: 199–208

Tiersky L, Johnson S, Lange G et al 1997 Neuropsychology of chronic fatigue syndrome: a critical review. Journal of Clinical and Experimental Neuropsychology 19: 560–586

van der Linden G, Chalder T, Hickie I et al 1999 Fatigue and psychiatric disorder: different or the same? Psychological Medicine 29: 863–868

Vercoulen J, Bazelman S, Swanink C et al 1997 Physical activity in chronic fatigue syndrome: assessment and its role in fatigue. Journal of Psychiatry and Research 31: 661–673

Walker J 1985 Social problems of shift work. In: Folkard S, Monk T (eds) Hours of work: temporal factors in work-scheduling. John Wiley, Chichester, pp. 211–225

Welsh R, Woodhouse L 1992 Overuse syndromes. In: Shepard R, Astrand P (eds) Endurance in sport, vol 2. Blackwell Scientific, Oxford, pp. 505–515

Winningham M 1996 Fatigue. In: Groenwald S, Hansen F, Goodman M, Yarbro C (eds) Cancer symptom management. Jones & Barlett, Boston, MA, pp. 42–58

Winningham M, Nail L, Burke M et al 1994 Fatigue and the cancer experience: the state of the knowledge. Oncology Nursing Forum 21: 23–36

Woo B, Dibble S, Piper B et al 1998 Differences in fatigue by treatment methods in women with breast cancer. Oncology Nursing Forum 25: 915–920

Wool M 1990 Understanding depression in medical patients. Part I: diagnostic considerations. Social Work and Health Care 14: 25–38

Wright J, Beverly D 1998 Chronic fatigue syndrome. Archives of Disease in Childhood 79: 368–374

Grief – an analysis of the concept as it relates to bereavement

Kate Sullivan

EDITORIAL

Few credible nursing scholars would make the claim that grief is a concept exclusive to the discipline of nursing. Yet, given the nature of much of nursing work, it is hardly surprising that nurses need a thorough knowledge of how to help patients (and their families) with their grief. The truth of the matter is that death, loss and bereavement are an inextricable aspect of health care and there is a wealth of evidence that shows the crucial role nurses play in dealing with these issues. Nurses often remember their first encounter with death and, more often than not in contemporary society, this experience occurs within some kind of clinical setting. Death, and concomitantly grief, are subsequently realities that nurse will have to face. The truism so aptly and eloquently expressed by the poet Samuel Beckett in the words below, that death is inevitable, may lose meaning in a technologically driven health care world and, at the same time, this raises something of a dichotomy. Despite the frequency with which nurses are faced with matters pertaining to grief (often arising from death), there can be few concepts encountered in nursing that are, if you will forgive the pun, shrouded in so much mystery; this warrants attention.

Many nursing models mention death and dealing with death, and thus issues of dealing with grief. Furthermore, some attention to dealing with dying, death and grief occurs within nursing programmes. Yet, irrespective of this theoretical and educational attention, dealing with death and grief are still areas of nursing practice that many nurses have great difficulty with. As we are reminded in Kate's chapter, attitudes towards death and grief have not been consistent over time. Additionally, for our contemporary generation exposure to death and dying is very different from the exposure our forefathers experienced. Consequently, many nurses have little or no personal exposure to death (and grief resulting from death) until they encounter it in a clinical situation.

One might speculate that this lack of experiential exposure to death adds to the mystery and, subsequently, the discomfort. Furthermore, there is a substantial literature that highlights how, mainly during the last century, death has become more medicalized. More and more individuals are dying in hospitals rather than their homes, decisions about when people die are sometimes made not by the individual or their families but by physicians, and death (and grief) remains something of a taboo subject in many healthcare settings. Accordingly, nurses would benefit from an increased understanding of grief as one means to demystify the concept and help overcome any difficulty they have in dealing with death and/or grief.

INTRODUCTION

In *Waiting for Godot*, one of his more profound pieces of writing, Samuel Beckett, winner of the 1969 Nobel Prize for Literature, reminded the reader of the tenuous grip human beings have on life:

> *One day we were born, one day we shall die. They (women) give birth astride of a grave, the light gleams an instant, then it's night once more*
>
> *Beckett 1965*

For most people, the death of someone they love produces an emotional reaction of grief. For grief to occur certain events or incidents, usually referred to as antecedents, must be present. Once the concept is present other events or incidents, referred to as consequences, may result (Walker & Avant 1995). While the feelings associated with grief may be similar among humans, grief is manifest in a number of different ways and varies enormously both across and within societies (Cutcliffe 1998, Walter 1999). It may be present for short or long periods of time and, in some cases, has the potential to disable the sufferer for life. Sometimes the term 'grief' is used interchangeably with 'bereavement' or 'mourning'. In this chapter a clear distinction is drawn between bereavement – the objective state of having lost someone or something; grief – the emotions that accompany bereavement; and mourning – the behaviour that social groups expect following bereavement (Walter 1999, Cutcliffe 2002).

According to Walter (1999), theoreticians have attempted to draw distinction between models, which describe the observed phenomena associated with grief, and theories, which attempt to explain and find causes of grief. Published work on grief often refers to the grief process. Categorizing grief in this way, Walter (1999) reminds us, has frequently been criticized because it seems to suggest that there is only one way to grieve. While accepting that some of this criticism is justified, it is also evident that grief has the potential to create chaos in the life of the person experiencing it. Consequently, the psychological construct of the grief process has been introduced in order to ameliorate some of the chaos created (Walter 1999).

Another area within the debates around the concept of grief that has evoked criticism is the notion of grief work. This approach, popular in the USA, is seen as a more proactive and positive aid to recovery from grief. Rather than sit and wait for the chaos caused by grief to overcome them, the bereaved actively work towards regaining control of their lives (Walter 1999). However, critics of grief work conclude that the evidence of its efficacy is equivocal (Wortman & Silver 1989, Stroebe et al 1994). The purpose of this concept analysis is to attempt to clarify the definitions, properties and attributes of grief experienced as a consequence of bereavement.

CONCEPTUAL ANALYSIS

Grief is frequently referred to in nursing and health-related publications, yet no single, universal definition of the concept exists. While it is accepted that the concept of grief is difficult to define or even understand, it has been suggested that one way to clarify and understand a term is to conduct a concept analysis (Morse et al 1992). Conceptual analysis has been described as a technique or mental activity that requires critical approaches in uncovering subtle elements of meaning that can be embedded in abstract concepts (Chinn & Kramer 1995). McKenna (1997) argued that concepts are the building blocks of theory; he noted that if the concepts are poorly understood then the theory will be built on shaky foundations.

Different approaches to concept analysis are commonly used in nursing. Exponents of the logical positivist movement, such as Walker and Avant (1995) and Chinn and Kramer (1995), follow the 'entity' view of concepts and apply this perspective not only to the sciences but also to concepts that involve human emotions and feelings (Lacey 1976). Others have been critical of this approach and contend that bringing scientific equations to bear on understanding human feelings and relationships is to demean them because concepts are by nature evolutionary and dynamic and should be valued as such (Rodgers 1994, Morse 1995). Both broad approaches to concept analysis have strengths and weaknesses. Consequently, in this chapter, it is proposed to use a combination of approaches (Bevan 1991) as a basis for the analysis of the concept grief.

According to Cowles and Rodgers (1991), fundamental to any concept analysis is a review of relevant literature. For the purpose of writing this chapter, both classic and contemporary literature was accessed. Inclusion of the former was undertaken to facilitate examination of the concept over time and accessing alternative forms of literature, in addition to theoretical and empirical literature, is encouraged by Chinn and Kramer (1995).

The chapter commences by identifying uses of the concept, proceeds to examine issues relevant to the concept in its different manifestations and over time, and concludes by outlining the critical attributes and empirical referents associated with the concept.

IDENTIFYING USES OF THE CONCEPT

The *Oxford English Dictionary* suggests two uses of the word grief. The first entry refers to 'deep or violent sorrow, keen regret; cause of this; come to grief, meet with disaster, fail, fall'. The second usage relates to an exclamation of surprise or alarm, 'good grief', or 'great grief'. Considering the first definition, other dictionaries and thesauruses have variously defined grief as: anguish, suffering, agony, misery, distress, wretchedness, pain, hurt, sadness, unhappiness, torment, desolation, heartache, heartbreak, mourning. Based on these definitions, grief is considered an abstract concept because it exists in thought rather than in matter. It is also suggested that, in this context, the only other concept that has a meaning similar to grief, is sorrow.

GRIEF: THE HISTORICAL CONTEXT WITHIN CERTAIN CLASSIC LITERATURE

One suggestion that has been made is that when people lose the social interaction basis for defining events, feelings and meanings in their lives, they often feel compelled to seek alternative means of defining self and situations (Rosenblatt 1993). When grief is considered, exploration of writings on loss may be one way in which a bereaved person is enabled to find meaning in their life (Rosenblatt 1993).

This, of course, is not a new phenomenon but something that has existed for thousands of years. Plays and poetry written by two of the most celebrated literati in history, Homer and Shakespeare, are replete with themes of death and grief. It has been suggested that, in the period of Greek history that Homer dealt with, both death and grief were accepted with stoical resolve (Sourvinou-Inwood 1981). Homer's depiction of grief is markedly different to that portrayed by the 16th-century English dramatist and poet William Shakespeare. Themes of death and grief are evident throughout Shakespeare's sonnets and plays – Richard III, King John, King Lear and Hamlet. Various intellectuals have made suggestions as to the deeper meaning of Shakespeare's intense interest in, if not obsession with, death and grief (Lewis 1942, Grinstein 1973, Pollock 1975, Oremland 1983, Silver 1983, Shaughnessy 1985).

In a later period of history the concept of creative writing was hypothesized as one means of achieving a catharsis of grief. The idea that repressed emotions could be freed by literal expression was put forward as the motivation behind the poetry of the 19th-century American poet Emily Dickinson. One of Dickinson's biographers implied that the poet had an unhealthy preoccupation with thoughts of death and grief (Cody 1959). On the other hand, McDermott and Porter (1989), who did a content analysis of word frequency in nine of her death poems, challenged this assumption and suggested that, rather than her poetry demonstrating the presence of personal difficulty with death, it emphasized a mastery of her personal struggle with grief and her recovery from it.

Some researchers have suggested that the whole concept of grief has changed in Western society within the last 100 years (Gorer 1965, Aries 1974). These writers have argued that during the 19th century, in Britain at least, most members of society were exposed to death and grief as an integral part of life. Children often witnessed the deaths of their siblings and, perhaps, one or both parents at an early age. As the vast majority of these deaths took place at home, the dying person was surrounded by their loved ones, death and grief were integrated into family life and the grieving received support from their extended family and from the community in which they lived.

The image created of this very structured and almost idyllic end to life during the 19th century has been argued to be in sharp contrast to death in the latter part of the 20th century. In a study of grief and mourning in Britain, Gorer (1965) suggested that, during this time, there was very little support for the bereaved. No longer did individuals die in the bosom of their family, with the attendant support available to those who were grieving. No longer was an elaborate ritual of mourning observed, which helped the grieving process. Indeed, in modern society death, bereavement and grief are characterized by isolation and loneliness.

However, this point of view has been challenged by Cannadine (1981) and Richardson (1987) who point to the fact that the whole ritual attached to grief and mourning in earlier times was not so much a way of helping the bereaved as a well-orchestrated attempt at their exploitation for commercial purposes. The perfunctory wearing of mourning clothes and all the impedimenta that accompanied this was frequently an added stress for the bereaved, and often added to their grief.

Which of these assertions is the most accurate will no doubt continue to be debated. However, what does appear to be commonly accepted by researchers is that a reaction of grief usually follows the death of a loved person.

TYPES AND CONSEQUENCES OF GRIEF

Identification of the characteristics of a concept that arise again and again whenever the concept is present is seen as an integral component of Walker and Avant's (1995) approach to concept analysis. Furthermore, these authors, in addition to Rodgers (1994), advise the analyst to first identify the critical attributes for the concept and then consider the consequences. On the other hand, Chinn and Kramer (1995) suggested that criteria for the concept emerge gradually; they emerge only when it has been defined and other sources and circumstances surrounding it have been examined. In this chapter the consequences of grief are examined first.

Since Freud's famous essay on mourning and melancholia in 1915, a number of researchers have investigated the concepts and paradigms surrounding grief (Lindemann 1944, Engel 1961, Hinton 1967, Parkes 1976, Bowlby 1980, Kalish 1985, Worden 1991). Freud's psychoanalytic perspective on grief described grief as the process of gradual withdrawal of the love and energy that tied the bereaved person to the deceased. The bereaved person was then thought to replace the loved one with someone or something else. Other researchers who described the events that occurred when a loss was sustained proffered a developmental process model (Kavanaugh 1972, Parkes 1976, Backer et al 1982). In an authoritative study of widows (Parkes 1976), a number of events that occurred following bereavement were described. The first reaction was one of alarm. This was manifested by physiological symptoms usually associated with fear. Often, the alarm was accompanied by searching for the lost person. While most adults were aware that this was a futile exercise, some perhaps innate response motivated them to search. Searching was described as a restless activity in which one moves towards possible locations of a lost object. Bowlby (1980) asserted that this searching was a response to the loss of attachment experienced when a loved person dies.

Having considered the work related to attachment and loss in animals, Bowlby (1980) progressed to posit the idea of attachment theory in humans. Attachment theory suggested that primitive biological processes were responsible for the reactions of human beings to the loss of a loved person. It was noted in British and American studies that the bereaved, particularly grieving parents and spouses, often had vivid dreams of the dead, hallucinations about them and conversations with them. Often they would visit places they had been to together to try and rekindle, or preserve, their relationship with the deceased.

One criticism of this work is its emphasis on the biological responses associated with grief, with very little attention being paid to the social context in which death and grief takes place. In research where the social context of death is acknowledged, Parkes (1976) found that many of the participants studied had a feeling or impression that their loved one was in their presence without actually seeing or hearing them. This was termed 'mitigation' and proved, for some, a positive experience because their search was over as they had now found their loved one, if only in their imagination.

Where anger, guilt and yearning were described as typical reactions to loss, anger (see, for example, Parkes 1976) was sometimes directed at the dead person for having died. Often it was directed at healthcare professionals, who might, realistically or unrealistically, be perceived to have in some way contributed to the loved one's suffering, and sometimes at 'God', who, like the doctors, was seen as having power over life and death. According to Parkes (1976), guilt was often centred on the self. Acts of omission, however seemingly trivial, were magnified. For many of the bereaved, anger, feelings of apathy and despair and a loss of heart displaced guilt. Finally, the concept of gaining a new identity was described. This concept had its roots in the phenomenon of identification with the dead person and in the feeling that the bereaved person had lost part of themselves.

In an attempt to explain the grief process, stage models of grief were constructed (Kavanaugh 1972). In a seven-stage model bereaved individuals were said to experience: initial shock, unstable emotions, guilt, anger, loneliness, relief and, eventually, re-establishment of their lives. Similarly, Bowlby (1980) identified four phases associated with the grieving process. The first phase was one of numbness that usually lasted from a few hours to a week. Sometimes this numbness was interrupted by outbursts of extremely intense distress and/or anger. The second phase was one of yearning and searching for the lost figure. This lasted for some months and often for years. The third phase consisted of disorganization and despair. The fourth and final phase was one of reorganization of the individual's life without their loved one.

One difficulty with using stage models of grief is that the stages tend to overlap. If the models were true stage models, then each step in the process would be separate and identifiable. More contemporary understandings posit that grief is not a mechanistic process and view it as both an experience that is unique to each individual and one that can be more chaotic. Individuals react in a way that is consistent with their character and their previous methods of coping and people's emotions are 'mosaic' in form and thus convoluted (Buckman 1993, Solari-Twadell et al 1995, Cutcliffe 1998, 2002). Furthermore, it has been postulated that bereavement outcome is unequivocally bound up with hope and hopelessness. Where there is the re-emergence of hope there is a completed bereavement process (Cutcliffe 2004). However, when the grieving person feels a continued sense of hopelessness the bereavement process may become complicated (Cutcliffe 1998, 2004).

INSTRUMENTS USED TO MEASURE GRIEF

In order to provide empirical evidence of the phenomenon of grief, instruments have emerged to measure both the process and outcome of grief (Zisook et al 1982, Remondet & Hansson 1987, Stroebe & Stroebe 1991). Based on the literature of normative and atypical grief reactions, as well as their clinical experience, Zisook et al (1982) undertook a study of 211 bereaved individuals to assist with the development of an instrument to measure grief. While the researchers recognized that several investigators had elucidated normal and pathological grief processes, several pertinent questions remained unanswered. They categorized these as: the time course of normal grief; knowledge of the importance of unresolved grief; the frequency and manifestations of unresolved grief; and the morbidity and mortality associated with bereavement. They concluded that long after death occurred most bereaved people continued to feel upset, empty or tearful, with several grief-related feelings continuing indefinitely.

Several limitations are evident within this study. The researchers used a convenience sample. The data examined were gathered from friends and neighbours of one of the investigators. The study population, therefore, had a similar social and educational background, i.e. adult, white, professional and middle-class. There was no evidence that issues of validity and reliability were addressed. The researchers concluded by defining 'unresolved grief' in terms of the respondent's answer to one item on the inventory – their perception of whether or not they have 'gotten over the loss'. While this study suffered from a number of weaknesses it was one of the first steps taken by researchers to measure adjustment to grief over time.

Stroebe and Stroebe (1991) conducted a longitudinal study over a 2-year period following bereavement. They provided information on the health status of participants, assessed those who were likely to be at greatest risk from bereavement and evaluated participants' recovery from grief. Participants in this study were samples of widows ($n = 30$) and widowers ($n = 30$) who were assessed three times over the period of the study. In addition, measures of their health and well-being were compared to those of a matched sample of married individuals ($n = 60$). This study used a wide variety of scales to measure the different risk factors and outcomes associated with bereavement and grief. The findings of this study were that, while the majority of people had made a reasonable recovery from their grief, about one-third of participants showed few signs of recovery at the end of the 2 years. Findings indicated that the poor bereavement outcome evident among the latter group could be attributed to a combination of personality and situational factors that were common among those respondents who were classified as being in the 'high-risk' bereavement group.

ISSUES THAT MAY INFLUENCE THE COURSE OF GRIEF

Because grief is a complex phenomenon some researchers have suggested that its course can be influenced by a number of issues, including whether or not the bereaved person has had time to prepare for the loss (Parkes 1976). When a death is expected, as in the case of a terminal illness, the bereaved may be better prepared to deal with their loss as they may have started to grieve long before the death takes place. If, however, the person has a sudden illness, the situation is more complex, and those close to them live with two sets of contingency plans, one for the person continuing to live and one for the possibility of their imminent death. In this situation the loved ones may or may not be grieving in anticipation of their loss. Also referred to in this study was the timeliness or untimeliness of the loss, which differentiated between the quiet slipping away of an old man and the tragic cutting-off of a young one in his prime. Widows who were in the over-65 age group did not appear to experience the same grief-related problems as did widows in the under-65 age group. One example of this was the sevenfold increase in sedative consumption among the latter group, with only a slight decrease in their use over the 18 months following bereavement.

Another factor that may possibly influence how an individual deals with their grief is gender. In Shuchter and Zisook's (1993) study of spousal bereavement, specific gender differences in response to bereavement were identified 13 months after the spouse's death. Women were more likely to report debilitating health problems and feel a greater degree of helplessness than men. Men showed less acceptance of the death, were less likely to express their feelings, drank more and formed new attachments more quickly than women. Based on empirical evidence it seems appropriate to suggest that for most individuals the loss of a loved person causes a 'normal' grief reaction.

COMPLICATED GRIEF

While accepting that bereavement is experienced uniquely by each individual, and is influenced by their personal biography and the cultural norms of the society of which they are part, there is also recognition that two distinct types of grief reaction exist (Cutcliffe 1998, 2002). There are those people who resolve to work through their grief experience to a state of peace without intervention from formal healthcare services, and there are those who fail to return to their prebereavement level of emotional well-being, performance or level of hope (Glick et al 1974, Scruby & Sloan 1989, Kim & Jacobs 1991, Marwitt 1991, Worden 1991, Lendrum & Syme 1992, Lloyd 1992, Dimond et al 1994, Prigerson et al 1995, Cowles 1996). It is probable that persons in the latter group are experiencing complicated grief.

Complicated or unresolved grief has been categorized or described in a number of ways, including delayed grief (Littlewood 1992), distorted or absent grief (Raphael 1984) and chronic grief (Gorer 1965, Marris 1986). Delayed grief occurs when the recognition of the loss and associated expression of grief is postponed. Typically, grief is experienced with particular severity at a later date. In distorted grief there is a priority attached to one aspect of the grief, usually anger or guilt, to the exclusion of all other emotions. In order to illustrate chronic grief, I have decided to draw on two individuals; one is factual – the bereaved British monarch Queen Victoria (Gorer 1965) – and one is fictional – the lovelorn Miss Havisham in Dickens's *Great Expectations* (Marris 1986). Both of these exemplars, albeit for different reasons, personify what could be described as complicated grief and might, in the present context, be analogous to 'model cases'.

A number of theoretical frameworks have tried to explain the difference between complicated and 'normal' grief. However, no consensus has been reached among researchers and no universally accepted definition of complicated grief exists (Prigerson et al 1995). Parkes' (1976) study analysed the major presenting symptoms in 35 individuals, some of whom had more than one major symptom, of what was described as atypical grief. A total of 26 suffered from depression, six from alcoholism, five had hypochondriacal symptoms, four had phobic symptoms and two had frank psychosis. Other symptoms such as asthma, panic attacks, alopecia, fainting and headaches were also noted. While it was recognized that none of these symptoms was a sign of pathology per se, when a comparison was made between this group and a group of widows not having psychiatric treatment, two important differences were apparent – the intensity and the duration of the symptoms.

In the disturbed group, one feature that was noted was that grief tended to be prolonged; the other tendency was for the reaction to the bereavement to be delayed. Years after their bereavement, many of the group were still severely distressed and any thoughts or reminders of the loved one caused uncontrollable crying. Intense pining, anger, aggression and withdrawal from friends and family were also evident. Four of the group admitted to having suicidal preoccupations. Eight of the study group had suffered from a delayed grief reaction. Three had not felt any grief at all until at least 2 weeks after the death and five had not even experienced a feeling of numbness in the period following their loss. Several subjects in the study group were clinically depressed and began to grieve intensely, making it difficult for the researcher to distinguish between delayed and chronic grief.

Fear, experienced as panic attacks and characterized by breathless attacks and choking sensations, was recognized as being caused by reminders of the death and by loneliness and loss of support. Parkes (1976) referred to this as separation anxiety and, while recognizing that defining complicated or, as it was then called, pathological grief was a complex issue, concluded that atypical forms of grief can precipitate mental health problems. Those individuals who were perceived as timid and clinging; had probably not dealt adequately with loss before; had a previous history of depressive illness; had difficulty expressing their feelings because of their cultural or family background; had either an over-reliant or an ambivalent relationship with the deceased; or were experiencing other losses were the most likely to be at high risk of developing complicated grief.

Other researchers, e.g. Raphael (1984), Clayton (1975) and Stylianos and Vachon (1993) recognized that when the bereaved are isolated their grief is intensified. Often this intensification of grief occurs because the bereaved do not have others to help them define their loss or to assist them to invest in the future. Indeed, they could be described as experiencing a sense of hopelessness (Cutcliffe 1998, 2004). Hopelessness may well be a consequence when, for whatever reason, the significance of the bereaved person's loss cannot be shared with others.

GRIEF IN 'NON-TRADITIONAL' RELATIONSHIPS

The majority of studies of grief and bereavement have concentrated on the impact of death and bereavement on the immediate family and close relations of the deceased person, the assumption being that the individual's legal relationship with and attachment to the deceased determines the intensity of their grief. Where other relationships, described as non-traditional relationships, exist, little consideration has been given to the impact of grief on the survivor. Non-traditional relationships have been defined as those involving extramarital affairs, heterosexual cohabitation and homosexual relationships. While these relationships differ in a number of ways, in one respect they are similar in that they are less likely to have public acceptance or recognition (Doka 1987).

A study undertaken to examine the grief experienced by the survivor in a non-traditional relationship (Doka 1987) recognized 'normal' grief reactions – the same grief reactions described by other researchers (e.g. those documented by Parkes 1976 and Worden 1991). However, among this group of people these reactions appeared to be intensified. Adding to the feelings associated with a grief reaction, feelings of embarrassment and shame frequently existed. These feelings were usually caused by the negative sanction to which the relationship had been exposed. Often, restricted access to the dying partner intensified the grief experienced. Social support for the bereaved is often considered an important factor in facilitating effective grief work. Yet a lack of social support for the survivor in a non-traditional relationship was evident in the data presented.

Doka stated:

> In cases in which the relationship is secret, there naturally is no recognition or even knowledge of grief within that relationship. In some cases the exclusion is total. Sometimes due to the clandestine and sporadic nature of the relationship, the survivor may not even become aware of the death until weeks after the event.
>
> *Doka 1987, p. 461*

As alluded to earlier, bereavement and grief know no bounds (Beckett 1969). Various writers have estimated that approximately between 5% and 10% of the population can be identified as homosexual (Kinsey et al 1948, Ramsey et al 1974, Whitam 1983, Fay 1989). While many studies have been carried out into the grief experienced on the loss of a spouse (e.g. Parkes 1976, Hampe 1979, Bowlby 1980, Raphael 1984), little recognition has been given to the intense difficulty and grief suffered by the bereaved partner in a same-sex relationship (Doka 1987). Because of perceived social attitudes towards homosexual coupling, the relationship may not have been disclosed, resulting in the couple living in relative isolation. Ultimately, when one of the couple dies, there may be few people available to support the grieving partner.

In a study that described the impact of AIDS on a group of homosexual men (Klein & Fletcher 1986) the researchers observed normal grief reactions, but also new paradigms of grief that appeared to be unique to the gay population. They noted that the majority of those in the group were men, frequently below the age of 45. There was evidence of them having low self-esteem and guilt feelings, often exacerbated by introjected homophobic attitudes. They often felt abandoned and isolated and lacked a support network. For these men there was no societal approval for their grieving and no descriptive title to identify them as a significant other of the deceased. Some had suffered severe financial disadvantage when their partner died, including the loss of their home. Some were excluded from, or made to feel unwelcome in, the healthcare setting. If they were in a position to visit their loved one in hospital they felt unable to display affection towards him as they believed this aroused hostility among staff and other patients. Often they were excluded from their partner's funeral by blood relations who did not wish to give any recognition to his true lifestyle.

Other writers in this area (Murphy & Perry 1988) have asked how these men, referred to as 'hidden grievers', who have been censored by both lay people and professionals in all walks of life, could be expected to be anything other than hidden in a society that is uncomfortable in the face of death and grief.

For the person who has lost a same-sex partner, their grief may be intensified because of the secret nature of their partnership. They may have little opportunity to engage in actions that are often helpful to the bereaved. If their partner has died suddenly they may not have been officially notified about the death because the partnership was not recognized. Items that were meaningful to the couple may be given to the deceased's family and the partner may be unable to ask for their return. If they are permitted to attend to the legal requirements necessary when their partner dies, they may experience problems with funeral directors and government officials because they are not legally defined as a relative of the deceased (Sullivan 1997). At their partner's funeral they may not be accorded their rightful place as the chief mourner. And it is possible that the person conducting the funeral rite will avoid mentioning their relationship with the deceased. Indeed, if their partner's close family are aware of the relationship they may ask the bereaved partner either not to attend the funeral or, if attending, to sit with the general congregation and not make themselves known to the wider family circle (Sullivan 1997).

The privileges of grief (Averill & Nunley 1993) extended to the spouse in a heterosexual marriage may not be available to the partner in a same-sex relationship. These privileges include the public display of otherwise private emotions, being excused from work for an extended period of time and having the right to expect care and support from others. When the significance of the bereaved partner's loss is not recognized by others, they may have little opportunity to reminisce about life with their partner, something that is recognized as a normal and helpful part of the grieving process. The only source of social support available to them has to come from those few people who recognize the significance of their grief. Many of the difficulties experienced by these individuals may be related to the social stigma attached to homosexuality, which adds to the stress experienced by bereaved partners (Siegal & Hoefer 1981). Because of perceived stigmatization many people feel unable to declare their partnership and consequently experience loneliness and isolation when their partner dies (Sullivan 1997).

GRIEF: WHAT IT IS AND WHAT IT IS NOT

In order to promote further understanding of a concept, case examples are included in the analysis (Walker & Avant 1995). In this analysis two such examples are presented. The first, an example from 'real life', includes all the critical attributes of the concept grief. The second is a constructed case in which there is complete absence of the critical attributes of the concept. The first example is taken from a British study of same-sex bereavement (Sullivan 1997).

Case study 11.1
A model case of grief

Charles and Clive met at a promenade concert in 1946 and shared a home from 1947 until Clive's death in 1990. Charles described their initial encounter as 'love at first sight'. He spoke of how they shared a love of literature, theatre, classical music and travel and of the 'wonderful life' they had together and of how things had changed since Clive's death. More than 3 years after Clive's death Charles articulated his feelings thus:

'But there are lots and lots of hours and hours and hours and I still can't get used to it. I can't sit in this room at night on my own. Once I have had my evening meal, about seven, and I have washed up, I go to bed. I don't sleep. Even now (summer) the sun will still be shining when I go to bed. We always sat here together after dinner. I can hardly play music. I have all the Wagners and we used to listen to them. I have tried it, but I can't.

'We did everything together. We thought the same things. We didn't used to have to speak or ask things. I suppose I was too close to him really. But my life is very, very much changed since then. It will never be the same again, and I realize that. I used to weep until I went to sleep. Also, I suppose part of me was dead and I couldn't help thinking, well, this is the end. I mean, almost 44 years is a hell of a long time. I just couldn't reconcile this shutting off so quickly. My life finished that morning, the 22nd of May. My life finished then.'

In this interview Charles illustrates clearly the depth of love he felt for his partner Clive. He also reminds the reader of the investment he, and no doubt Clive, made in their relationship and the grief he continues to experience 3 years after Clive's death. All of what have been described as the critical attributes of the concept grief are contained in the feelings expressed by Charles.

The second example shows that grief is not always experienced when a relative or close family member dies. As part of a concept analysis of grief that sought to illustrate what grief was not (Jacob 1993) a case was constructed about Linda, a 16-year-old girl who had been sexually abused by her stepfather. Both Linda and her stepfather were involved in a serious car accident that resulted in the stepfather's death. When told of her stepfather's death Linda did not experience any of the defining attributes that are associated with grief, but experienced a feeling of joy and relief. It was suggested that this reaction happened because Linda did not value or cherish her stepfather and, indeed, may have considered his death beneficial as it marked an end to her suffering. The use of a constructed case in this situation has been criticized for two reasons. First, how typical is the example given (Messer & Meldrum 1995)? Second, being fictitious, the example used may be divorced from reality. However, other writers (Robinson & McKenna 1998) suggested that the reader should remain open to such examples as they have the potential to provide valuable perspectives on life.

CRITICAL ATTRIBUTES

The critical attributes or underlying assumptions of grief, i.e. the characteristics of the concept that appear over and over again (Walker & Avant 1995), may be gleaned from the above discussion. Each attribute must be present in a valid instance of grief. As a result of this analysis, I posit three critical attributes of grief, experienced as a consequence of bereavement.

- Grief is a normal emotional response experienced on the death of a person who is valued and loved.
- Grief is a complex phenomenon, the meaning of which is determined individually, subjectively and contextually by the person experiencing it. For some individuals the trajectory of grief may become complicated and may never be resolved.
- Grief impacts on all aspects of the bereaved person's life and produces physiological, emotional and sociological sequelae.

The first attribute links the death of a loved person with an emotional response that we term grief. The second attribute stresses the individualized nature of the grief experience and the possible difficulties inherent in that experience. The multifaceted nature of grief, as exemplified by the range of symptomatology it produces, is determined by the third defining attribute.

The identification of these attributes has provided a basis for the following definition. Grief is a normal, yet highly complicated, deeply distressing and very personal reaction to the death of someone we love. Grief has the potential to permeate through all aspects of a bereaved person's life.

EMPIRICAL REFERENTS

Empirical referents are classes or categories of actual phenomenon that by their existence demonstrate the occurrence of the concept (Walker & Avant 1995). The second critical attribute outlined above suggests that grief is a complex, subjective experience the meaning of which is determined by the person experiencing it. As such, grief is a unique and traumatic event, the pain of which cannot be quantified by others and is either experienced or is not. For most individuals the death of someone they love causes a normal grief reaction. However, for some people the grieving process may become prolonged, complicated and unresolved. Therefore, rather than seeking to measure different dimensions of grief it is better to determine whether it exists or whether it does not and how it is affecting the person who is experiencing it.

As mentioned above, a number of instruments have been developed to measure the process and outcome of grief. The results of these measures, while not demonstrating classes or categories of grief, can help to provide information on the health status and well-being of the grieving person.

CONCLUSION

This chapter has explored the concept of grief experienced as a consequence of bereavement. It has highlighted the multifaceted and complex nature of grief and demonstrated that the death of a loved person has the potential to cause great distress and suffering. It is hoped that these deliberations may be helpful to health and social care professionals, and others, who provide support and care to those who are grieving. Of particular significance is the experience of Charles. This example of grief should alert care providers to the significance of this man's loss and help them to recognize and validate the experience of others in similar situations. The analysis may also provide a basis for further exploration of how professional carers assess the needs of those who are experiencing grief and help them to determine how best to meet their needs. The results of this analysis are not intended to be conclusive but rather seek to precipitate further consideration and investigation.

REFERENCES

Aries P 1974 Western attitudes towards death from the Middle Ages to the present. Johns Hopkins University Press, Baltimore, MD

Averill JR, Nunley EP 1993 Grief as an emotion and as a disease. In: Stroebe MS, Stroebe W, Hansson RO (eds) Handbook of bereavement. Cambridge University Press, Cambridge

Backer BA, Hannon N, Russell NA 1982 Death and dying: individuals and institutions. John Wiley, New York

Beckett S 1965 Waiting for Godot, 3rd edn. Faber & Faber, London

Bevan W 1991 Contemporary psychology: a tour inside the onion. The American Psychologist 46: 475–483

Bowlby J 1980 Attachment and loss: loss, sadness and depression. Hogarth Press, London

Buckman R 1993 Communication in palliative care: a practical guide. In: Doyle D, Hanks GWC, MacDonald N (eds) Oxford textbook of palliative medicine. Oxford Medical Publications, Oxford, pp 51–70

Cannadine D 1981 War and death, grief and mourning in modern Britain. In: Whaley J (ed) Mirrors of mortality: studies in the social history of death. Europa Publications, London

Chinn PL, Kramer MK 1995 Theory and nursing: a systematic approach, 4th edn. Mosby, London

Clayton PJ 1975 The effect of living alone on bereavement symptoms. American Journal of Psychiatry 132: 133–137

Cody J 1959 After great pain: the inner life of Emily Dickinson. Harvard University Press, Boston, MA

Cowles KV 1996 Cultural perspectives of grief: an expanded concept analysis. Journal of Advanced Nursing 23: 287–294

Cowles KV, Rodgers BL 1991 The concept of grief: a foundation for nursing research and practice. Research in Nursing and Health 14: 119–127

Cutcliffe JR 1998 Hope, counselling and complicated bereavement reactions. Journal of Advanced Nursing 28: 754–761

Cutcliffe JR 2002 Understanding and working with bereavement. Mental Health Practice 6: 29–37

Cutcliffe JR 2004 The inspiration of hope in bereavement counselling. Jessica Kingsley, London

Dimond M, Caserta M, Lund D 1994 Understanding depression in bereaved older adults. Clinical Nursing Research 3: 253–268

Doka KJ 1987 Silent sorrow: grief and the loss of significant others. Death Studies 11: 455–469

Engel G 1961 Is grief a disease? Psychosomatic Medicine 23: 18–22

Fay RE, Turner CF, Klassen AD et al 1989 Prevalence and patterns of same-gender sexual contact among men. Science 243: 38–348

Glick IO, Weiss RS, Parkes CM 1974 The first year of bereavement. John Wiley, New York

Gorer G 1965 Death, grief and mourning in contemporary Britain. Cresset Press, London

Grinstein A 1973 King Lear's impending death. The American Imago 30: 121–141

Hampe SO 1979 Needs of the grieving spouse in a hospital setting. Nursing Research 24: 113

Hinton J 1967 Dying. Penguin, Harmondsworth

Jacob SR 1993 An analysis of the concept of grief. Journal of Advanced Nursing 18: 1787–1794

Kalish RA 1985 Death, grief and caring relationships, 2nd edn. Brooks-Cole, Monterey, CA

Kavanaugh R 1972 Facing death. Penguin, Baltimore, MD

Kim K, Jacobs S 1991 Pathological grief and its relationship to other psychiatric disorders. Journal of Affective Disorders 21: 257–263

Kinsey AC, Pomeroy WB, Martin CE 1948 Sexual behaviour in the human male. WB Saunders, London

Klein SJ, Fletcher W 1986 Gay grief: an examination of its uniqueness brought to light by the AIDS crisis. Journal of Psychosocial Oncology 4: 15–25

Lacey AR 1976 A dictionary of philosophy. Routledge & Kegan Paul, London

Lendrum S, Syme G 1992 Gift of tears: a practical approach to loss and bereavement counselling. Routledge, London

Lewis CS 1942 Hamlet: the prince or the poem. In: Hoy C (ed) William Shakespeare, Hamlet. Norton, New York

Lindemann E 1944 Symptomatology and management of acute grief. American Journal of Psychiatry 101: 141–148

Littlewood J 1992 Aspects of grief bereavement in adult life. Routledge, London

Lloyd M 1992 Tools for many trades: reaffirming the use of grief counselling by health, welfare and pastoral workers. British Journal of Guidance Counselling 20: 150–163

McDermott JF, Porter D 1989 The efficacy of poetry therapy: a computerized content analysis of the death poetry of Emily Dickinson. Psychiatry 4: 462–468

McKenna HP 1997 Nursing models and theories. Routledge, London

Marris P 1986 Loss and change. Routledge & Kegan Paul, London

Marwitt SJ 1991 DSM 3, grief reactions, and a call for revision. Professional Psychology: Research and Practice 22: 75–79

Messer D, Meldrum C 1995 Psychology for nurses and health care professionals. Prentice-Hall, London

Morse JM 1995 Exploring the theoretical basis of nursing using advanced techniques of concept analysis. Advances in Nursing Science 17: 31–46

Morse JM, Anderson G, Bottorff JL et al 1992 Exploring empathy: a conceptual fit for nursing practice. Image 24: 273–280

Murphy P, Perry K 1988 Hidden grievers. Death Studies 12: 451–462

Oremland JD 1983 Death and transformation in Hamlet. Psychoanalytical Inquiry 3: 485–511

Parkes CM 1976 Bereavement studies of grief in adult life. Penguin, Harmondsworth

Pollock GH 1975 Mourning and memorialization through music. Annals of Psychoanalysis 3: 423–436

Prigerson HG, Frank E, Kasl SV et al 1995 Complicated grief and bereavement-related depression as distinct disorders: preliminary empirical validation in elderly bereaved spouses. American Journal of Psychiatry 152: 22–30

Ramsey RW, Heringa PM, Boorsma I 1974 A case study: homosexuality in the Netherlands. In: Loraine JA (ed) Understanding homosexuality: its biological and psychological bases. American Elsevier, New York

Raphael B 1984 The anatomy of bereavement: a handbook for the caring professions. Hutchinson, London

Remondet JH, Hansson RO 1987 Assessing a widow's grief: a short index. Journal of Gerontological Nursing 13: 31–34

Richardson R 1987 Death dissection and the destitute. Routledge & Kegan Paul, London

Robinson DS, McKenna HP 1998 Loss: an analysis of a concept of particular interest to nursing. Journal of Advanced Nursing 27: 779–784

Rodgers BL 1994 Concepts, analysis and the development of nursing knowledge: the evolutionary cycle. In: Smith PJ (ed) Models, theories and concepts. Blackwell Scientific, Oxford

Rosenblatt PC 1993 Grief: the social context of private feelings. In: Stroebe MS, Stroebe W, Hansson RO (eds) Handbook of bereavement. Cambridge University Press, Cambridge

Scruby LS, Sloan JA 1989 Evaluation of bereavement interventions. Canadian Journal of Public Health 80: 394–398

Shaughnessy MF 1985 The best kept secret in creativity. Creative Child and Adult Quarterly 10: 223–232

Shuchter SR, Zisook S 1993 The course of normal grief. In: Stroebe MS, Stroebe W, Hansson RO (eds) Handbook of bereavement. Cambridge University Press, Cambridge

Siegal RA, Hoefer DD 1981 Bereavement counselling for gay individuals. American Journal of Psychotherapy 35: 517–525

Silver D 1983 The dark lady: sibling loss and mourning in the Shakespearean sonnets. Psychoanalytical Inquiry 3: 513–527

Solari-Twadell PA, Bunkers S, Wang C et al 1995 The pinwheel model of bereavement. IMAGE: Journal of Nursing Scholarship 27: 323–326

Sourvinou-Inwood C 1981 to die and enter the house of Hades: Homer, before and after. In: Whaley J (ed) Mirrors of mortality: studies in the social history of death. Europa Publications, London

Stroebe M, van den Bout J, Schut H 1994 Myths and misconceptions about bereavement: the opening of a debate. Omega 29: 187–203

Stroebe MS, Stroebe W 1991 Does 'grief work' work? Journal of Consulting and Clinical Psychology 59: 479–482

Stylianos SK, Vachon MLS 1993 The role of social support in bereavement. In: Stroebe MS, Stroebe W, Hansson RO (eds) Handbook of bereavement. Cambridge University Press, Cambridge

Sullivan KA 1997 The grief that dare not speak its name: issues of openness and support in homosexual bereavement. Unpublished PhD Thesis, University of Ulster

Walker LO, Avant KC 1995 Strategies for theory construction in nursing, 3rd edn. Appleton & Lange, Norwalk, CT

Walter T 1999 On bereavement: the culture of grief. Open University Press, Buckingham

Whitam F 1983 Culturally invariable properties of male homosexuality. Archives of Sexual Behavior 12: 207–226

Worden JW 1991 Grief counselling and grief therapy, 2nd edn. Tavistock, London

Wortman C, Silver R 1989 The myths of coping with loss. Journal of Consulting and Clinical Psychology 57: 349–357

Zisook S, Devaul RA, Click MA 1982 Measuring symptoms of grief and bereavement. American Journal of Psychiatry 139: 1590–1593

Diversity or divisiveness? A critical analysis of hope

Cheryl L. M. Nekolaichuk

EDITORIAL

Arguments about the centrality of concepts to nursing are not new; neither is the claim made in this book that the concepts focused herein are representative of the 20 most crucial or central concepts to nurses and nursing. Nevertheless, if we were to select concepts that are 'close to our hearts' and/or concepts that can be regarded as the 'raison d'être' for nurses, then hope would be selected without a moment's hesitation. In search of a deeper understanding, if one were to trace the etymological origins of these central concepts, then incidents of them in historical, mythological and theological literature should be examined. One might speculate that the concepts that occur throughout and within these literatures might have an inherent importance and thus centrality to human existence. It follows a reasonable chain of logical reasoning, then, given the inextricably human nature of nursing, that the centrality of these concepts would be translated into nursing. Cheryl's chapter reminds us that, despite this centrality, conceptualizations of hope are far from consistent or unequivocal. Furthermore, and importantly, Cheryl's chapter also reminds us that this conceptual confusion not only presents challenges to nurses (and nursing epistemologists/theorists) but, perhaps paradoxically, may also lead to a deeper understanding of hope.

Two critical caveats arise here. First, the literature is consistent in showing the (critical) therapeutic value of hope in clinical scenarios and lived experiences, and is beginning to illustrate the variety of ways in which hope can be inspired and maintained in patients. Accordingly, one needs to ask, does the inspiration of hope then become a duty of the nurse? Is it and would it be considered remiss of nurses to be ignorant of such a duty? Second, and accepting the cogency of the first caveat, given the emerging literature that speaks to hope as a finite resource within the nurse, there is a parallel duty upon the individual practitioner and, equally importantly, upon the employing organization to ensure that mechanisms, processes and time are provided for nurses to maintain their own hope level. Unfortunately, the theory in this area is very underdeveloped and these processes are not well understood (although a tentative relationship between engaging in clinical supervision and maintaining hope in the practitioner has been purported). This obviously points to some of the key research questions that need to be asked next in the substantive area of hope and hope inspiration.

INTRODUCTION

> Hope is an expectation greater than zero of achieving a goal.
> Stotland 1969, p. 2

> I guess hope is the art of living to me, hope is to get to the point... to kick that field goal that wins the game... hope is just to keep on going.
> Dave – a cancer patient

What does hope mean to you? This question has enticed and puzzled many people in their search for the definitive answer. Both Ezra Stotland (1969) and Dave, a cancer patient, quoted above, provide their unique perspectives about hope. They each describe a link between hope and goals, yet they speak about them in very different ways: Stotland describes the link between hope and goal attainment in abstract terms, while Dave uses a football metaphor to describe his personal experience. Two contrasting questions emerge in response to these different perspectives:

- Who is ultimately right?
- How might these different perspectives help us better understand the concept of hope?

The first question stems from the philosophical orientations of positivism and postpositivism, positions that emphasize the delineation or approximation of a single objective reality and subsequently the development of a unifying framework for a concept. The second question stems from the interpretive/constructivist perspective, in which reality is socially constructed; a concept may be based upon multiple personal constructions, resulting in different meanings for different people. Constructivists further suggest that the major goal is to understand these multiple constructions, rather than to search for an objective reality (Mertens 1998).

These philosophical differences underpin different approaches for conducting concept analyses. Proponents of a unifying framework for concepts, such as Walker and Avant (1988, 1995), essentially fall within the positivist/postpositivist camps. Opponents to this perspective, such as Wuest (1994) and Morse (1995), with apparent interpretive/constructivist leanings, question the validity of providing a unifying framework for complex concepts such as hope. Rather, they argue for the need to examine concepts within a context that reflects the diversity of human experience.

The purpose of this chapter is to provide a conceptual analysis of hope. This analysis is based on a review of the hope literature, with a primary focus on *how hope is conceptualized in research*. Rather than using a traditional concept analysis approach, a critical analysis of current understandings about hope in research will be presented, integrating ideas proposed by Wuest (1994) and Morse (1995). This critique is not intended to provide an exhaustive summary of all research in this area. Rather, using a sampling of publications, three key points will be highlighted:

- **Conceptual differences regarding hope are inevitable, given the complexity of the concept. These differences can enrich, yet also complicate, understandings about hope.**
- **A complex concept such as hope cannot be simplified to a universal definition or conceptual framework. Thus, it is imperative to situate oneself amidst the complexity of perspectives.**
- **Current hope definitions and frameworks have varying origins and degrees of rigour. There is an urgent need to develop systematic approaches for evaluating the hope literature and selecting appropriate frameworks for the intended research context(s).**

To highlight these key points, this analysis will be presented within three primary subsections: trends within hope research 1983–2004; synthesis of hope frameworks; and dichotomies of hope. Prior to this discussion, the methods used for this critique will be presented. This chapter will close with a synopsis of current understandings, outlining challenges for conceptualizing hope in research as well as questions for further reflection.

PARAMETERS AND METHODS USED FOR THE LITERATURE REVIEW

The types of publications included in this review were:

- research studies using quantitative, qualitative or combined research methods, including journal articles, books and monographs
- publications focusing on concept development and analysis, including both deductive and inductive approaches.

Publications were identified primarily through library holdings, as well as three major databases (MEDLINE, PsycINFO and CINAHL). The following criteria were used for the selection of these publications:

- 'hope' as a key search term and/or inclusion of the word 'hope' in the publication title or abstract (other hope derivatives, such as hopefulness, were not intentionally searched but may be included where pertinent)
- predominant focus on hope
- published between 1983 and 2004.

References published before 1983, as well as theoretical/philosophical publications, were not included in the sample but may be referred to in the discussion where relevant. Unpublished research and research focusing on 'hopelessness' were not included. An analysis of other linguistic derivatives of hope (e.g. hopeful, hoping, hopefully) is beyond the scope of this review (see Elliott & Olver 2002 for discussion of discursive properties of hope). A review of the different ways that hope is used in non-research settings, such as clinical practice, the creative arts or different cultures, is an important area for further exploration but is also beyond the scope of this discussion.

SEARCHING FOR THE 'DEFINITIVE ANSWER'? TRENDS WITHIN HOPE RESEARCH 1983–2004

> *It isn't answers that make a scientist, it's questions. ... Science is a way of making more and more meaningful questions. The answers are important mainly in leading us to new questions.*
>
> *Wald 1961*

The concept of hope is not new, its importance being traced back to ancient times (see, for example, Averill et al 1990 for a historical overview of hope). Despite this long-term interest, it is only within the past two decades that hope has become a focal point of disciplined inquiry. This renewed interest in hope as a field of inquiry has resulted in a proliferation of research studies across a wide spectrum of populations. Initial studies focused on people with illness, including cancer patients

(Stoner & Keampfer 1985, Hinds & Martin 1988, Herth 1989, Owen 1989), the critically ill (Miller 1989, 1991, Perakyla 1991, Cutcliffe 1996), terminally ill (Dufault & Martocchio 1985, Hall 1990, Herth 1990a, Cutcliffe 1995), and chronically ill (Foote et al 1990, Raleigh 1992, Cutcliffe & Grant 2001). This body of research, focusing on hope in illness, has continued to expand (Kylma et al 2001, Ebright & Lyon 2002, Elliott & Oliver 2002, Lin et al 2003). Paralleling this growth, the net has widened to capture non-illness populations, such as healthy adults (Benzein et al 1998, Nekolaichuk et al 1999), college students (Averill et al 1990, Brackney & Westman 1992, Range & Penton 1994, Irving et al 1998, Onwuegbuzie & Snyder 2000), people from different cultures (Parse 1999, Benzein et al 2000) and children (Hicks & Holden 1994). More recently, the net has widened further still to include hope in certain lived experiences (e.g. bereavement counselling – Cutcliffe 2004).

Similar to sampling, the focal points and methodological approaches of research studies have also varied. A sample of studies published between 1983 and 2004 appears in Tables 12.1 and 12.2. Table 12.1 provides an overview of hope research themes and corresponding studies, organized under three methodological categories: quantitative, qualitative and combined approaches. Table 12.2 highlights the diversity of quantitative studies focusing on the relationships between hope and other concepts.

As shown in Table 12.1, within the *quantitative* realm there are five major research themes: concept development/analysis; descriptive; correlational; interventions; and biology of hope. In the first theme, measurement is a predominant focus, advancing concept development primarily through instrument development. This has resulted in a proliferation of measurement tools, with diverse theoretical underpinnings and varying degrees of psychometric soundness (see Farran et al 1995 for a detailed description of hope instruments). Apart from this predominant theme, most studies have been either descriptive, focusing on diverse populations such as the elderly (Farran & McCann 1989, Beckerman & Northrop 1996), adolescents with cancer (Hinds et al 1999) and caregivers (Borneman et al 2002), or correlational, exploring the relationships between hope and other concepts (Table 12.2). Within the past decade, researchers have begun to focus on the development and evaluation of hope-oriented interventions, despite being limited by the developmental infancy of hope instruments. The fifth theme, the biological basis of hope, has remained a relatively underdeveloped field of interest.

Within the *qualitative* realm, there are four major themes: concept development/analysis; descriptive; interventions; and relationships with other concepts (Table 12.1). Researchers have primarily focused on understanding and clarifying hope through concept development and analysis (see Table 12.5). Some have attempted to gain greater clarity by focusing on the meaning, lived experience or process-oriented nature of hope. Most studies on meaning have focused on either the individual (non-caregiver) or caregiver perspectives. A few researchers have moved beyond the individual to focus on the experience of hope within relationships (Wong-Wylie & Jevne 1997, Cutcliffe 1995, 2004; Cutcliffe & Grant 2001) or social contexts (Perakyla 1991), two areas in need of further research. As in the quantitative realm, some researchers have recently focused on hope-oriented interventions through the delineation of assessment frameworks and hope-enhancing strategies. A few researchers have attempted to explore relationships between hope and other concepts using qualitative methods. Other researchers have attempted to use complementary triangulated approaches, *combining quantitative and qualitative methods,* to deepen their understanding of hope (Table 12.1). These studies, although limited, have focused on four primary themes: concept development/analysis; descriptive; interventions; and relationships with other concepts. Given the complexity of hope, future research combining methodological approaches is warranted.

Across all three methodological categories, researchers have used a variety of conceptual frameworks to delineate the concept of hope. These vary from theoretical unidimensional frameworks, such as those of Stotland (1969) and Snyder (1995) to deductively derived (Farran et al 1995) and inductively derived (Dufault & Martocchio 1985) multidimensional frameworks. Some theoretical frameworks were developed through literature reviews (Miller 1983), while others were based on personal, philosophical and/or clinical perspectives (Stotland 1969) or adapted from existing theoretical frameworks (Snyder 1995). In some studies, the authors did not describe the conceptual framework that informed their research, making it difficult to evaluate the findings.

Accompanying this conceptual diversity, researchers have used numerous approaches for measuring and assessing hope. These approaches were often based on different conceptual frameworks, resulting in a proliferation of instruments and assessment guides (Table 12.3). This measurement diversity is most apparent within the quantitative correlational research theme (Table 12.2). As shown in this table, researchers have used a vast array of instruments to explore the relationships between hope and other concepts. In some cases, the number of different hope measures was almost as profuse as the number of studies (e.g. quality of life, social support, well-being).

The use of different conceptual frameworks and instruments makes it difficult, if not impossible, to conduct comparisons across studies. Despite this major shortcoming, cross-study comparisons are often made in the hope literature without clarifying the conceptual frameworks and/or hope measures that were used in each study. Further, links between hope and other concepts may be made on the basis of theoretical or personal frameworks that lack empirical support. **Although conceptual diversity can stimulate new thinking, it can also impede the research process, with careless interpretations and overgeneralizations.**

SUMMARY

Over the past 20 years, the field of hope research has grown substantially, in both the quantitative and qualitative realms. The use of combined approaches, though less frequent, is an interest for some researchers. Regardless of methodological approach, most research studies have been primarily descriptive in nature. Concept and instrument development have remained the primary areas of focus. The lack of psychometrically sound instruments has hampered the move towards intervention and outcome studies, despite a recent growth in this area.

This wealth of research has enriched, yet also complicated, our understanding of this complex phenomenon. Accompanying this growth in research, approaches for conceptualizing and operationalizing hope have grown exponentially, resulting in an overwhelming diversity of definitions, conceptual frameworks and measurement tools. This next section will further highlight these diverse conceptual approaches, to illustrate both the richness in and complexity of conceptualizing hope in research.

CONCEPTUAL CLARITY OR CONCEPTUAL CONFUSION? SYNTHESIS OF HOPE FRAMEWORKS

The most creative thinking occurs at the meeting places of disciplines. At the centre of any tradition, it is easy to become blind to alternatives. At the edges, where the lines are blurred, it is easier to imagine that the world might be different. Vision cam sometimes arise from confusion (Bateson 1989, p. 73, cited in Sandelowski 1994).

Many people have attempted to develop definitions, critical attributes and conceptual frameworks for hope (see Fowler 1995, for a sampling of hope definitions; also see Cutcliffe & Herth 2002 and Elliott & Olver 2002, for a review of publications delineating hope attributes). The terminology for describing hope frameworks has varied from models (Ersek 1992, Haase et al 1992, Bunston et al 1995) to concepts (Stephenson 1991, Hendricks-Ferguson 1997, Benzein & Saveman 1998b) to theories (Stotland 1969, Snyder 1995). For the purposes of this discussion, 'conceptual framework' will be used as an umbrella term for capturing these different perspectives.

Not only are the frameworks diverse, the approaches for conceptualizing hope have also varied, including both deductive (Table 12.4) and inductive (Table 12.5) methods. The publications included in Tables 12.4 and 12.5 encompass the continuum from initial concept development to analysis (see Morse 1995 for discussion of different concept analysis approaches based on concept maturity) and were limited to literature reviews, concept analyses and research studies. A discussion of theoretical, philosophical, theological and personal descriptions of hope was beyond the scope of this review (see Pilkington 1999 for detailed discussion of these perspectives; also see Jacoby 1993 for excellent description of psychological theories of hope). A summary of these approaches follows.

DEDUCTIVE APPROACHES

A number of people have used deductive approaches for concept development and analysis (Table 12.4). Initially, informal approaches, using non-specific literature reviews based on theoretical frameworks, were most common, given the limited research on hope (Miller 1983, McGee 1984). The use of informal deductive approaches for conceptualizing hope has continued to grow with the expansion of hope research, focusing on specific areas such as the critically ill (Brown 1989), nursing/nursing research (Kindleman 1993, Kylma et al 1997), oncology (Yates 1993), neuroscience nursing (Fowler 1995) and psychiatry (Nunn 1996). Apart from one study using meta-analysis (Kylma et al 1997), most of these reviews did not specify the approach for synthesizing the literature, making it difficult to assess the credibility of findings.

Since 1990, a number of people have conducted formal concept analyses to further clarify the concept. As shown in Table 12.4, all of these analyses were either based on or adapted from the work of Walker and Avant (1983, 1988, 1995). In keeping with this method, originally developed by Wilson (1963), a stepwise approach was used to develop a unifying definition and critical attributes for hope (Stephenson 1991, Forbes 1994, O'Connor 1996, Cutcliffe 1997, Hendricks-Ferguson 1997). Haase et al (1992) extended Walker and Avant's (1983) approach by creating a simultaneous concept analysis method, analysing hope concurrently with three other concepts: spiritual perspective, acceptance and self-transcendence. As a further modification, Benzein and Saveman (1998b) identified seven critical attributes without developing an operational definition.

INDUCTIVE APPROACHES

In contrast to these deductive approaches, a number of researchers have used inductive methods for conceptualizing hope (Table 12.5). These methods have primarily included qualitative approaches, such as grounded theory, ethnography, ethnonursing and interviews/document analysis. Morse and Doberneck (1995) used their own method for concept development, while Wang (2000) adopted a human science perspective using Parse's (1998, 1999) theory of human becoming. Some authors used quantitative approaches, such as surveys (Bunston et al 1995) and questionnaires (Farran & Popovich 1990), while others have used combined methods, integrating survey designs with qualitative approaches (Averill et al 1990, Nekolaichuk et al 1999). Regardless of method, all of these conceptual frameworks were derived from empirical data with different samples, ranging from adolescence to the elderly, the ill to the well, and patients to caregivers; as well as across different cultural groups. The specificity of these samples, as well as the limited sample size in many cases (particularly qualitative studies), limits the nomothetic generalizability of these frameworks without further validation studies.

SUMMARY

Regardless of conceptual framework, most researchers share a common goal of deepening our understanding of this complex concept. Despite this common vision, a universal definition for hope does not exist. Rather, a diversity of approaches for conceptualizing hope has emerged. Deductive approaches vary in their rigour, as many informal analyses do not explicitly state the methods used for the analysis, making it difficult to evaluate the credibility of findings. Formal deductive approaches exclusively used Walker and Avant's (1983, 1988, 1995) method for concept analysis, which may be limiting. Inductive approaches, though varied, were primarily based on qualitative methods using small and specific samples, thus limiting nomothetic generalizability of findings.

Regardless of conceptual approach, further validation is required to enhance the credibility and utility of these frameworks. This conceptual diversity offers considerable flexibility in research design directions. At the same time, however, it presents a noble challenge to anyone pursuing an interest in this area. A substantial challenge is to be able to position oneself amidst these diverse frameworks without becoming disoriented or discouraged. The following section will provide an overview of some competing perspectives about hope.

LIVING IN THE 'SPACE BETWEEN': DICHOTOMIES OF HOPE

> *As we move between the dichotomies of life, we feel the pulse of life, the pull homeward. We feel the tension between giving up and going on. ... Hope happens in the space between. ... Between the concrete and the intangible. Between evidence and intuition. Between religion and spirituality. Between doubt and faith.*
>
> *Jevne 1994, pp. 134–135*

As a result of these diverse frameworks, differences in opinion about hope abound in the literature. These differences can be characterized by the following questions:

- Is hope a universal or a uniquely personal experience?
- Is hope a unidimensional or a multidimensional concept?
- Is hope a tangible or an intangible experience?
- Is hope time-bound or time-free?
- Is hope predictable or unpredictable?
- Is hope valuable or worthless?
- Is hope realistic or unrealistic?

IS HOPE A UNIVERSAL OR A UNIQUELY PERSONAL EXPERIENCE?

Many people have strived to develop a unifying hope definition or framework that would accurately depict this complex concept (Stephenson 1991, Haase et al 1992, Cutcliffe 1997, Hendricks-Ferguson 1997). Recently, some people have questioned this notion, suggesting that hope is grounded in personal experience and therefore defies a singular definition or framework (Jevne 1991, 1994, Yates 1993, Fowler 1995, Morse 1995, Benzein & Saveman 1998b, Nekolaichuk et al 1999, Parse 1999, Wang 2000, Elliott & Olver 2002). Proponents of this perspective argue for the need to understand hope 'as a process of human understanding' (Wang 2000, p. 251), by using 'phenomenological descriptions or ethnographic accounts' (Yates 1993, p. 702) and uncovering 'as many different interpretations as possible' (Benzein & Saveman 1998b, p. 327). Similarly, Elliott and Olver (2002, p. 189) have developed a preliminary taxonomy of hope, in place of a single framework, in which hope may be located within a set of 'dualist constructs'.

Others have described this tension between universal (abstract) and unique (personal) frameworks (Herth & Cutcliffe 2002), which, in the social science field, can be traced back to the mid-1950s. At that time, Charles Osgood and his associates (1957) challenged their contemporaries, who were in the throws of behaviourism, by proposing an innovative method (the semantic differential technique) for capturing the connotative meaning of stimuli (e.g. concepts). Osgood et al contrasted *connotative meaning*, the personal meaning that individuals attribute to stimuli, with *denotative meaning*, which is the abstract, universal attributes assigned to stimuli. For example, the denotative meaning for the word 'apple' may include universal descriptions such as red- or yellow-skinned fruit with white pulp. In contrast, the connotative meaning for the word 'apple' would be based on a person's experience. If a person bites into a rotten apple, then the connotative meaning may involve descriptions such as unpleasant, distasteful and upsetting. Thus, concepts may have both universal (denotative) and personal (connotative) meanings.

Many of the deductively derived conceptual frameworks in this review represent the denotative meaning of hope. Inductively derived frameworks may be more representative of the connotative meaning of hope, although many of these frameworks are abstractions of personal experience. Regardless of its derivation, any given framework provides an orientation for understanding the complex phenomenon of hope. Within research communities, it is important to have some way to structure a concept, even if that structure is a non-structured orientation (e.g. a 'personally embedded' or socially constructed perspective).

IS HOPE A UNIDIMENSIONAL OR A MULTIDIMENSIONAL CONCEPT?

Initial conceptualizations depicted hope as a unidimensional concept. Stotland (1969), for example, proposed a hope theory that focused primarily on the cognitive realm, emphasizing goal attainment. Snyder (1995) extended Stotland's original theory by suggesting that hope consists of two distinct cognitive components, agency (will) and pathways (ways). Although Snyder did not discount the role of emotions in the experience, he clearly viewed emotions as a 'by-product' of effective goal setting. McGee (1984) also proposed a linear, probability-based model apparently influenced by Stotland's work. She conceptualized hope along a continuum, ranging from 'unjustifiably hopeful' to 'unrealistically hopeless'.

In contrast to these unidimensional frameworks, most people have conceptualized multidimensional frameworks for hope (see, for example, Cutcliffe & Herth 2002). As an example, Dufault and Martocchio (1985) developed one of the most frequently cited inductively derived frameworks. They suggested that hope consists of two spheres (generalized and particularized hope) and six dimensions (affective, cognitive, behavioural, affiliative, temporal and contextual). Farran et al (1995) described a deductively derived multidimensional model consisting of four critical processes: experiential, spiritual/transcendent, rational (cognitive) and relational. Although most people view hope as a multidimensional concept, it is important to acknowledge that, for some people, hope may essentially be a unidimensional experience or that the emphasis on different dimensions may change over time.

In a recent telephone survey (Nekolaichuk et al 2002; $n = 1203$), when people were asked to choose the single best descriptor of hope from seven possible choices, the three most frequent responses were 'having a positive outlook' (39.3%), 'having a deep inner faith' (16.1%) and 'having goals or plans' (13.5%). In a subanalysis by age group, young adults (18–24 years) selected 'having goals or plans' more often than any other age group (23.4% of young adults). In contrast, older people (65+ years) were more likely to describe their hope as 'having a deep inner faith' (24.8%) than young adults (7.2%). One possible reason for these observed differences is that younger people may be more focused on specific goals, such as furthering their education or developing a career, than older people. As people age, they may shift their emphasis from one dimension of hope (e.g. goal-orientation) to another (e.g. faith orientation). Further research is warranted to explore people's perceptions about hope across different age groups and time.

IS HOPE A TANGIBLE OR AN INTANGIBLE EXPERIENCE?

To operationalize the concept, a number of people have developed hope measures based on differing conceptual frameworks. Instrument development is still in its infancy; this is a perspective that is shared by others in the field (e.g. Jacoby 1993, Farran et al 1995, Pilkington 1999, Herth & Cutcliffe 2002). Some people, such as Wang (2000, p. 249), have questioned whether hope should be measured at all. Rather, Wang believes that hope is uniquely structured by each individual and should thus be 'understood and supported rather than assessed, measured, and intervened on'.

There are at least three inherent problems with current hope measurement approaches. First, some measures may be more relevant to and representative of the underlying concept than others. For example, the use of a tool to measure hopelessness (as an indirect measure of hope) may be less valid than one specifically targeted to hope. Second, many of these measures vary in psychometric soundness, often being validated on restricted samples. Despite this limitation, some measures may be used in contexts for which they were not intended, further compromising the validity of findings. Third, all these instruments are only an approximation of the underlying concept. No instrument will ever be able to completely capture the concept in its entirety. Unfortunately, findings based on these instruments are often interpreted as if the instrument were measuring the complete concept.

These inherent problems regarding measurement relate to the intangibility of the hope concept. The experience of hope is comprised of both tangible (visible) and intangible (invisible) components. Measurement tools have succeeded, to some degree, in capturing the tangible components of hope (e.g. people's expressed hopes, hopeful behaviours, hopeful thoughts, hopeful feelings). They have not succeeded, and perhaps never will, in capturing the inner, intangible hope experience. Nekolaichuk et al (1999) attempted to do this with the development of a research tool for measuring the personal (connotative) meaning of hope. Intangible components of hope may be better accessed or made visible through the symbolic realm, such as artful questioning, story, metaphor and symbolism (Jevne 1993, Edey & Jevne 2003). To obtain a comprehensive understanding of the experience, hope measures are best combined with qualitative approaches, bearing in mind the limitations of any measurement tool or assessment framework. It is also important to acknowledge that there may be some intangible aspects of hope that may never be uncovered, regardless of the approach used.

IS HOPE TIME-BOUND OR TIME-FREE?

One of the most commonly cited attributes of hope is that it is future-oriented (Nowotny 1989, Owen 1989, Herth 1991, 1992, Haase et al 1992, Rustoen 1995, Cutcliffe 1997, Hendricks-Ferguson 1997, Benzein & Saveman 1998b). A number of people have suggested an alternative perspective, conceptualizing hope as being influenced by the past, the present and the future (Dufault & Martocchio 1985, Stephenson 1991, Nekolaichuk & Bruera 1998, Jevne et al 1999). Others have proposed the notion of non-time-specific hopes (Dufault & Martocchio 1985, Yates 1993) or generalized hopes that provide a protective intangible umbrella without being connected to specific goals or time (Dufault & Martocchio 1985). In contrast, Post-White et al (1996) described the temporal relationship of hope as living in the present, one of five central themes identified by cancer patients ($n = 32$). Based on a sample of 45 people living with HIV/AIDS, Ezzy (2000) offered yet another perspective in which the relationship between hope and time varied, depending upon individual illness narratives. Clearly, this area warrants further research.

IS HOPE PREDICTABLE OR UNPREDICTABLE?

There are two competing perspectives regarding the relationship between hope and predictability (uncertainty). From the first perspective, uncertainty is viewed as an inherent part of the hope experience. Some have theoretically conceptualized uncertainty as an antecedent to hope, suggesting that hope only arises from adversity (Marcel 1962, Fromm 1968, Moltmann 1975). Others have described uncertainty or related terms, such as anticipation, probability or control, as an element (Stotland

1969, Miller & Powers 1988) or attribute (Miller 1989, Nowotny 1991, Stephenson 1991, Haase et al 1992, Farran et al 1995) of hope. From the second perspective, some people have theorized that certainty, as opposed to uncertainty, is an integral component of the hope experience. Korner (1970), for example, has suggested that hope is associated with an 'assumed certainty' that the dreaded will not happen, much like the concept of faith. Snyder (1995) has further proposed that hope is associated with clear goals and definite pathways for achieving these goals.

The question arises as to whether or not these two seemingly opposing views might be integrated. Based on Nekolaichuk et al's (1999) three-dimensional hope model, predictability in some aspects of a person's life may influence uncertainty in other parts of life. If, for example, a person is experiencing uncertainty due to an illness, then there may be other predictable aspects that could enhance a person's willingness to risk and potentially facilitate the coping process. Although some preliminary work has been done through theory development (Mishel 1988, 1990), concept analysis (Morse & Penrod 1999, Penrod 2001) and empirical studies (Wonghongkul et al 2000), further research to advance our understandings of this complex relationship is needed.

IS HOPE VALUABLE OR WORTHLESS?

Throughout the centuries, people have debated the value of hope. From the ancient Greek myth of Pandora's box to Nietzsche's view of hope as the 'worst of evils' (Nietzsche 1878/1986, cited in Averill et al 1990), many have questioned its value. Kant (1781/1966, cited in Averill et al 1990, p. 5) offered a compromise view of hope as 'a disease only if it leads one to act immorally or imprudently, but that it is good if it inspires one to lead a moral, rational life'. Others have philosophically affirmed its worth, describing hope as an indispensable factor in treatment (Menninger 1959) and a curative factor (Yalom 1985). Although not explicitly stated, most hope studies in the past 20 years share a common assumption that hope has an underlying goodness factor.

Despite this resounding endorsement, it is important to acknowledge that not everyone experiences or values hope in the same way. As Osgood et al's (1957) framework for understanding connotative meaning suggests, personal experiences shape the way in which individuals interpret personal meanings of concepts. It is possible that some people may view hope in a negative light, as illustrated by one elderly gentleman with a terminal illness who described hope as 'a mother of fools' (Nekolaichuk 2003). This case example, although seemingly rare, reinforces the need to explore hope from the individual's perspective.

IS HOPE REALISTIC OR UNREALISTIC?

Many of the concept analyses of hope identified a reality-based attribute for hope (Miller & Powers 1988, Morse & Doberneck 1995, Hendricks-Ferguson 1997, Benzein & Saveman 1998b). Despite this frequent endorsement, a number of questions, which others have also raised (Jevne 1993, Yates 1993), need to be considered:

- How do we assess whether or not a person's hope is realistic or unrealistic?
- Upon whose reality do we base our assessment?
- Can hope ever be unrealistic?

Depending upon the philosophical orientation, people may find themselves responding to these questions in different ways. For example, from the positivist/postpositivist perspectives, an objective reality (or an approximation of one) may be used as a guide for evaluating realistic and unrealistic hopes. In contrast, from a social constructivist perspective, it might be argued that hope is grounded in each person's unique experience or reality.

SUMMARY

Based on these guiding questions, debates regarding the nature of hope may be categorized according to the following seven themes: universality, dimensionality, intangibility, temporality, predictability, value-based and reality-based. For each theme, a working assumption about hope can be identified (Table 12.6). **These underlying assumptions, provide a guide for conceptualizing hope yet also pose enormous challenges to people interested in pursuing research in this area.** The final section of this review will highlight three challenges for conceptualizing hope, as well as provide questions for further reflection.

NAVIGATING THE FIELD: THE CHALLENGES OF CONCEPTUALIZING HOPE IN RESEARCH

> *The proof for you is in the things I have made – how they look to your mind's eye, whether they satisfy your sense of style and craftsmanship, whether you believe them, and whether they appeal to your heart.*
>
> *Sandelowski 1994, p. 61*

At the outset of this chapter, three key points were highlighted. These key points may be rephrased as three primary challenges for conceptualizing hope in research.

1. To be aware of the vast amount of hope research, encompassing diverse conceptual frameworks and methods, recognizing their strengths and limitations
2. To be able to situate yourself amid the diverse opinions regarding the conceptualization of hope rather than identifying a universal framework
3. To develop a systematic approach for selecting a credible, rigorous conceptual framework that meets the needs of the context in which you practise (do

research), acknowledging that no framework will ever completely capture the concept in its totality.

A discussion of each of these challenges follows.

CHALLENGE 1: EXPLORING THE POSSIBILITIES

The first challenge is to be aware of the diverse conceptual frameworks for hope, acknowledging both their strengths and limitations. Despite the overwhelming growth in hope research over the past 20 years, a number of limitations were identified earlier in this chapter:

- the varying degrees of rigour for conceptual frameworks
- the lack of well-developed psychometrically sound instruments
- the inability to make cross-study comparisons because of differing conceptual frameworks and instruments, despite the tendency to do so
- the potential for overgeneralization of findings and the lack of clarity, in some studies, regarding the conceptual framework(s) used.

Pilkington (1999) raises a serious concern regarding the number and variety of borrowed theories for guiding hope research, which she described as 'theoretical eclecticism'. In contrast, Paley (1996) advocates the need to examine concepts within the context of theories. He implies that theoretical eclecticism is a natural evolution of studying complex phenomena. He further suggests that lines of research evolve from specific theories, the longevity of a theory often being determined by its credibility or the interest that it generates. **Although theoretical eclecticism has broadened our views of hope, a primary concern in the hope literature is the proliferation and use of diverse conceptual frameworks that have varying degrees of rigour.**

CHALLENGE 2: FINDING YOUR PLACE IN THE FIELD

To work effectively in this area, a second challenge is to be able to position yourself amid differing opinions about hope. To illustrate these differing perspectives, each of the themes outlined earlier in this chapter may be characterized by distinct polarities or dichotomies of hope (Table 12.7). As you read through the list in Table 12.7, consider the following questions:

- To which side of the polarity are you drawn?
- What are some of your reasons for selecting one end of the continuum over the other?

In some cases your choice may be very clear, while in other cases it may be more difficult. The clearer you are about your position, the easier it will be for you to select a conceptual framework that fits your needs and the context in which you work. Once you have articulated your assumptions about hope, the selection of a conceptual framework still presents a noble challenge.

CHALLENGE 3: EVALUATING THE OPTIONS

Given the multiplicity of frameworks, a third substantive challenge is to be able to critique the literature to discern the types and merit of frameworks that informed the research. As shown in Table 12.8, there are a number of factors to consider when selecting a conceptual framework. Some of these revolve around the underlying assumptions of the framework, as previously discussed. Others refer to the nature of derivation, transferability, validation and contributions to the literature. Ultimately, the selection of a framework is dependent upon your personal orientation, as well as its appropriateness for the context and population in which it is being applied.

CONCLUSION

Diversity or divisiveness? Does the proliferation of conceptual frameworks contribute to the literature by offering a variety of unique perspectives or does it create divisions, dissonance and potential chaos? The complexity of hope eludes simplification, inevitably leading to diverse frameworks and opinions. Exposure to diverse perspectives can stimulate new thought and serve as a catalyst for further research. It can also lead to confusion and chaos, especially when frameworks have varying degrees of rigour. Rather than searching for a universal framework, systematic approaches for sifting through and evaluating these differing perspectives need to be developed, to properly inform researchers and ensure a continuation of disciplined inquiry in the hope research field. Despite recent advances, there are still many questions to be answered. In closing, the following questions are offered for further thought and reflection:

- Should hope be defined? Is it even possible to define it? Are there some parts of the experience that are undefinable?
- By striving to define hope, do we lose its essence? Can we find a balance between defining/operationalizing hope and preserving its essence?
- How can we live with the ambiguity of a concept that appears to have such a vital role in life, yet remains elusive even after all these years of inquiry?

ACKNOWLEDGEMENTS

I would like to gratefully acknowledge the many patients, clients, students and participants in my clinical, teaching and research practices who have helped shape my thoughts about hope over the past 15 years. A special thanks to my colleagues on the Hope Research Advisory Committee, Hope Foundation of Alberta, for our countless discussions and debates about this complex concept:

Drs Jeanette Boman, Ceinwen Cumming, Ronna Jevne, Dianne Kieren, Sharon Moore, Carol Vogler and Ms Sharon Matthias. An additional thanks to Dr Ronna Jevne for initially enticing me into the field of hope and for her ongoing mentorship..

REFERENCES

Adams VH, Jackson JS 2000 The contribution of hope to the quality of life among aging African Americans: 1980–1992. International Journal of Aging and Human Development 50: 279–295

Averill JR, Caitlin G, Chon KK 1990 Rules of hope. Springer–Verlag, New York

Ballard A, Green T, McCaa A, Logsdon MC 1997 A comparison of the level of hope in patients with newly diagnosed and recurrent cancer. Oncology Nursing Forum 24: 899–904

Bateson MC 1989 Composing a life. Plume, New York

Bays CL 2001 Older adults' descriptions of hope after a stroke. Rehabilitation Nursing 26: 18–27

Beck A, Weissman A, Lester D, Trexler L 1974 The measurement of pessimism: the hopelessness scale. Journal of Consulting and Clinical Psychology 42: 861–865

Beckerman A, Northrop C 1996 Hope, chronic illness and the elderly. Journal of Gerontological Nursing 22 19–25

Benzein E, Saveman BI 1998a Nurses' perception of hope in patients with cancer: a palliative care perspective. Cancer Nursing 21: 10–16

Benzein E, Saveman BI 1998b One step towards the understanding of hope: a concept analysis. International Journal of Nursing Studies 35: 323–329

Benzein E, Norberg A, Saveman B 1998 Hope: future imagined reality. The meaning of hope as described by a group of healthy Pentecostalists. Journal of Advanced Nursing 28: 1063–1070

Benzein E, Saveman B, Norberg A 2000 The meaning of hope in healthy, non-religious Swedes. Western Journal of Nursing Research 22: 303–319

Benzein E, Norberg A, Saveman BI 2001 The meaning of the lived experience of hope in patients with cancer in palliative home care. Palliative Medicine 15: 117–126

Bland R, Darlington Y 2002 The nature and sources of hope: perspectives of family caregivers of people with serious mental illness. Perspectives in Psychiatric Care 38: 61–68

Borneman T, Stahl C, Ferrell BR, Smith D 2002 The concept of hope in family caregivers of cancer patients at home. Journal of Hospice and Palliative Nursing 4: 21–33

Brackney BE, Westman AS 1992 Relationships among hope, psychosocial development, and locus of control. Psychological Reports 70: 864–866

Brockopp D 1982 Cancer patients' perceptions of five psychosocial needs. Oncology Nursing Forum 9: 31–35

Brockopp DY, Hayko D, Davenport W, Winscott C 1989 Personal control and the needs for hope and information among adults diagnosed with cancer. Cancer Nursing 12: 112–16

Brown P 1989 The concept of hope: implications for care of the critically ill. Critical Care Nursing 9: 97–105

Bunston T, Mings D, Mackie A, Jones D 1995 Facilitating hopefulness: The determinants of hope. Journal of Psychosocial Oncology 13: 79–103

Cantrill H 1965 The pattern of human concerns. Rutgers University Press, New Brunswick, NJ

Carifio J, Rhodes L 2002 Construct validities and the empirical relationships between optimism, hope, self-efficacy, and locus of control. Work 19: 125-136

Carson V, Soeken KL, Grimm PM 1988 Hope and its relationship to spiritual well-being. Journal of Psychology and Theology 16: 159–167

Carson V, Soeken KL, Shanty J, Terry L 1990 Hope and spiritual well-being: essentials for living with AIDS. Perspectives in Psychiatric Care 26: 28–34

Chang LC, Li IC 2002 The correlation between perceptions of control and hope status in home-based cancer patients. Journal of Nursing Research 10: 73–81

Chapman KJ, Pepler C 1998 Coping, hope, and anticipatory grief in family members in palliative home care. Cancer Nursing 21: 226–234

Chen ML 2003 Pain and hope in patients with cancer. Cancer Nursing 26: 61–67

Christman NJ 1990 Uncertainty and adjustment during radiotherapy. Nursing Research 39: 17–20

Cousins N 1989 Head first: the biology of hope. EP Dutton, New York

Curry LA, Snyder CR, Cook DL et al 1997 The role of hope in academic and sport achievement. Journal of Personality and Social Psychology 73: 1257–1267

Cutcliffe JR 1995 How do nurses inspire and instill hope in terminally ill HIV patients? Journal of Advanced Nursing 22: 888–895

Cutcliffe J 1996 Critically ill patients' perspectives of hope. British Journal of Nursing 5: 674, 687–690

Cutcliffe JR 1997 Towards a definition of hope. International Journal of Psychiatric Nursing Research 3: 319–332

Cutcliffe JR 2004 The inspiration of hope in bereavement counselling. Jessica Kingsley Publishing, London

Cutcliffe JR, Grant G 2001 What are the principles and processes of inspiring hope in cognitively impaired older adults within a continuing care environment? Journal of Psychiatric and Mental Health Nursing 8: 427–436

Cutcliffe JR, Herth K 2002 The concept of hope in nursing. 1: Its origins, background and nature. British Journal of Nursing 11: 832–840

Daly J, Davidson PM, Jackson D 1999 The experience of hope for survivors of acute myocardial infarction (AMI): a qualitative study. Australian Journal of Advanced Nursing 16: 38–44

Davies H 1993 Hope as a coping strategy for the spinal cord injured individual. Axon 15: 40–46

Delvecchio Good MJ, Good BJ, Schaffer C, Lind SE 1990 American oncology and the discourse on hope. Culture, Medicine and Psychiatry 14: 59–79

Dufault K, Martocchio BC 1985 Hope: its spheres and dimensions. Nursing Clinics of North America 20: 379–391

Ebright PR, Lyon B 2002 Understanding hope and factors that enhance hope in women with breast cancer. Oncology Nursing Forum 29: 561–568

Edey W, Jevne RF 2003 Hope, illness and counselling practice: making hope visible. Canadian Journal of Counselling 37: 44–51

Elliott J, Olver I 2002 The discursive properties of 'Hope': a qualitative analysis of cancer patients' speech. Qualitative Health Research 12: 173–193

Elliott TR, Witty TE, Herrick S, Hoffman JT 1991 Negotiating reality after physical loss: hope, depression, and disability. Journal of Personality and Social Psychology 61: 608–613

Ersek M 1992 The process of maintaining hope in adults undergoing bone marrow transplantation for leukemia. Oncology Nursing Forum 19: 883–889

Ezzy D 2000 Illness narratives: time, hope and HIV. Social Science and Medicine 50: 605–617

Farran CJ 1985 A survey of community-based older adults: stressful life events, mediating variables, hope and health. Doctoral dissertation, Rush University, Chicago. Dissertation Abstracts International 46: 113B

Farran CJ, McCann J 1989 Longitudinal analysis of hope in community-based older adults. Archives in Psychiatric Nursing 3: 272–276

Farran CJ, Popovich JM 1990 Hope: a relevant concept for geriatric psychiatry. Archives of Psychiatric Nursing 4: 124–130

Farran CJ, Wilken C, Popovich JM 1992 Clinical assessment of hope. Issues in Mental Health Nursing 13: 129–138

Farran CJ, Herth KA, Popovich JM 1995 Hope and hopelessness: critical clinical constructs. Sage, Thousand Oaks, CA

Fehring RJ, Miller JF, Shaw C 1997 Spiritual well–being, religiosity, hope, depression, and other mood states in elderly people coping with cancer. Oncology Nursing Forum 24: 663–671

Flemming K 1997 The meaning of hope to palliative care cancer patients. International Journal of Palliative Nursing 3: 14–18

Foote AW, Piazza D, Holcombe J, Paul P, Daffin P 1990 Hope, self-esteem and social support in persons with multiple sclerosis. Journal of Neuroscience Nursing 22: 155–159

Forbes SB 1994 Hope: an essential human need. Journal of Gerontological Nursing 20: 5–10

Forsyth GL, Delaney KD, Gresham ML 1984 Vying for a winning position: management style of the chronically ill. Research in Nursing and Health 7: 181–188

Fowler SB 1995 Hope: implications for neuroscience nursing. Journal of Neuroscience Nursing 27: 298–304

Franken RE, Brown DJ 1996 The need to win is not adaptive: the need to win, coping strategies, hope and self-esteem. Personality and Individual Differences 20: 805–808

Fromm E 1968 The revolution of hope: toward a humanized technology. Harper & Row, New York

Gelling L 1999 The experience of hope for the relatives of head injured patients admitted to a neurosciences critical care unit: a phenomenological study. Nursing in Critical Care 4: 214–221

Gibson PR 1999 Hope in multiple chemical sensitivity: social support and attitude towards healthcare delivery as predictors of hope. Journal of Clinical Nursing 8: 275–283

Gottschalk LA, Gleser GC 1969 The measurement of psychological states through the content analysis of verbal behavior. University of California Press, Berkley, CA

Gottschalk LA, Fronczek J, Buchsbaum MS 1993 The cerebral neurobiology of hope and hopelessness. Psychiatry 56: 270–281

Grimm P 1984 The State–Trait Hope Inventory: a measurement project. Unpublished manuscript, University of Maryland School of Nursing

Haase JE, Britt T, Coward DD, Leidy NK, Penn PE 1992 Simultaneous concept analysis of spiritual perspective, hope, acceptance and transcendence. Image – the Journal of Nursing Scholarship 24: 141–147

Hall BA 1990 The struggle of the diagnosed terminally ill person to maintain hope. Nursing Science Quarterly 3: 177–184

Hall BA 1994 Ways of maintaining hope in HIV disease. Research in Nursing and Health 17: 283–293

Hatcher D, Macdonald J, Bauer C, Wilson C 1999 Hope, who needs it? A study of hope in older people in a residential care facility. Geriaction 17: 6–12

Hendricks-Ferguson VL 1997 An analysis of the concept of hope in the adolescent with cancer. Journal of Pediatric Oncology Nursing 14: 73–80

Herth K 1989 The relationship between level of hope and level of coping response and other variables in patients with cancer. Oncology Nursing Forum 16: 67–72

Herth K 1990a Fostering hope in terminally-ill people. Journal of Advanced Nursing 15: 1250–1259

Herth K 1990b Relationship of hope, coping styles, concurrent losses, and setting to grief resolution in the elderly widow(er). Research in Nursing and Health 13: 109–117

Herth K 1991 Development and refinement of an instrument to measure hope. Scholarly Inquiry for Nursing Practice: an International Journal 5: 39–51

Herth K 1992 Abbreviated instrument to measure hope: development and psychometric evaluation. Journal of Advanced Nursing 17: 1251–1259

Herth K 1993a Hope in the family caregiver of terminally ill people. Journal of Advanced Nursing 18: 538–548

Herth K 1993b Hope in older adults in community and institutional settings. Issues in Mental Health Nursing 14: 139–156

Herth K 2000 Enhancing hope in people with a first recurrence of cancer. Journal of Advanced Nursing 32: 1431–1441

Herth KA, Cutcliffe JR 2002 The concept of hope in nursing 6: research/education/policy/practice. British Journal of Nursing 11: 1404–1411

Heszen-Niejodek I, Gottschalk LA, Januszek M 1999 Anxiety and hope during the course of three different medical illnesses: a longitudinal study. Psychotherapy and Psychosomatics 68: 304–312

Hicks D, Holden C 1994 Tomorrow's world: children's hopes and fears for the future. Educational and Child Psychology 11: 63–70

Hinds PS 1984 Inducing a definition of 'hope' through the use of grounded theory methodology. Journal of Advanced Nursing 9: 357–362

Hinds PS 1988 Adolescent hopefulness in illness and health. Advances in Nursing Science 10: 79–88

Hinds PS, Gattuso J 1991 Measuring hopefulness in adolescents. Journal of Pediatric Oncology Nursing 8: 92–94

Hinds PS, Martin J 1988 Hopefulness and the self–sustaining process in adolescents with cancer. Nursing Research 37: 336–340

Hinds P, Quargnenti A, Fairclough D et al 1999 Hopefulness and its characteristics in adolescents with cancer. Western Journal of Nursing Research 21: 600–620

Holdcraft C, Williamson C 1991 Assessment of hope in psychiatric and chemically dependent patients. Applied Nursing Research 4: 129–134

Holt J 2000 Exploration of the concept of hope in the Dominican Republic. Journal of Advanced Nursing 32: 1116–1125

Irving LM, Snyder CR, Crowson JJ 1998 Hope and coping with cancer by college women. Journal of Personality 66: 195–214

Jacoby R 1993 'The miserable hath no other medicine, but only hope': some conceptual considerations on hope and stress. Stress Medicine 9: 61–69

Jakobsson A, Segesten K, Nordholm L, Oresland S 1993 Establishing a Swedish instrument measuring hope. Scandinavian Journal of Caring Science 7: 135–139

Jensen KP, Back-Pettersson S, Segesten K 2000 The meaning of 'not giving in' – lived experiences among women with breast cancer. Cancer Nursing 23: 6–11

Jevne RF 1991 It all begins with hope: patients, caregivers and the bereaved speak out. LuraMedia, San Diego, CA

Jevne R 1993 Enhancing hope in the chronically ill. Humane Medicine 9: 121–130

Jevne RF 1994 The voice of hope: heard across the heart of life. LuraMedia, San Diego, CA

Jevne RF, Nekolaichuk CL 2002 Dichotomies of hope. Hope and the helping relationship manual (revised), Hope Foundation of Alberta, Edmonton, Alberta

Jevne RF, Nekolaichuk C, Boman J 1999 Experiments in hope: blending art and science with service. Hope Foundation of Alberta, Edmonton, Alberta

Kant I 1781/1966 Critique of pure reason (trans FM Muller). Doubleday, Garden City, NY (Original work published 1781).

Kennett CE 2000 Participation in a creative arts project can foster hope in a hospice day centre. Palliative Medicine 14: 419–425

Kindleman B 1993 The concept of hope: implications for nursing. CAET Journal 12: 7–10, 29

Kirkpatrick H, Landeen J, Byrne C et al 1995 Hope and schizophrenia: clinicians identify hope-instilling strategies. Journal of Psychosocial Nursing 33: 15–19

Kirkpatrick H, Landeen J, Woodside H, Byrne C 2001 How people with schizophrenia build their hope. Journal of Psychosocial Nursing and Mental Health Services 39: 46–53

Koopmeiners L, Post-White J, Gutknecht S et al 1997 How healthcare professionals contribute to hope in patients with cancer. Oncology Nursing Forum 24: 1507–1513

Korner IN 1970. Hope as a method of coping. Journal of Consulting and Clinical Psychology 34: 134–139

Kylma J, Vehvilainen-Julkunen K 1997 Hope in nursing research: a meta-analysis of the ontological and epistemological foundations of research on hope. Journal of Advanced Nursing 25: 364–371

Kylma J, Vehvilainen–Julkunen K, Lahdevirta J 2001 Hope, despair and hopelessness in living with HIV/AIDS: a grounded theory study. Journal of Advanced Nursing 33: 764–775

Landeen J, Pawlick J, Woodside H et al 2000 Hope, quality of life, and symptom severity in individuals with schizophrenia. Psychiatric Rehabilitation Journal 23: 364–369

Laskiwski S, Morse JM 1993 The patient with spinal cord injury: the modification of hope and expressions of despair. Canadian Journal of Rehabilitation 6: 143–153

Leydon GM, Boulton M, Moynihan C et al 2000 Faith, hope, and charity: an in-depth interview study of cancer patients' information needs and information-seeking behavior. Western Journal of Medicine 173: 26–31

Lin C, Tsai H, Chiou J et al 2003 Changes in level of hope after diagnostic disclosure among Taiwanese patients with cancer. Cancer Nursing 26: 155–160

McGee R 1984 Hope: a factor influencing crises resolution. Advances in Nursing Science 6: 34–44

Magaletta PR, Oliver JM 1999 The hope construct, will and ways: their relations with self-efficacy, optimism, and general well-being. Journal of Clinical Psychology 55: 539–551

Marcel G 1962 Homo viator: introduction to a metaphysics of hope (trans E Crauford). Harper & Row, New York (Original publication 1951)

Menninger K 1959 The academic lecture: Hope. American Journal of Psychiatry 116: 481–491

Mercier M, Fawcett J, Clark D 1984 Hopefulness: a preliminary examination. Unpublished manuscript, Rush-Presbyterian-St. Lukes Medical Center, Chicago, IL

Mertens DM 1998 Research methods in education and psychology: integrating diversity with quantitative and qualitative approaches. Sage, Thousand Oaks, CA

Mickley J, Soeken K 1993 Religiousness and hope in Hispanic- and Anglo-American women with breast cancer. Oncology Nursing Forum 20: 1171–1177

Mickley JR, Soeken K, Belcher A 1992 Spiritual well-being, religiousness and hope among women with breast cancer. Image – the Journal of Nursing Scholarship 24: 267–272

Miller JF 1983 Inspiring hope. In: Miller J (ed) Coping with chronic illness: overcoming powerlessness. FA Davis, Philadelphia, PA, pp 287–289

Miller JF 1989 Hope-inspiring strategies of the critically ill. Applied Nursing Research 2: 23–29

Miller JF 1991 Developing and maintaining hope in families of the critically ill. AACN: Critical Issues 2: 307–315

Miller JF, Powers MJ 1988 Development of an instrument to measure hope. Nursing Research 37: 6–10

Mishel MH 1988. Uncertainty in illness. Image – the Journal of Nursing Scholarship 20: 225.–232

Mishel MH 1990. Reconceptualization of the uncertainty in illness theory. Image – the Journal of Nursing Scholarship 22: 256–262

Moadel A, Morgan C, Fatone A et al 1999 Seeking meaning and hope: self-reported spiritual and existential needs among an ethnically-diverse cancer patient population. Psycho-Oncology 8: 378–385

Moltmann J 1975. The experiment hope. Fortress Press, London

Morse J 1995 Exploring the theoretical basis of nursing using advanced techniques of concept analysis. Advances in Nursing Science 17: 31–46

Morse JM, Doberneck B 1995 Delineating the concept of hope. Image – the Journal of Nursing Scholarship 27: 277–285

Morse JM, Penrod J 1999 Linking concepts of enduring, uncertainty, suffering and hope. Image – the Journal of Nursing Scholarship 31: 145–150

Nekolaichuk CL 2003 The experience of hope in people who are terminally ill. Unpublished research data

Nekolaichuk CL, Bruera E 1998 On the nature of hope in palliative care. Journal of Palliative Care 14: 36–42

Nekolaichuk CL, Bruera E 2005 Assessing hope at end-of-life: validation of an experience of hope scale in advanced cancer patients. Palliative and Supportive Care, in press

Nekolaichuk CL, Jevne RF, Maguire TO 1999 Structuring the meaning of hope in health and illness. Social Science and Medicine 48: 591–605

Nekolaichuk CL, Boman J, Cumming C et al 2002 Fact sheet 1: The Alberta experience of hope. Hope Foundation of Alberta, Edmonton, Alberta

Nietzsche F 1878/1986 Human, all too human, vol 1 (trans RJ Hollingdale). Cambridge University Press, Cambridge (Original work published in 1878)

Nowotny ML 1989 Assessment of hope in patients with cancer: development of an instrument. Oncology Nursing Forum 16: 57–61

Nowotny ML 1991 Every tomorrow, a vision of hope. Journal of Psychosocial Oncology 9: 117–126

Nunn KP 1996 Personal hopefulness: a conceptual review of the relevance of the perceived future to psychiatry. British Journal of Medical Psychology 69: 227–245

O'Connor P 1996 Hope: a concept for home care nursing. Home Care Provider 1: 175–179

O'Malley P, Menke E 1988 Relationship of hope and stress after MI. Heart and Lung 17: 184–190

Onwuegbuzie AJ, Snyder CR 2000 Relations between hope and graduate students' coping strategies for studying and examination taking. Psychological Reports 86: 803–806

Osgood CE, Suci GJ, Tannenbaum PH 1957 The measurement of meaning. University of Illinois Press, Urbana, IL

Owen DC 1989 Nurses' perspectives on the meaning of hope in patients with cancer: a qualitative study. Oncology Nursing Forum 16: 75–79

Paley J 1996 How not to clarify concepts in nursing. Journal of Advanced Nursing 24: 572–578

Parse RR 1990 Parse's research methodology with an illustration of the lived experience of hope. Nursing Science Quarterly 3: 9–17

Parse RR 1998 The human becoming school of thought: a perspective for nurses and other health professionals. Sage, Thousand Oaks, CA

Parse RR 1999 Hope: an international human becoming perspective. Jones & Bartlett, London

Patel CTC 1996 Hope-inspiring strategies of spouses of critically ill adults. Journal of Holistic Nursing 14: 44–65

Penrod J 2001 Refinement of the concept of uncertainty. Journal of Advanced Nursing 34: 238–245

Penrod J, Morse JA 1997 Strategies for assessing and fostering hope: the hope assessment guide. Oncology Nursing Forum 24: 1055–1063

Perakyla A 1991 Hope work in the care of seriously ill patients. Qualitative Health Research 1: 407–433

Piazza D, Holcombe J, Foote A et al 1991 Hope, social support and self-esteem of patients with spinal cord injuries. Journal of Neuroscience Nursing 23: 224–230

Pilkington FB 1999 The many facets of hope. In: Parse RR (ed) Hope: an international human becoming perspective. Jones & Bartlett, Sudbury, MA, pp. 9–44

Plummer EM 1988 Measurement of hope in the elderly institutionalized person. Journal of the New York State Nurses Association 19: 8–11

Popovich JM 1991 Hope, coping and rehabilitation outcomes in stroke patients. Doctoral dissertation, Rush University, Chicago. Dissertation Abstracts International 52: 750B

Popovich JM, Fox PG, Burns KR 2003 'Hope' in recovery from stroke in the US. International Journal of Psychiatric Nursing Research 8: 905–920

Post-White J, Ceronsky C, Kreitzer MJ et al 1996 Hope, spirituality, sense of coherence, and quality of life in patients with cancer. Oncology Nursing Forum 23: 1571–1579

Rabkin J, Neugebaur R, Remien R 1990 Maintenance of hope in HIV-spectrum homosexual men. American Journal of Psychiatry 147: 1322–1326

Raleigh EDH 1992 Sources of hope in chronic illness. Oncology Nursing Forum 19: 443–448

Raleigh EH, Boehm S 1994 Development of the multidimensional hope scale. Journal of Nursing Measurement 2: 155–167

Range LM, Penton SR 1994 Hope, hopelessness, and suicidality in college students. Psychological Reports 75: 456–458

Rideout E, Montemuro M 1986 Hope, morale and adaptation in patients with chronic heart failure. Journal of Advanced Nursing 11: 429–433

Rustoen T 1995 Hope and quality of life, two central issues for cancer patients: a theoretical analysis. Cancer Nursing 18: 355–361

Rustoen T, Moem T 1997 Reliability and validity of the Norwegian version of the Nowotny Hope Scale. Scandinavian Journal of Caring Science 11: 33–41

Rustoen T, Wiklund I, Hanestad BR, Moum T 1998 Nursing intervention to increase hope and quality of life in newly diagnosed cancer patients. Cancer Nursing 21: 235–245

Salander P, Bergenheim T, Henriksson R 1996 The creation of protection and hope in patients with malignant brain tumors. Social Science and Medicine 42: 985–996

Salerno EM 2002 Hope, power and perception of self in individuals recovering from schizophrenia: a Rogerian perspective. Visions 10: 23–36

Sandelowski M 1994 The proof is in the pottery: toward a poetic for qualitative inquiry. In: Morse J (ed) Critical issues in qualitative research methods. Sage, Thousand Oaks, CA, pp. 46–63

Sardell AN, Trierweiler SJ 1993 Disclosing the cancer diagnosis: procedures that influence patient hopefulness. Cancer 72: 3355–3365

Snyder CR 1989 Reality negotiation: from excuses to hope and beyond. Journal of Social and Clinical Psychology 8: 130–157

Snyder CR 1995 Conceptualizing, measuring, and nurturing hope. Journal of Counseling and Development 73: 355–360

Snyder CR, Harris C, Anderson JR et al 1991 The will and the ways: development and validation of an individual-differences measure of hope. Journal of Personality and Social Psychology 60: 570–585

Staats S 1987 Hope: expected positive affect in an adult sample. Journal of Genetic Psychology 148: 357–364

Staats S 1989 Hope: a comparison of two self-report measures for adults. Journal of Personality Assessment 53: 366–375

Staats S 1991 Quality of life and affect in older persons: hope, times frames, and training effects. Current Psychology: Research and Reviews 10: 21–30

Stanton AL, Danoff-Burg S, Huggins ME 2002 The first year after breast cancer diagnosis: hope and coping strategies as predictors of adjustment. Psycho-Oncology 11: 93–102

Stephen-Haynes J 2002 The concept of hope – a phenomenological study. Journal of Community Nursing 16: 28–32

Stephenson C 1991 The concept of hope revisited for nursing. Journal of Advanced Nursing 16: 1456–1461

Stoner M 1982 Hope and cancer patients. Dissertation Abstracts International 43 1983B–2592B (University Microfilms No. 83–12:243)

Stoner MH, Keampfer SH 1985 Recalled life expectancy information, phase of illness and hope in cancer patients. Research in Nursing and Health 8: 269–274

Stotland E 1969 The psychology of hope. Jossey-Bass, San Francisco, CA

Tollett JH, Thomas SP 1995 A theory-based nursing intervention to instill hope in homeless veterans. Advances in Nursing Science 18: 76–90

Tracy J, Fowler S, Margarelli K 1999 Hope and anxiety of individual family members of critically ill adults. Applied Nursing Research 12: 121–127

Udelman DL, Udelman HD 1985a A preliminary report on anti-depressant therapy and its effects on hope and immunity. Social Science and Medicine 20: 1069–1072

Udelman HD, Udelman DL 1985b Hope as a factor in remission of illness. Stress Medicine 1: 291–294

Udelman DL, Udelman HD 1991 Affects, neurotransmitters, and immunocompetence. Stress Medicine 7: 159–162

Volume CI, Farris KB 2000 Hoping to maintain a balance: the concept of hope and the discontinuation of anorexiant medications. Qualitative Health Research 10: 174–187

Wald G 1961 Forward. In: Ames G, Wyler R (eds) Biology: an introduction to the science of life. Golden Press, New York

Walker L, Avant K 1983 Strategies for theory construction in nursing. Appleton-Century-Crofts, Norwalk, CT

Walker LO, Avant KC 1988 Strategies for theory construction in nursing, 2nd edn. Appleton-Century-Crofts, Norwalk, CT

Walker LO, Avant KC 1995 Strategies for theory construction in nursing 3rd edn. Appleton & Lange, Norwalk, CT

Wall LM 2000 Changes in hope and power in lung cancer patients who exercise. Nursing Science Quarterly 13: 234–242

Wang C 2000 Developing a concept of hope from a human science perspective. Nursing Science Quarterly 13: 248–251

Weil CM 2000 Exploring hope in patients with end stage renal disease on chronic hemodialysis. Nephrology Nursing Journal 27: 219–224

Wilson J 1963 Thinking with concepts. Cambridge University Press, New York

Wong-Wylie G, Jevne RF 1997 Patient hope: exploring the interactions between physicians and HIV seropositive individuals. Qualitative Health Research 7: 32–56

Wonghongkul T, Moore SM, Musil C et al 2000 The influence of uncertainty in illness, stress appraisal, and hope in coping in survivors of breast cancer. Cancer Nursing 23: 422–429

Wuest J 1994 A feminist approach to concept analysis. Western Journal of Nursing Research 16: 577–586

Yalom ID 1985. The theory and practice of group psychotherapy. Basic Books, New York

Yates P 1993 Towards a reconceptualization of hope for patients with a diagnosis of cancer. Journal of Advanced Nursing 18: 701–706

Table 12.1 Research themes involving the concept of hope

Research theme	Sampling of research studies
Quantitative	
Concept development/analysis	
Measurement	Stoner and Keampfer 1985, Staats 1987, 1989, Miller and Powers 1988, Plummer 1988, Nowotny 1989, Snyder 1989, 1995, Herth 1991, 1992, Holdcraft and Williamson 1991, Snyder et al 1991, Jakobsson et al 1993, Raleigh and Boehm 1994, Rustoen and Moum 1997
Non-measurement	See Table 12.5
Descriptive	Farran and McCann 1989, Raleigh 1992, Beckerman and Northrop 1996, Ballard et al 1997, Hinds et al 1999, Borneman et al 2002
Correlational	See Table 12.2
Interventions	Staats 1991, Tollett and Thomas 1995, Rustoen et al 1998, Herth 2000, Wall 2000
Biology of hope	Udelman and Udelman 1985a, b, 1991, Cousins 1989, Gottschalk et al 1993
Qualitative	
Concept development/analysis	See Table 12.5
Descriptive	
Meaning	
Individual (non-caregiver)*	Dufault and Martocchio 1985, Hall 1990, 1994, Cutcliffe 1996, Flemming 1997, Daly et al 1999, Hatcher et al 1999, Benzein et al 1998, 2000, Volume and Farris 2000, Weil 2000, Bays 2001, Elliott and Olver 2002
Caregiver†	Owen 1989, Delvecchio Good et al 1990, Benzein and Saveman 1998a, Gelling 1999, Bland and Darlington 2002, Stephen-Haynes 2002
Within relationships	Wong-Wylie and Jevne 1997
Within social contexts	Perakyla 1991
Lived experience	Parse 1990, 1999, Jensen et al 2000, Benzein et al 2001
Hoping process	Hinds and Martin 1988, Salander et al 1996, Kylma et al 2001
Interventions	
Individuals (non-caregivers)*	Miller 1989, Kirkpatrick et al 1995, 2001, Cutcliffe 1995, Koopmeiners et al 1997, Penrod and Morse 1997, Kennett 2000, Cutcliffe and Grant 2001
Caregivers†	Patel 1996
Relationships with other concepts	Forsyth et al 1984, Dufault and Martocchio 1985, Hinds and Martin 1988,
Coping	Perakyla 1991, Ersek 1992, Davies 1993, Leydon et al 2000
Combined: quantitative/ qualitative	
Concept development/analysis	See Table 12.5
Descriptive:	
Individual (non-caregiver)*	Herth 1990a, 1993b, Post-White et al 1996
Caregiver†	Herth 1993a
Hoping process	Herth 1990a
Interventions	
Hope strategies	Herth 1990a, 1993b, Kirkpatrick et al 1995, 2001, Post-White et al 1996
Impact of relationships	Sardell and Trierweiler 1993
Relationships with other concepts	Post-White et al 1996, Ezzy 2000

*Consumers, clients, patients, healthy adults
†Healthcare professionals, family members, spouses
See Farran et al 1995 and Pilkington 1999 for a detailed literature review on hope research

Table 12.2 A sampling of quantitative studies comparing hope with other concepts

Related concept	Author	Hope framework/instrument
Achievement, academic	Curry et al 1997	Hope Scale (Snyder et al 1991)
	Irving et al 1998	Hope Scale (Snyder et al 1991)
Achievement, general	Franken and Brown 1996	Hope Scale (Snyder et al 1991)
Adjustment	Stanton et al 2002	Hope Scale (Snyder et al 1991)
Appraisal	Ebright and Lyon 2002	Herth Hope Index (Herth 1992)
Anxiety	Heszen-Niejodek et al 1999	Gottschalk-Gleser Content Analysis Scales: Hope and Anxiety (Gottschalk & Gleser 1969)
	Tracy et al 1999	Herth Hope Index (Herth 1992)
Attitudes toward health care delivery	Gibson 1999	Herth Hope Scale (Herth 1991)
Control (locus of)	Brockopp et al 1989	Needs Assessment Inventory (Brockopp 1982)
	Foote et al 1990	Miller Hope Scale (Miller & Powers 1988)
	Rabkin et al 1990	Beck Hopelessness Scale (Beck et al 1974)
	Brackney and Westman 1992	Single 10-point rating scale; Miller Hope Scale (Miller & Powers 1988); Beck Hopelessness Scale (Beck et al 1974)
	Carifio and Rhodes 2002	Hope Scale (Snyder et al 1991)
Control (perception of)	Snyder et al 1991	Hope Scale (Snyder et al 1991)
	Bunston et al 1995	Herth Hope Index (Herth 1992)
	Chang and Li 2002	Nowotny Hope Scale (Nowotny 1989)
Coping (central role)	Rideout and Montemuro 1986	Beck Hopelessness Scale (Beck et al 1974)
	Christman 1990	Beck Hopelessness Scale (Beck et al 1974)
	Popovich et al 2003	Modified Stoner Hope Scale (Farran 1985); Hopefulness Scale I (Mercier et al 1984); Hope and Coping Questionnaire (Popovich 1991)
	Irving et al 1998	Snyder Hope Scale (Snyder et al 1991)
	Wonghongkul et al 2000	Herth Hope Index (Herth 1992)
	Herth 1990b	Herth Hope Scale (Herth 1991)
	Onwuegbuzie and Snyder 2000	Hope Scale (Snyder et al 1991)
Coping (predictor of hopefulness)	Bunston et al 1995	Herth Hope Index (Herth 1992)
Coping (prerequisite of)	Herth 1989 Chapman and Pepler 1998	Herth Hope Scale (Herth 1991) Herth Hope Index (Herth 1992)
Depression	Rabkin et al 1990	Beck Hopelessness Scale (Beck et al 1974)
	Elliott et al 1991	Hope Scale (Snyder et al 1991)

Continued

Table 12.2 A sampling of quantitative studies comparing hope with other concepts—cont'd

Related concept	Author	Hope framework/instrument
	Snyder et al 1991	Hope Scale (Snyder et al 1991)
	Fehring et al 1997	Miller Hope Scale (Miller & Powers 1988)
Diagnostic disclosure	Lin et al 2003	Herth Hope Index (Herth 1992)
Functional status	Popovich 1991	Stoner Hope Scale (Stoner 1982), Hopefulness Scale I (Mercier et al 1984)
Grief (anticipatory)	Chapman and Pepler 1998	Herth Hope Index (Herth 1992)
Grief (resolution)	Herth 1990b	Herth Hope Scale (Herth 1991)
Hopelessness	Snyder et al 1991	Hope Scale (Snyder et al 1991)
	Range and Penton 1994	Hope Scale (Snyder et al 1991); Beck Hopelessness Scale (Beck et al 1974)
Mood	Fehring et al 1997	Miller Hope Scale (Miller & Powers 1988)
Optimism	Snyder et al 1991	Hope Scale (Snyder et al 1991)
	Magaletta and Oliver 1999	Hope Scale (Snyder et al 1991)
	Carifio and Rhodes 2002	Hope Scale (Snyder et al 1991)
Pain	Chen 2003	Herth Hope Index (Herth 1992)
Phase of illness	Stoner and Keampfer 1985	Stoner Hope Scale (Stoner 1982)
Power	Salerno 2002	Miller Hope Scale (Miller & Powers 1988)
Problem solving	Snyder 1995	Hope Scale (Snyder et al 1991)
Psychosocial development	Brackney and Westman 1992	Single 10-point rating scale; Miller Hope Scale (Miller & Powers 1988); Beck Hopelessness Scale (Beck et al 1974)
Psychosocial impairment	Elliott et al 1991	Hope Scale (Snyder et al 1991)
Quality of life	Stoner and Keampfer 1985	Stoner Hope Scale (Stoner 1982)
	Staats 1991	Hope Index (Staats 1989)
	Post-White et al 1996	Herth Hope Scale (Herth 1991); Hope interview (Hinds 1984)
	Adams and Jackson 2000	Questions from the National Survey of Black Americans (for hope and life satisfaction)
Religiosity	Mickley et al 1992	Nowotny Hope Scale (Nowotny 1989)
	Mickley and Soeken 1993	Nowotny Hope Scale (Nowotny 1989)
	Fehring et al 1997	Miller Hope Scale (Miller & Powers 1988)
	Ebright and Lyon 2002	Herth Hope Index (Herth 1992)
Self-efficacy	Magaletta and Oliver 1999	Hope Scale (Snyder et al 1991)
	Carifio and Rhodes 2002	Hope Scale (Snyder et al 1991)

Table 12.2 A sampling of quantitative studies comparing hope with other concepts—cont'd

Related concept	Author	Hope framework/instrument
Self-esteem	Foote et al 1990	Miller Hope Scale (Miller & Powers 1988)
	Piazza et al 1991	Miller Hope Scale (Miller & Powers 1988)
	Snyder et al 1991	Hope Scale (Snyder et al 1991)
	Franken and Brown 1996	Hope Scale (Snyder et al 1991)
	Ebright and Lyon 2002	Herth Hope Index (Herth 1992)
Self-perception	Salerno 2002	Miller Hope Scale (Miller & Powers 1988)
Sense of coherence	Post-White et al 1996	Herth Hope Scale (Herth 1991); Hope interview (Hinds 1984)
Social desirability	Snyder et al 1991	Hope Scale (Snyder et al 1991)
Social support	Farran and Popovich 1990	Stoner Hope Scale (Stoner 1982); Hopefulness Scale I (Mercier et al 1984)
	Foote et al 1990	Miller Hope Scale (Miller & Powers 1988)
	Rabkin et al 1990	Beck Hopelessness Scale (Beck et al 1974)
	Piazza et al 1991	Miller Hope Scale (Miller & Powers 1988)
	Raleigh 1992	Sources of Support Interview Guide (by author)
	Gibson 1999	Herth Hope Scale (Herth 1991)
	Ebright and Lyon 2002	Herth Hope Index (Herth 1992)
Spirituality	Post-White et al 1996	Herth Hope Scale (Herth 1991); Hope interview (Hinds 1984)
	Moadel et al 1999	Needs Assessment Survey (developed by authors)
Sports performance	Curry et al 1997	Hope Scale (Snyder et al 1991)
Stressful life events	O'Malley and Menke 1988	Beck Hopelessness Scale (Beck et al 1974)
Suicidality	Range and Penton 1994	Hope Scale (Snyder et al 1991); Beck Hopelessness Scale (Beck et al 1974)
Symptom severity	Landeen et al 2000	Miller Hope Scale (Miller & Powers 1988); Cantrill's Ladder (Cantrill 1965)
Uncertainty	Wonghongkul et al 2000	Herth Hope Index (Herth 1992)
Wellbeing, general	Magaletta and Oliver 1999	Hope Scale (Snyder et al 1991)
Wellbeing, spiritual	Carson et al 1988	State-Trait Hope Scale (Grimm 1984)
and/or existential	Miller and Powers 1988	Miller Hope Scale (Miller & Powers 1988)
	Carson et al 1990	Beck Hopelessness Scale (Beck et al 1974)
	Mickley et al 1992	Nowotny Hope Scale (Nowotny 1989)
	Mickley and Soeken 1993	Nowotny Hope Scale (Nowotny 1989)
	Fehring et al 1997	Miller Hope Scale (Miller & Powers 1988)

Table 12.3
Examples of conceptual frameworks and corresponding instruments/assessment guides

Conceptual framework	Instruments and assessment guides
Stotland 1969	Beck's Hopelessness Scale (Beck et al 1974) Stoner Hope Scale (Stoner & Keampfer 1985) Hope Index (Staats 1989) Multidimensional Hope Scale (Raleigh & Boehm 1994)
Miller 1983	Miller Hope Scale (Miller & Powers 1988)
Hinds 1984, Hinds and Martin 1988	Hopefulness Scale for Adolescents (Hinds & Gattuso 1991)
Dufault and Martocchio 1985	Herth Hope Scale (Herth 1991); Herth Hope Index (Herth 1992)
Nowotny 1989	Nowotny Hope Scale (Nowotny 1989)
Farran et al 1995	Guidelines for the Clinical Assessment of Hope (Farran et al 1992)
Morse and Doberneck 1995	Hope Assessment Guide (Penrod & Morse 1997)
Snyder 1995	Snyder's Hope Scale (Snyder et al 1991)
Nekolaichuk et al 1999	Hope Framework-Palliative Care (Nekolaichuk & Bruera 1998); Hope Differential-Short (Nekolaichuk & Bruera 2005)

Table 12.4
A sampling of deductive approaches for conceptualizing hope

Author(s)	Approach	Focal point of analysis
Informal approaches		
Miller 1983	Non-specific, theoretical	Non-specific
McGee 1984	Non-specific, theoretical	Non-specific
Brown 1989	Nursing, theology, philosophy, psychology	Critically ill
Nowotny 1989	Psychology, psychiatry, theology, nursing	Non-specific
Kindleman 1993	Non-specific	Nursing
Yates 1993	Non-specific	Cancer patients
Farran et al 1995	Non-specific	Multidisciplinary, clinical, research
Fowler 1995	Non-specific	Neuroscience
Rustoen 1995	Non-specific	Link with quality of life
Nunn 1996	Non-specific	Psychiatry
Kylma et al 1997	Meta-analysis: articles 1975–1993 ($n = 46$)	Nursing research

Continued

Table 12.4
A sampling of deductive approaches for conceptualizing hope—cont'd

Author(s)	Approach	Focal point of analysis
Formal approaches		
Stephenson 1991	Walker and Avant 1988, 1995	Nursing
Haase et al 1992	Simultaneous concept analysis (adapted from Wilson 1963, Walker and Avant 1983)	Analysis with spiritual perspective, acceptance and self-transcendence
Forbes 1994	Walker and Avant 1995	Elderly
O'Connor 1996	Walker and Avant (non-specific)	Home care nursing
Cutcliffe 1997	Walker and Avant 1988	Non-specific
Hendricks-Ferguson 1997	Walker and Avant 1995	Adolescents with cancer
Benzein and Saveman 1998b	Wilson 1963, Walker and Avant 1995	Approx 100 references: articles (1970–1996) + books (1965–1991)

Table 12.5
A sampling of inductive approaches for conceptualizing hope

Author(s)	Approach	Focal point of analysis
Qualitative methods		
Hinds 1984	Grounded theory	Well and ill adolescents ($n = 25$)
Dufault and Martocchio 1985	Participant observation	Elderly cancer patients ($n = 35$) and terminally ill ($n = 47$)
Hinds 1988	Grounded theory	Healthy & ill adolescents ($n = 117$)
Hinds and Martin 1988	Grounded theory	Adolescent oncology patients ($n = 58$)
Owen 1989	Grounded theory	Oncology nurse specialists ($n = 6$)
Ersek 1992	Grounded theory	Adults undergoing bone marrow transplantation ($n = 20$)
Jacoby 1993	Interviews, document analysis (e.g. reports, stories, poems, songs)	Patients in surgical ward coping with surgery, terminal illness, etc. + people who survived severe danger and threats (e.g. Holocaust, war, prison)
Laskiwski and Morse 1993	Ethnography	Patients with spinal cord injuries on a rehabilitation unit ($n = 31$)
Cutcliffe 1995	Grounded theory	Nurses' perspectives of inspiring hope in terminally ill HIV patients
Cutcliffe 1996	Phenomenology	Critical care perspectives of hope
Cutcliffe 2004	Grounded theory	The inspiration of hope in bereavement counselling

Continued

Table 12.5

A sampling of inductive approaches for conceptualizing hope—cont'd

Author(s)	Approach	Focal point of analysis
Cutcliffe and Grant 2001	Grounded theory	The principles and processes of inspiring hope in cognitively impaired older adults within a continuing care environment
Morse and Doberneck 1995	Qualitative analysis using authors' own concept development method	Four samples: transplant patients, people with spinal-cord injuries, breast cancer survivors, breastfeeding mothers
Morse and Penrod 1999	Method to qualitatively explore concepts simultaneously developed by authors	Relationship between hope, enduring and suffering based on three previous qualitative studies
Holt 2000	Ethnonursing method: observation, participation research methods, interviews	People living in the Dominican Republic (nurses, villagers)
Wang 2000	Human science perspective – Parse's (1998) theory of human becoming	Use of 'mending a torn fish net' as a metaphor for hope
Quantitative methods		
Farran and Popovich 1990	Questionnaire: development of a hope intervention model using general linear models procedure	People living in senior citizens' housing ($n = 126$)
Bunston et al 1995	Theoretical model confirmed with cross-sectional survey and path analysis	Cancer patients: head and neck, ocular melanoma ($n = 194$)
Combined: quantitative–qualitative methods		
Averill et al 1990	Four studies: 1 Questionnaires + open response 2 Questionnaires + open response 3 Metaphors of hope 4 Questionnaires + open response	Four studies: 1 College students ($n = 150$) 2 College students ($n = 150$) 3 College students ($n = 59$) 4 American ($n = 100$) and Korean ($n = 100$) college students
Nekolaichuk et al 1999	Quantitative/qualitative: survey design, qualitative responses, factor analysis	Healthy adults, adults with chronic or life threatening illness and nurses ($n = 550$)

This list is not exhaustive. Rather it provides a sampling of articles. It could also be argued that all research in this area helps in the conceptualization of hope. For the purposes of this review, articles were included that had a specific focus on conceptualizing hope and/or provided specific definitions, attributes or conceptual frameworks.

Table 12.6
Working assumptions about hope based on hope themes

Theme	Working assumption
Universality	1. Hope is both a universal and an intensely personal experience
Dimensionality	2. Hope is a complex concept ranging from unidimensional to multidimensional aspects of a person's experience
Intangibility	3. Hope has both tangible and intangible components, some of which may never be elucidated
Temporality	4. Hope appears to imply some sense of temporality, although this may not necessarily be limited to a *future orientation*. It is also possible that some components of hope may not be bound by time
Predictability	5. Hope may have both predictable and unpredictable components to the experience
Value-based	6. The value of hope appears to be embedded in personal experience
Reality-based	7. Hope appears to be connected with some sense of realism, although the viewpoints of reality remain unclear

Table 12.7 Dichotomies of hope
The following pairs of statements have intentionally been grouped as dichotomies of hope. As you read each pair, choose the one statement with which you are in most agreement. Notice to which end of the dichotomy you are drawn. Write down some of your thoughts about your choice.

Theme	Polarity	Dichotomy
Universality	Universal	Hope is universally experienced as an inherent part of the human condition
	Unique	Hope is uniquely structured and experienced
Dimensionality	Unidimensional	Hope is most directly linked to goal attainment and problem solving
	Multidimensional	Hope is a complex experience that encompasses many facets of a person's experience, including behavioural, cognitive, emotional, spiritual and relational dimensions
Intangibility	Definable	Hope can be clearly and specifically defined
	Undefinable	Hope is a virtue (intangible) that will never be defined
	Measurable	Hope can be measured
	Immeasurable	Hope is not directly observable; thus, it cannot be measured
Temporality	Time-bound	Hope lives in the future
	Time-free	Hope is not restricted by time
Predictability	Certainty	To be hopeful, I must have clear goals and a well-defined pathway for meeting these goals
	Uncertainty	To be hopeful, I must learn to live with uncertainty and vague goals
Value-based	Valuable	Hope is always positive and good
	Worthless	Hope is a necessary evil
Reality-based	Reality-bound	Hope is appropriate only if it is realistic
	Reality-free	Hope is always appropriate

Adapted from Jevne and Nekolaichuk 2002

Table 12.8   Guiding questions for evaluating a hope model

What constitutes a 'good model?' What would a 'good model' of hope look like? These are some key themes and corresponding questions to ask yourself when comparing models.

Theme	Guiding question
Underlying assumptions	
Universality	Does this model represent the commonalty (universality) or the uniqueness of the hope experience?
Dimensionality	Is the model unidimensional or multidimensional? Which dimensions of hope are emphasized?
Intangibility	Does the model include a definition of hope? A measurement tool? Does it address the intangible components of hope?
Temporality	How is time portrayed within this model? Is the model static or dynamic?
Predictability	How does this model deal with the issue of predictability (uncertainty)?
Value-based	Is there an underlying goodness factor to this model?
Reality-based	Is there a reality-base to this model? If so, then how is it described?
Nature of derivation	How was this model derived? Is there a theoretical underpinning to this model? Was this model derived empirically? If so, then what type of sample was used as a data source? What type of method was used? Does this model balance the theoretical and clinical perspectives of hope? Does this model integrate previous learnings regarding hope within its design?
Transferability across disciplines and contexts	Who proposed this model? Upon which philosophical school of thought is this model based? Is this model discipline-specific or is it interdisciplinary in nature? Is it applicable across different contexts?
Validation of framework	How, if at all, has this model been validated? What are the strengths of this model? What are its limitations?
Contribution to understandings of hope	How has this model contributed to our understandings about hope? What, if any, are the implications for practice?
Personal orientation	How does this model fit with your own conceptions about hope, your philosophical orientation? How does this model fit within your 'practice' (the contexts in which you work)?

Adapted from Jevne and Nekolaichuk 2002

Taking 'humour' seriously – an analysis of the concept 'humour'

Kristiina Hyrkäs

EDITORIAL

The value of humour as a therapeutic entity, while perhaps lacking in unequivocal empirical evidence (though the body of evidence is growing), is one of those phenomena that have immense experiential credibility. That is to say, each of us who has experienced humour and laughter has an experiential knowledge of how good it can make us feel. We each have an intuitive sense that humour helps. Nevertheless, in the days of evidence-based practice, it still behoves nursing academics and scholars to undertake additional research in order to have the required empirical underpinnings upon which to base their practice. While it would be conceptually difficult to separate many of the concepts in this book from the lived experiences of being human, few credible nursing scholars would disagree that humour is essentially a human experience. This in no way upholds the 'Hollywood'-perpetuated myth that life should be personified by happiness, laughter and joy. (Interestingly, this myth then leads to the perception that there is something wrong with each of us if we are not experiencing this kind of life and therefore that we need some pharmacological intervention to 'fix us'.) Life, as the Holocaust survivor and psychotherapist Victor Frankl points out, is often about struggle and suffering.

Kristiina's chapter reminds us that in these clinical situations where patients are likely to be enduring a degree of suffering and/or experiencing a struggle, the therapeutic value of humour should not be underestimated or ignored. Whether instigated by the nurse as a purposeful act or arising in response to patient-initiated humour, therapeutic humour appears to be a most powerful tool, although it is worth adding a cautionary note that, if handled inappropriately and insensitively, humour can also be harmful. In her chapter, Kristiina also reminds us that humour is quite clearly culturally bound and determined, and anyone who has nursed in a culture different from their culture of origin will attest to this.

The need for personal and cultural sensitivity in the use of humour raises a number of questions for the editors. How much attention and focus is given to the concept of therapeutic humour within nursing education programmes? How, if at all, are nurses trained/educated in the use of therapeutic humour? Given that some people appear to have a more natural or innate capacity for humour, how do we help those with less of this innate ability to develop it? And, lastly, are nurses with a more natural or innate sense of humour attracted to certain nursing specialty areas rather than others? What is clear is that a deeper understanding of humour (hopefully arising from this chapter) could help with answering many of these questions.

INTRODUCTION

Humour has fascinated mankind for centuries. The first attempts to define humour were recorded in 340 BC in the writings of Plato and Aristotle (Cassell 1985, Kruger 1996, Struthers 1999). Throughout history, different schools of thought have developed and produced theories of humour that reflect the knowledge base and philosophical underpinnings of the discipline involved. The theories of humour most often referred to in the literature are Freud's psychoanalytic views, found in *Jokes and Their Relation to the Unconscious*, Lorenz's perceptions of humour and behaviour and Zijderveld's sociological theory of humour (see, for instance, Sumners 1990, Struthers 1994, Sheldon 1996, Ziegler 1998, Goldin & Bordan 1999). In nursing literature, humour and its association with health and well-being, have been discussed for a century. Many studies of humour in nursing have focused on specific aspects of humour such as nurses' attitudes and perceptions of humour (Sumners 1990, Åstedt-Kurki & Liukkonen 1994), humour between nurses and patients, humour among staff (Åstedt-Kurki & Isola 2001), the importance of humour for patients (Åstedt-Kurki et al 2001), and nurses' perspective on humour in the nurse–patient relationship (Beck 1997).

Despite the existence of this literature, however, and the significance of humour for enhancing health and well-being, our understanding of humour is incomplete and there is clearly room for additional scrutiny of the concept. Accordingly, the purpose of this paper is to examine and analyse the concept of humour and its contemporary use in health care. The method employed in this paper to analyse and thus facilitate a degree of clarity is the technique advocated by Rodgers (1989). This technique is used because it is one of the commonly applied approaches to concept analysis in nursing literature.

DICTIONARY DEFINITIONS OF HUMOUR – SURROGATE TERMS AND RELEVANT USE OF THE CONCEPT

In order to identify the concept, its relevant use, and explore the surrogate terms, a dictionary definition was chosen as a starting point. The *New International Webster's Dictionary and Thesaurus of English Language* (2002, p. 471) gives the following definition of humour.

1. Disposition of mind or feeling, caprice, freak, whim
2. A facetious turn of thought, playful fancy, jocularity, drollery
3. The capacity to perceive, appreciate or express what is funny, amusing, incongruous, ludicrous etc.; also the capacity to make something seem funny, amusing, ludicrous etc.; especially in the literature the expression of this in speech or action
4. Moisture: specifically an animal fluid: the serous humour. In medieval times, the humours consisting of blood, phlegm, yellow bile, and black bile were supposed to give rise to the sanguine, phlegmatic, choleric and melancholic temperaments respectively
5. Pathology: any chronic cutaneous eruption supposed to be due to disorder of the blood [See synonyms under: fancy, temper, whim, wit]
6. Out of humour: irritated, annoyed (verb transitive) (a) to comply with the moods or caprices of; (b) to accommodate or adapt oneself to [See synonym under: indulge]

The etymological origins of the term 'humour' are interesting. Originally, the term derives from the Latin meaning of the word as 'a fluid'. In medieval times it was thought that the body was composed of four humours or types of fluid: choler, melancholy, blood and phlegm. It was thought that these fluids determined a person's health, temperament or mood. If all the humours were in balance, the individual had a 'good humour/sense of humour' (Struthers 1994, Sheldon 1996, Ziegler 1998).

ATTRIBUTES OF HUMOUR – THE CORE OF THE CONCEPT

Humour is individual, unique to each person (Åstedt-Kurki & Liukkonen 1994, Åstedt-Kurki & Isola 2001). In other words, humour is an elusive concept and means different things to different people. What one person finds humorous may be shocking to someone else (Sumners 1990, Åstedt-Kurki & Liukkonen 1994, Struthers 1994, Sheldon 1996, Åstedt-Kurki & Isola 2001). Humour is evolutionary over time; that is to say, the context of humour (e.g. what is regarded as funny) is not static. For example, Johnson's (2002) findings show that breast cancer women do not find anything funny in the beginning, after hearing the diagnosis or during the crisis situation. However, later they found more and more to make them laugh and see humour in the events going on in their life (see also Dowling 2002). The studies have also shown that there appear to be cultural, ethnic and age differences and diversity in the use of humour and its appreciation (Mallett & A'Hern 1996, Åstedt-Kurki & Isola 2001, Maples et al 2001, Minden 2002). According to Docking et al (1999, 2000), the essence of humour relies heavily on cognitive–communicative skills. For example, humour involves understanding words, metaphors and idioms, detecting ambiguity, perceiving incongruity and the appreciation of the possibility of a sudden or unexpected shift of perspective (i.e. morphological, semantic and syntactic elements of language).

Humour is related to a mood, or state of mind, or to a quality in a person that is conducive to producing laughter and fun (Åstedt-Kurki & Liukkonen 1994, Crapanzano 1999). In a particular situation, someone's words or acts, a film or a book become humorous (Isola & Åstedt-Kurki 1997). This mood, state of mind or quality in a person has also been described as a sense of humour (Newton & Dowd 1990, Åstedt-Kurki & Liukkonen 1994, Åstedt-Kurki et al 2001). Sense of humour consists of: humour production, comprehension, humour appreciation and humour attitude. In other words, a sense of humour includes recognition of one-self as humorous, recognition of others' humour, a propensity to laugh and a per-spective that allows an appreciation of life's absurdities. It incorporates a general attitude of playfulness and a coinciding ability to play on ideas. Some authors (e.g. Moran & Massam 1999) have regarded sense of humour as a personality disposi-tion. The ability to manipulate and reframe ideas playfully enables individuals with a sense of humour to view unpleasant events as funny instead of frightening, annoying or stressful. The predisposition towards humour, seeking out humour stimuli or making jokes, is seen to influence sense of humour (Åstedt-Kurki & Liukkonen 1994, Moran & Massam 1999, Åstedt-Kurki et al 2001, Franzini 2001, Kelly 2002). The sense of humour, however, varies depending on, for example, the stage of illness. Studies have shown that, when the most difficult stage of illness is over, humour begins to figure more prominently in the patient–nurse relationship.

An important attribute of humour is that it is related to communication. This communication can be written, verbal, drawn or otherwise displayed. The content may be formed of jokes, witticism, cartoons, puns or physical humour (Sheldon 1996, Ziegler 1998, Crapanzano 1999, Åstedt-Kurki & Isola 2001, Åstedt-Kurki et al 2001, Bennett 2003). Through humour, patients and nurses communicate and interact openly and they are able to create a relationship that is supportive emotionally and physically. There is some evidence to indicate that, when patients feel supported, they also feel empowered (Greenberg 2003). Humour is seen to narrow interpersonal gaps as well as communicating a sense of caring and humanness (Bennett 2003). Humour is spontaneous and it is characterized by sportive behaviour that connotes kindness and geniality (i.e. good, healthy humour) and carries a message of affection, caring and humanness (Sumners 1990, Crapanzano 1999).

Berk (2001) has argued that humour involves a cognitive shift, allowing one to distance oneself from the immediate threat of a problem situation. In other words, humour offers a different frame of reference and reduces the negative feelings that normally occur. Humour is like a 'buffer' to negative emotional responses, such as feelings of shame, fear, embarrassment, loneliness, anger and hostility. According to Berk (2001), humour can reduce the impact and possibly paralysing effect of those negative reactions.

Humour is a context-bound phenomenon and many times it is not easy to discern who has originally initiated the humour; the nurse or patient (Mallett & A'Hern 1996, Åstedt-Kurki & Isola 2001). This means that humour occurs in relation to various incidents or mishaps preceding and related to nursing procedures, or in verbal nurse–patient communication (Mallett & A'Hern 1996, Åstedt-Kurki & Isola 2001). The use of humour requires sensitivity, 'good taste', intuition and knowledge of the patient's attitudes and ability to deal with humour (Dewane 1978, Åstedt-Kurki & Liukkonen 1994, Åstedt-Kurki et al 2001, Olsson et al 2002). **Humour needs to respect patients' values and not to be used at the expense of patients. The purpose is to laugh with one another, not at one another (Dowling 2002).**

Studies have shown that patients employ humour for many different reasons. For example, they use it to highlight feelings of anxiety, difficulties they have encountered or in order to avoid conflict (Åstedt-Kurki & Isola 2001) Humour may function as a means of forgetting unpleasant things (e.g. pain), accepting things that have happened, providing new, positive perspectives and the opportunity for pleasure, happiness and relaxation. According to Crapanzano (1999), humour also has social functions. It can serve as a means of building, maintaining and developing individual relationships and group solidarity by blurring differences or removing barriers between and within social groups (e.g. handicapped wheelchair students among college students). It can also serve as an instrument for social reform and expressing/signalling or dealing with social tension/aggression, fear and despair in an acceptable way.

ANTECEDENTS, EMPIRICAL REFERENTS AND CONSEQUENCES OF HUMOUR

ANTECEDENTS

Humour has been associated with empathic understanding and empathy has been seen as a perquisite for the use of humour (Sumners 1990, Olsson et al 2002).

Various kinds of incidents can precede humour. Such sources have been reported as everyday happenings, people, entertainment (e.g. movies, jokes, comedies, funny stories) and pets. Different kinds of mishaps related to nursing care, or in the verbal interactions between nurse and patient, were described, especially in the studies related to nursing (Mallett & A'Hern 1996, Åstedt-Kurki & Isola 2001, Westburg 2003). This means that patients as well as nurses can act as initiators of humour and that 'humour' occurs between nurses, between nurses and patients, and between patients (Åstedt-Kurki & Isola 2001). Several studies related to nursing clearly explain that humour was always used in appropriate situations and the initiatives came primarily from patients (Åstedt-Kurki & Liukkonen 1994, Åstedt-Kurki & Isola 2001, Dowling 2002).

In verbal communication humour may follow when the patient and nurse speak jokingly to one another, express themselves in metaphors, use a dialect or speak in proverbs. Humour may also manifest itself when there are misunderstandings between nurse and patient, misunderstandings of verbal instructions or other factors complicating communication, such as poor knowledge of a language (Åstedt-Kurki & Isola 2001). Patients' observations may precede 'humour', focusing on for example self-irony, cheekiness, witticism and quips (Åstedt-Kurki & Isola 2001). In these situations, words can be used to express their opposite meaning; thus patients can be regarded as engaging in satire and litotes. Nurses' mishaps and forgetfulness may lead to funny situations and humour. For example, a nurse may pick and bring the completely wrong instrument (a kidney basin) and give it to the patient (instead of a bedpan).

REFERENTS – MANIFESTATION OF 'HUMOUR'

Situations involving humour are characterized by mirth, different kinds of verbal and a variety of facial expressions (Van Wormer & Boes 1997, Åstedt-Kurki & Isola 2001, Berk 2001). Van Wormer and Boes (1997) and Berk (2001) have specified that mirth is the emotional response and laughter the physical response to humour. Humour and jocularity make people laugh and the most common empirical referents of humour are laughter and laughing (Åstedt-Kurki & Liukkonen 1994, Ziegler 1998, Åstedt-Kurki et al 2001, Franzini 2001, Olsson et al 2002). Humour can evoke such indications of amusement, joy, or mirth as a smiling, grinning or giggling response (Franzini 2001, Minden 2002). Berk (2001) has described, in an interesting way, how the intensity of laughing can vary, and has listed 15 different stages of laughing as follows: smirk, smile, grin, snicker, giggle, chuckle, chortle, laugh, cackle, guffaw, howl, shriek, roar, convulse and die laughing. Humorous communication is often accompanied by twinkling eyes and voice inflection or exaggerated hand motions. Motions may be used to underscore jokes and playfulness but sometimes the whole body/body movements can express humour (Åstedt-Kurki & Liukkonen 1994, Greenberg 2003).

Laughing can occur, however, when a person is confused, embarrassed or as a result of tickling (Ziegler 1998, Åstedt-Kurki et al 2001) and humour may even exist apart from laughter (van Wormer & Boes 1997). **This means that laughter is not a sufficient characteristic to demonstrate the presence of humour**. The manifestation of humour may vary among people. Olsson et al (2002) have found that the effects of humour are, above all, an emotional experience and that it may initiate different kinds of reaction ranging from laughter to tears (i.e. tears of joy – see also Sheldon 1996). Verbal humour has been classified in the literature in several different ways (van Wormer & Boes 1997, Ziegler 1998, Lowis & Nieuwould 1995, Maples et al 2001, De Koning & Weiss 2002, Olsson et al 2002). Commonly used categories are:

- political humour
- workplace humour
- sexual humour
- male-dominated humour
- female-dominated humour
- illness/misfortune humour (van Wormer & Boes 1997, Ziegler 1998, Lowis & Nieuwould 1995).

Other studies indicate that the categorizations are more oriented around the domain or specialty of the profession. For example, the web pages for nursing humour (www.nursinghumour.com) have such titles as: general nursing humour, bedside humour, geriatric and nursing home humour, mental health and psychiatric humour, emergency department humour and 'Viagra jokes'. Nelson (1992) has categorized the verbal humour in paediatric emergency departments according to how it is manifest in three generic situations: chief complaints, telephone inquiries or encounter situations. Van Wormer and Boes's (1997) study described the verbal humour in emergency rooms using five categories:

- tension-relieving nonsense
- play on words
- sense of the preposterous and incongruous
- gallows humour
- foolish jest.

In summary, the types of verbal humour in nursing studies seem to focus on developing humour around health and illness issues, providing emotional support and humorous visioning.

CONSEQUENCES

In concept analysis, consequences mean those events or incidents that occur as a result of the occurrence of the concept (Rodgers 1989). In the studies reviewed for this concept analysis the consequences of humour were described in several different ways and, during the analysis process, these were classified in the following categories:

- psychological and physical health benefits
- collaboration

- coping
- possibilities for showing emotions.

PSYCHOLOGICAL AND PHYSICAL HEALTH BENEFITS

The effects of humour on physical health have been a focus of several empirical studies since early 1950s and these benefits have been referred to in several studies of nursing (Åstedt-Kurki & Liukkonen 1994, Åstedt-Kurki & Isola 2001, see also Kelly 2002). Berk (2001) has published an interesting paper based on an extensive analysis and synthesis of the studies of the psycho-physiological benefits and risks of humour. **This meta-analysis seems to confirm that the psychological benefits of humour are as follows: it reduces anxiety, tension, stress, depression, self-destructiveness and loneliness; it improves self-esteem; it restores hope and energy; and it provides a sense of empowerment and control. The described physiological benefits of 'humour' are described as: improved mental functioning, muscle exercise and relaxation, improved respiration, stimulated circulation, decreased stress-hormone levels, increased immune system defences and increased production of endorphins.**

Other studies have described gender differences in the beneficial effects of humour. For example, Abel's (1998) study indicated that humour has a moderating, buffering effect between stress and anxiety and this was statistically significant among men, but not among women. Åstedt-Kurki et al (2001) have described a similar kind of finding in the study exploring the importance of humour among patients.

Within medical journals humour and its physiological effects are described from a more critical perspective (Larkin 1998, Ziegler 1998, Bennett 2003, see also Mallett & A'Hern 1996). For example, Bennett (2003) has commented that humour as treatment modality has not gained wide acceptance in mainstream medicine. The author criticizes most of the studies in the field, claiming that the majority of the human research either negates the effects/benefits or is insufficient to support the stated claims. The main problems referred to are that the studies were often poorly designed, they had inadequate controls or they involved sample populations that were too small to support their conclusions.

COLLABORATION AND HUMOUR

The findings of reviewed empirical studies indicated that skilful, conscious use of humour on the part of a nurse can contribute and improve nurse–client collaboration aimed at promoting a client's well-being (Beck 1997, Åstedt-Kurki et al 2001, Johnson 2002). Several studies have indicated that the use of humour facilitates communication between nurse and patient (Mallett & A'Hern 1996, Beck

1997, Åstedt-Kurki et al 2001, Dowling 2002). Studies have found that humour brings people closer to one another, adds togetherness and increases closeness, warmth, friendliness and a sense of cohesion (Sheldon 1996, Beck 1997, Åstedt-Kurki & Liukkonen 1994, Olsson et al 2002). **Humour also helps to create a closer sense of rapport and foster a deeper relationship between client and nurse. (Åstedt-Kurki & Liukkonen 1994, Johnson 2002).** Johnson's (2002) study confirms these consequences and provides details that nurses who use humour appear more human, sensitive and trustworthy to patients. Nurses' use of humour has been found to motivate clients and strengthen their confidence in life and survival, e.g. in rehabilitation situations. The use of humour has further been described to stimulate acceptance, commitment and a positive sense of working together (Dowling 2002).

Olsson et al (2002) and Åstedt-Kurki and Liukkonen (1994) have described the effects of 'positive humour' and 'negative humour' on collaboration. They describe negative humour as 'laughing at' and positive humour as 'laughing with'. 'Positive humour' was found to increase familiarity and the use of 'negative humour' was found to distance individuals, and to hurt and damage not only collaboration between nurses and patients but also collaboration among nurses.

COPING AND HUMOUR FROM PATIENTS' PERSPECTIVE

Many studies have indicated how humour can help patients to cope with difficult situations, how it helps patients continue from one situation and one day to the next, get on with life and retain a sense of control without becoming overwhelmed by stressful events (Sheldon 1996, Witkin 1999, Cowley et al 2000, Mäkinen et al 2000, Åstedt-Kurki et al 2001, Dowling 2002, Fortune et al 2002, Johnson 2002). Åstedt-Kurki et al (2001) have argued that humour provides patients with a moment to rest and to forget unpleasant things for a while, it helps lift the patient's spirit and increases their hope and belief in survival. Humour helps also to draw attention away from minor ailments and pain for a while and gives an opportunity for pleasure, happiness and relaxation. Bennett (2003) sees humour as a coping mechanism that can reduce the anxiety and frustration associated with being in hospital, the insecurity of being ill, having to deal with hospital routines and submission to authority figures, and loss of control over bodily functions. The use of humour can also promote patients' coping through decreasing embarrassment and maintaining dignity (Walsh & Kowanko 2002).

Dowling (2002) has reported the importance of humour for paediatric patients. In fact, paediatric nurses can use this strategy among their patients and thus help children to cope with illness and hospitalization. Humour may enable a child to view a stressful event from an alternative perspective and reappraise it as less threatening and more of an opportunity or challenge. It may also lessen associated feelings of anxiety, fear, frustration and pain (Dowling 2002, see also Nelson 1992). Humour seems to play an important part in helping patients to cope with rehabilitation, to pull through and to carry on with life. Humour makes patients feel better and provides motivation for rehabilitation, as well as strengthening confidence in survival. A nurse's sense of humour motivates patients to try harder and look after themselves (Åstedt-Kurki et al 2001).

COPING AND HUMOUR AMONG NURSING STAFF

Humour has been described as important to nurses, helping them to alleviate and cope with job-related stress (Åstedt-Kurki & Liukkonen 1994, Åstedt-Kurki et al 2001). Humour seems to relieve tensions, improve the climate in the workplace, facilitate working, foster good working relationships among colleagues, improve morale and help nurses cope with difficult situations (Åstedt-Kurki & Liukkonen 1994, Bennett 2003). However, opposing findings have also been described. For example, Dorz et al (2003) have, studied predictors of burnout among HIV/AIDS and oncology healthcare workers. The study revealed that the negative aspects of burnout (i.e. emotional exhaustion and depersonalization) were predicted primarily by professional status (i.e. being a doctor), type of unit (oncology) and high depression scores, but also by the use of humour as a coping strategy. The use of humour seemed to be an inadequate coping strategy but the study does not describe whether the individuals who were experiencing high burnout were using 'black humour'. The other study describing the opposing perspective of humour as a coping strategy was reported by Healy and McKay (2000). No evidence was found that the use of humour had a moderating effect on the relationship between stress and mood but there was support for the influence of job satisfaction upon this relationship (Healy & McKay 2000).

Humour has been shown to promote coping through influencing the atmosphere on the ward, making it more relaxed (Sumners 1990, Åstedt-Kurki & Liukkonen 1994, Sheldon 1996, Åstedt-Kurki & Isola 2001). The use of appropriate humour has been found to be a very effective and efficient approach to assisting nurses caring for demanding, difficult, irritable patients or patients in severe pain and suffering (Beck 1997, Åstedt-Kurki & Isola 2001, Bennett 2003).

To sum up, humour between nurse and patient enables them both to cope with various unpleasant procedures (Åstedt-Kurki & Isola 2001). It helps to manage difficult situations and leads to an improvement in the working climate (Åstedt-Kurki & Isola 2001).

SHOWING AND DEALING WITH EMOTIONS

For patients, humour is a useful and acceptable outlet to express and communicate their emotions, attitudes and opinions (e.g. dissatisfaction, criticism, complaints of injustice). Nurses' humour, on the other hand, helps clients to 'save face' and maintain their dignity in difficult situations (Åstedt-Kurki & Liukkonen 1994, Åstedt-Kurki et al 2001, Walsh & Kowanko 2002). In difficult nursing situations both nurses and clients can use humour to show and deal with strong, otherwise suppressed emotions (e.g. fear, anxiety, anger and pain). Humour can function as a way of breaking the ice or resolving deadlocked or potential conflict situations. Humour may also be used to hide fears, anxiety, anger or extreme pain (Sumners 1990, Åstedt-Kurki & Liukkonen 1994, Mallett & A'Hern 1996, Sheldon 1996, Åstedt-Kurki et al 2001, Sayre 2001, Freeman 2002). **Struthers (1994) has suggested that sometimes it is very difficult to recognize hidden and persisting anger behind the 'mask of humour'. Similarly, Åstedt-Kurki and Liukkonen (1994) and Åstedt-Kurki et al (2001) have reported that sensitivity is required to understand when hidden fears or anxiety are behind humour**. The conflicting function of humour of allowing expression of hostile and aggressive feelings has, however, been seen to be beneficial because it helps the feelings to be expressed without, for example, fears of overt retaliatory attacks (Cassell 1985).

Studies have described that patients find it easier to discuss difficult matters and express their feelings if they know that nurse has a sense of humour. For the patients, a nurse who shows a sense of humour is easier to approach (Åstedt-Kurki & Liukkonen 1994). In these cases difficult matters can be discussed under the pretext of joking (Åstedt-Kurki & Liukkonen 1994, Åstedt-Kurki & Isola 2001) To sum up, humour provides a channel for expressing one's feelings and relieving anxiety, tension, fears and insecurity, and may serve as a defence mechanism with which a person deals with oppressive issues (Sheldon 1996, Åstedt-Kurki & Liukkonen 1994, Åstedt-Kurki & Isola 2001).

RELATED CONCEPTS

The concepts that are closely related to humour are 'therapeutic humour', 'inside humour', 'black humour' and 'aberrant humour'. Franzini (2001) has examined the definitions of therapeutic humour and described the emerging characteristics based on the literature (see also McGuire et al 1992, Minden 2002). Franzini's (2001) analysis is that therapeutic humour includes both intentional and spontaneous use of humour by, for example, a therapist or a healthcare professional. The special characteristic of therapeutic humour is that it can lead to improvements in the self-understanding and behaviour of clients and patients. Another interesting characteristic of therapeutic humour is that the humorous points or content of humour are assumed to have detectable relevance to client's own conflict situation or personal characteristics, and thus therapeutic humour is expected to be helpful. Therapeutic humour is expected to yield to a positive emotional experience shared by therapist and client. This can range anywhere from quiet empathic amusement to overt loud laughter. Minden (2002) has pointed out, however, that humour can be therapeutic but it does not necessarily always translate into achievement of treatment goals. Broader definitions of therapeutic humour have been introduced, for example by the American Association for Therapeutic Humour (www. AATH.org). According to this, therapeutic humour is any intervention that promotes health and wellness by stimulating a playful discovery, expression or appreciation of the absurdity or incongruity of one's life situation (see also Dewane 1978, Mooney 2000)

Inside humour is a form of humour manifesting among members of a profession (e.g. physicians, nurses), or a subgroup of professionals (e.g. emergency-room or operating-room staff). According to Åstedt-Kurki and Isola (2001), instances of inside humour are common in nursing and often rest upon common language, jargon or hospital slang. 'Outsiders' may find this kind of humour difficult to understand and sometimes even coarse. Among the members of profession or subgroup, however, 'inside humour' seems to serve an important function as a means of coping with difficult situations such as continuous illness or loss of patients (Åstedt-Kurki & Liukkonen 1994, Åstedt-Kurki & Isola 2001).

Black humour involves imagining horror stories related to, for example, care, or joking about others' incompetence. Black humour is a racy, insider style of humour that it is also characterized as 'postmortem-oriented humour' (Åstedt-Kurki & Isola 2001). The manifestation and content of black humour are interesting since this can be seen as inappropriate but, like inside humour, it still serves an important purpose for the individuals involved, defending against the feelings of horror, pain and fear experienced in situations of overwhelming stress. It is defined as a form of coping used to manage the numerous anxieties staff encounter, especially in high-stress areas such as operating and emergency rooms (Sayre 2001, see also Åstedt-Kurki & Liukkonen 1994, Åstedt-Kurki & Isola 2001).

Instead of black humour, Sayre (2001) has introduced a broader concept of 'aberrant humour' and described this as a way of coping within the context of erosive professionalism caused by having to deal with very ill patients in a compromised treatment setting. The resulting demoralization and resentment is expressed by cynicism and vengeful counteraction demonstrated in staff's jokes, ranging from benign forms to 'gallows humour'. Based on empirical findings Sayre (2001) describes aberrant humour as being composed of whimsical and sarcastic humour. Whimsical humour is characterized by 'playful joking or fun', which is minimally offensive to the object of the laughter. Sarcastic humour is distinguished from whimsical humour by its characteristic of intention to hurt by taunting, mocking or ridiculing. Sarcastic humour may also manifest in the form of 'satire', i.e. a form of ironic discourse exposing and attacking the vices and stupidities of others through communication, in which the intended meaning is opposite to what the statement actually means. Sarcastic humour differs from whimsical humour in the degree of hostility expressed and has additional goal of maliciously ridiculing a person, institution or object. Unlike whimsical humour, sarcastic humour intends to be damaging to the object of ridicule.

An interesting finding of this analysis is that several references specified different kinds of unacceptable or inappropriate forms and use of humour, for example racist, ethnic, sexist, religious and ridiculing humour. Timing, frequency, content and focus, receptiveness, respect, initiator of humour and context were identified as important factors for considering whether humour is appropriate or inappropriate (Dewane 1978, Åstedt-Kurki & Liukkonen 1994, Sheldon 1996, Goldin & Bordan 1999, Åstedt-Kurki & Isola 2001, Åstedt-Kurki et al 2001, Sayre 2001, Dowling 2002, Bennett 2003). Sayre's (2001) study was, however, the only one exploring more closely the negative forms and perspective on humour.

CONCLUSION

Humour is used in the literature to cover a variety of factors, for example sense of humour, generation of humour, humour appreciation and laughter. This reflects the complex, multifaceted, ubiquitous nature of the concept of humour. In this concept analysis humour was found to be a specific form of communication characterized by kindness and geniality. Humour is identified, interpreted and valued differently by individuals and thus it is an elusive but also context-bound concept. In addition, there are differences in the use and appreciation of humour between different professions, cultures, ethnic groups, ages and genders.

Almost anything (spontaneous or planned) can precipitate humour and the catalyst/stimulus may be 'internal' or 'external'. Humour can manifest in several different ways from verbal and facial expressions and tears to body movements. The congruence and conformity of verbal and non-verbal manifestations and a playful attitude/mood are, however, essential. It is possible to claim that, if the attitude/mood is not elated with happiness, humour has not been effective. This concept analysis has described and summarized the consequences of humour. The evidence indicates that humour is capable of enhancing health and well-being, collaboration and coping.

The nature of humour is, however, paradoxical. When used appropriately it can assist the development of trust, rapport and closeness. If humour is misinterpreted or used inappropriately, it is damaging and alienating. The challenge is thus how to judge when 'humour' or 'a humorous interaction' is beneficial to the client or among colleagues. Three important considerations for determining the appropriate and inappropriate use of humour emerged in the literature: right timing, receptiveness and context. In other words, humour is not appropriate, for example, at the time of crisis. Humour needs to respect the patient's/colleague's values, and the purpose is to laugh 'with one another' not 'at one another'. These characteristics are also important attributes of the concept, especially when describing its paradoxical nature.

REFERENCES

Abel M 1998 Interaction of humor and gender in moderating relationship between stress and outcomes. Journal of Psychology 132: 267–276

Åstedt-Kurki, P, Isola A 2001 Humour between nurse and patient, and among staff: analysis of nurses' diaries. Journal of Advanced Nursing 35: 452–458

Åstedt-Kurki P, Liukkonen A 1994 Humour in nursing care. Journal of Advanced Nursing 20: 183–188

Åstedt-Kurki P, Isola A, Tammentie T, Kervinen U 2001 Importance of humour to client-nurse relationships and clients' well-being. International Journal of Nursing Practice 7: 119–125

Beck CT 1997 Humour in nursing practice: a phenomenological study. International Journal of Nursing Studies 34: 346–352

Bennett H 2003 Humour in medicine. Southern Medical Journal 96: 1257–1261

Berk R 2001 The active ingredients in humour: psycho physiological benefits and risks for older adults. Educational Gerontology 27: 323–339

Cassell J 1985 Disabled humour: origin and impact. Journal of Rehabilitation Oct/Nov/Dec: 59–62

Cowley L, Heyman B, Stanton M, Milner S 2000 How women receiving adjuvant chemotherapy for breast cancer cope with their treatment: a risk management perspective. Journal of Advanced Nursing 31: 314–321

Crapanzano S 1999 The advancement of nursing competencies. The value of humour: a nursing perspective. Pelican News 55: 10–14

De Koning E, Weiss R 2002 The relational humour inventory: functions of humour in close relationships. American Journal of Family Therapy 30: 1–18

Dewane C 1978 Humour in therapy. Social Work Nov: 508–510

Docking K, Jordan F, Murdoch B 1999 Interpretation and comprehension of linguistic humour by adolescents with head injuries: a case-by-case analysis. Brain Injury 13: 953–972

Docking K, Murdoch B, Jordan M 2000 Interpretation and comprehension of linguistic humour by adolescents with head injuries: a group analysis. Brain Injury 14: 89–108

Dorz S, Novara C, Sica C, Sanavio E 2003 Predicting burnout among HIV/AIDS and oncology health care workers. Psychology and Health 18: 677–684

Dowling J 2002 Humour: a coping strategy for pediatric patients. Pediatric Nursing 28: 123–131

Fortune D, Richards H, Main C, Griffiths C 2002 Patients' strategies for coping with psoriasis. Clinical and Experimental Dermatology 27: 177–184

Franzini L 2001 Humour in therapy: a case for training therapists in its use and risks. Journal of General Psychology 128: 170–193

Freeman L 2002 Transcending circumstances: seeking holism at Auschwitz. Holistic Nursing 17: 32–39

Goldin E, Bordan T 1999 The use of humour in counseling: the laughing cure. Journal of Counseling and Development 77: 405–410

Greenberg M 2003 Therapeutic play: developing humour in the nurse-patient relationship. Journal of the New York State Nurses Association 34: 25–31

Healy C, McKay M 2000 Nursing stress: the effects of coping strategies and job satisfaction in a sample of Australian nurses. Journal of Advanced Nursing 31: 681–688

Isola A, Åstedt-Kurki P 1997 Humor as experienced by patients and nurses in aged nursing in Finland. International Journal of Nursing Practice 3: 29–33

Johnson P 2002 The use of humour and its influence on spirituality and coping in breast cancer survivors. Oncology Nursing Forum 29: 691–695

Kelly W 2002 An investigation of worry and sense of humour. Journal of Psychology 6: 657–666

Kruger A 1996 The nature of humour in human nature: cross-cultural commonalities. Counseling Psychology Quarterly 9: 235–241

Larkin M 1998 How humor heals ills. Lancet 352: 1562

Lowis M, Nieuwould J 1995 The use of a cartoon rating scale as a measure for the humour construct. Journal of Psychology 129: 133–144

McGuire F, Boyd R, James A 1992 Therapeutic humour with elderly. Haworth Press, New York

Mäkinen S, Suominen T, Lauri S 2000 Self-care in adults with asthma: how they cope. Journal of Clinical Nursing 9: 557–565

Mallett J A'Hern R 1996 Comparative distribution and use of humour within nurse–patient communication. International Journal of Nursing Studies 33: 530–550

Maples M, Dupey P, Torres-Rivera E et al 2001 Ethnic diversity and the use of humour in counseling: appropriate or inappropriate? Journal of Counseling and Development 79: 53–60

Minden P 2002 Humour as the focal point of treatment for forensic psychiatric patients. Holistic Nursing Practice 16: 75–86

Mooney N 2000 The therapeutic use of humour. Orthopedic Nurse 19: 88–92

Moran C, Massam M 1999 Differential influence of coping humour and humour bias on mood. Behavioral Medicine 25: 36–47

Nelson D 1992 Humor in the pediatric emergency department: a 20-year retrospective. Pediatrics 89: 1089–1090

New International Webster's Dictionary and Thesaurus of the English Language 2002. Trident Press International, Canada

Newton G, Dowd T 1990 Effects of client sense of humour and paradoxical interventions on test anxiety. Journal of Counseling and Development 68: 668–672

Olsson H, Backe H, Sörensen S, Kock M 2002 The essence of humour and its effects and functions: a qualitative study. Journal of Nursing Management 10: 21–26

Rodgers B 1989 Concepts, analysis and the development of nursing knowledge: the evolutionary cycle. Journal of Advanced Nursing 14: 330–335

Sayre J 2001 The use of aberrant medical humour by psychiatric unit staff. Issues in Mental Health Nursing 22: 669–689

Sheldon L 1996 An analysis of the concept of humour and its application to one aspect of children's nursing. Journal of Advanced Nursing 24: 1175–1183

Struthers J 1994 An exploration into the role of humour in the nursing student–nurse teacher relationship. Journal of Advanced Nursing 19: 486–491

Struthers J 1999 An investigation into community psychiatric nurses' use of humour during client interactions. Journal of Advanced Nursing 29: 1197–1204

Sumners A 1990 Professional nurses' attitudes towards humour. Journal of Advanced Nursing 15: 196–200

Van Wormer K, Boes M 1997 Humour in the emergency room: a social work perspective. Health and Social Work 22: 87–94

Walsh K, Kowanko I 2002 Nurses' and patients' perceptions of dignity. International Journal of Nursing Practice 8: 143–151

Westburg N 2003 Hope, laughter, and humour in residents and staff at an assisted living facility. Journal of Mental Health Counseling 25: 16–32

Ziegler J 1998 Use of humour in medical teaching. Medical Teacher 20: 341–348

An analysis of loneliness as a concept of importance for dying persons

Robert Brown

EDITORIAL

As editors, it strikes the two of us that, like some of the other concepts covered in this book (e.g. see the analysis of shame), loneliness can be regarded as an embodied, lived experience; an experience that nurses encounter more than they talk about. By way of an explanation, the editors were musing on how often we had seen 'addressing a patient's sense of loneliness' as a specific care objective. Additionally, Bob's chapter reminds us that the very nature of loneliness appears to exacerbate its inscrutability; the prohibitions, embarrassments and fear of loneliness contribute to avoidance and reluctance on the part of both sufferers and researchers to discuss the topic. Concomitantly, within the ever-changing context of heath care and healthcare provision, we wondered whether loneliness would be regarded as a 'healthcare' or a 'social care' need. These arbitrary distinctions and delineations might appear meaningless to many but a brief examination of some of the contemporary 'debates' and subsequent 'developments' within health care and, importantly, the growing influence of economics on a range of healthcare decisions gives these distinctions added meaning.

The UK government has recently commissioned a number of studies to attempt to separate 'healthcare' activities from 'social care' activities. Thus, by way of an example, applying a dressing to a person with a pressure sore would be regarded as 'health' (or nursing) care and helping somebody to bathe would be regarded as 'social care'. We will not belabour the obvious irony of this situation, given the therapeutic value of bathing in skin care and the many other dimensions of (and potentially therapeutic) engagement that occurs between the patient and nurse in such situations. The political and economic drivers underpinning such commissioning notwithstanding, the overlapping and holistic nature of a person and their needs renders many (if not all) of these studies moot. The UK government may relish the economic ramifications arising from a study that indicates that helping a person bathe or addressing a person's sense of loneliness are more 'social' than 'health'-related interventions. Yet experienced clinicians are very much aware that unmet needs (e.g. a pervasive sense of loneliness) can have a holistic impact on the person's health and well-being. Accordingly, accepting the well established and axiomatic position that nurses should offer holistic care means that nurses cannot ignore needs such as a person's sense of loneliness, irrespective of what the economically driven edicts of the current UK government are.

INTRODUCTION

In contemporary society, early and more accurate diagnosis, better treatments and advances occurring within palliative care during the last 30 years have led to improved management of the needs of patients with chronic illnesses and those of their relatives. Just over a decade ago, concern was expressed regarding the lack of available literature and research on the psychosocial needs of patients who are dying (Kellehear 1990). During the last 10 years, however, there has been a significant increase in the amount of work and publications in this area (Cocker et al 1994, Faulkner & Maguire 1994, Seale & Addington-Hall 1995, Lawton 1998, Thomas & Retsas 1999, Bolmsjo 2000, O'Leary & Nieuwstraten 2001, Dobratz 2002, Wright & Flemons 2002). A number of 'therapeutic innovations' have been reported in the literature (Davis & Sheldon 1997, Wilkinson et al 1999, Ernst 2001). These include the application of cognitive and behavioural therapies, image work, structured life review and other complementary processes and are increasingly being shown to be of value and of positive benefit to patients.

The *Oxford English Dictionary* (1993) defines loneliness as the quality or condition of being lonely; the want of society or company; the feeling of being alone; the sense of solitude; or dejection arising from want of companionship or society. Kurtz (1982) states that:

> *Because loneliness is within us and outside us, because each of us contains his own loneliness and also increases the loneliness of others, because there are characteristics of our society which exacerbate loneliness, and because we cannot hold loneliness or see it but only feel it, loneliness has become the cart horse for our misery.*

Loneliness can occur in people at any age, but may well represent a particular problem for persons with advanced disease, especially for those dying in an acute or cure-orientated setting. This chapter is based upon the assumption that a substantial number of persons experience periods of loneliness and social isolation during the weeks, months or years leading up to their death. This assumption is founded on communication between patients and professional colleagues within the author's local hospice and community palliative care settings.

By undertaking a thorough concept analysis of loneliness, it is hoped that a greater understanding of the dying experience will be generated, leading to relevant research, concept development and the eventual inductive construction of meaningful theory. In promoting conceptual clarity, the long-term aim will be to enhance communication within the discipline (Kemp 1985) and contribute to the development of nursing's knowledge base (Mason et al 1991) so that patient care will continue to improve.

APPROACH TO CONCEPT ANALYSIS

Nursing, as a discipline, has a societal mandate to provide health care for clients at different points in their development and in diverse settings (Hinshaw 1989). In order to fulfil this role, it is argued that the discipline must generate relevant, accurate and reliable knowledge to support practice (Cody 1997). The development of knowledge reflects the interface between nursing science and research, leading to the growth of frameworks and theories that provide guidance for practice. Walker and Avant (1995) argue that the starting point of theory involves concept analysis, which provides an opportunity to explain and describe phenomena of interest to practice. According to McKenna (1997) concepts are the building blocks of theory and are essential elements in the foundation of nursing science. An increasing number of concepts familiar to nursing, such as feeling, pain management, grief, challenging behaviour, loss and symptoms experience have been analysed in recent years (Beyea 1990, Davis 1992, Jacob 1993, Slevin 1995, Robinson & McKenna 1998, Armstrong 2003). Such analyses have employed the methods of Norris (1970), Smith and Medin (1981), Moody (1990), Rodgers (1994), Morse (1995) and Walker and Avant (1995).

Concept analysis is described as a technique or mental activity that requires critical approaches in uncovering subtle elements of meaning that can be embedded in abstract concepts (Chinn & Kramer 1995). This chapter uses the technique described by Walker and Avant (1995); however, in line with Rodgers' (1989a) critical view of this approach, it was decided to omit the contrary, invented and illegitimate cases. Instead, these functions will be addressed as related concepts, thus supporting Rodgers' use of a more qualitative approach in order to enhance the degree of clarification and credibility of the concept.

Concept analysis should begin with a comprehensive review of the literature. A rigorous search strategy was employed to uncover theoretical and research work in relation to loneliness and the meaning attributed to this concept. Medline, CINAHL, CancerLit, the Cochrane Research Databases and hand-searching of key cancer and palliative care journals were exploited using the following key words: loneliness, dying, palliative care, terminal care and chronic illness. While a large number of 'hits' were identified (173 published articles), the focus was directed at those sources that pertained to psychosocial aspects of chronic illness, palliative and terminal care. The following inclusion criteria were used in searching articles:

- patients with chronic and advanced illness such as cancer, HIV/AIDS and chronic obstructive pulmonary disease
- patients having palliative treatment
- adult patients
- articles published in peer-reviewed journals.

Exclusion criteria included:

- loneliness in elderly people without mention of specific chronic illness
- case reports and non-empirically-based articles.

The literature on loneliness reveals two related aspects (Wenger 1983). First, it is evident that, while the concept is often referred to (see Rodgers 1989b, Zack 1995, Donaldson & Watson 1996), research on the topic itself is scant (Fromm-Reichmann 1959, Weiss 1973, Donaldson & Watson 1996, Andersson 1998). **Second, many who have written about loneliness comment on the fear of loneliness and suggest that avoidance and reluctance on the part of both sufferers and researchers to discuss the topic is partly responsible for our lack of understanding.** According to Seabrook (1973) the subject of loneliness is surrounded by prohibitions and embarrassments. He argues that it is a vague term, presenting no definition; a position previously taken by Fromm-Reichmann (1959), who asserted that real loneliness defies description. At a basic level Moustakas (1961) has described it as a longing to be with others and to be loved, while Weiss (1973) argues that loneliness is caused not by being alone but by being without some definite needed relationship or relationships

Wenger (1983) claimed that the psychological literature appeared to be primarily concerned with existential loneliness. Almost 20 years prior to this claim, Berblinger (1968) defined loneliness as an unhappy compound of having lost one's points of reference, of suffering the fate of individual and collective discontinuity and of living through or dying from a crisis of identity to the point of alienation from oneself. Witzleben (1968), while admitting that there is no clear definition of loneliness, identifies two types: loneliness caused by loss of an object, which he calls secondary loneliness, and a loneliness 'inborn in everyone' characterized by the feeling of being alone and helpless in the world, which he calls 'primary loneliness'.

Lopata (1969) defines loneliness as a sentiment felt by a person when they define their experienced level or form of interaction as inadequate. Lopata considers one of the characteristics of loneliness to be its infusion in all three time dimensions – past, present and future. People may feel lonely for a person, object or event that has been experienced in the past. They may feel lonely when no one else is present, when a particular other is absent, when partners treat them differently than they deserve or when aspects of the situation make them feel alienated from those with whom they could develop different relations. Loneliness experienced in connection with the future can be called 'loneliness anxiety', characterized by a fear of losing companions and of being powerless to build satisfactory levels of new relations.

Younger (1995) states that the alienation of the 'sufferer' could be one of the great paradoxes of human existence: in fact, it is in suffering that the realization of one's aloneness becomes most acute. He describes a continuum of relatedness that exists from connectedness to solitude, inward turning, existential aloneness, loneliness and finally alienation. Each step on the continuum is a state of separateness from self and others, while each step toward connectedness reflects gradually increasing harmony in one's feeling of community. According to Younger, one step up from alienation is loneliness, where loneliness as a subjective state is distinguished from the objective states of social isolation and aloneness. Loneliness is the feeling of being alone in spite of longing for others. The lonely person experiences a sense of utter aloneness, often accompanied by aimlessness and boredom. It is argued that loneliness lies close to alienation but lacks its antipathy. While Younger's view is interesting, using a continuum to conceptualize such complex psychosocial aspects of human life is arguably too simplistic.

In his book *The Loneliness of the Dying*, Elias (1985) develops a powerful argument that reinforces the image of loneliness in older people and the chronically ill. For Elias, the development of a meaningful death is dependent upon people's specific pattern of 'individualization', with the image of death being bound up with people's image of themselves and the image of human beings prevalent in their society. The way a person dies depends not least on whether or how far they have been able to set goals and to reach them. It depends on how far the dying person feels that life has been fulfilled and meaningful or, alternatively, unfulfilled and meaningless.

For those who are dying, physical care by doctors and nurses may be planned appropriately and implemented but, at the same time, the separation of individual persons from normal life and their congregation in hospitals, hospices, or nursing homes with strangers may result in loneliness for the individual. As a result of this, Elias suggests that many old people's homes are 'deserts of loneliness'. Elias also describes how, in modern intensive care units, dying people can be cared for in accordance with the latest specialist knowledge but as regards feelings they may die in total isolation. Therefore, of great concern are not just the physical 'objective' symptoms but what dying people themselves subjectively experience.

In concluding, Kurtz (1982) reports that loneliness is a feeling and, like all other feelings, must be subjective and therefore difficult to measure, to weigh or to compare. Shame, solitude and romantic delusions are components of our loneliness; the key component is loss – loss of nature, loss of God, loss of each other and the apogee of loneliness is loss of self.

DEFINING ATTRIBUTES OF LONELINESS

Walker and Avant (1995) refer to 'defining attributes' as those particular aspects of a concept that characterize its meaning. Analysis of the findings from the literature review uncovered the following attributes about loneliness as it pertains to palliative care:

- It involves the social meaning of death
- It is based upon people's relationship with those around them
- It is an individualized process
- It is characterized by loss
- It is a subjective experience.

Based upon these defining attributes, and the literature reviewed, it is possible to give a tentative theoretical definition of loneliness: 'Loneliness is an individualized and subjective experience that is characterized by loss and people's attempt to construct meaning for their life or death process and the relationships that form it.'

CONSTRUCTION OF A MODEL CASE

Rodgers (1994) argues that, by providing a real life example that includes all the defining attributes, a model case enhances the degree of clarification and credibility of the concept. The following model case is constructed from a real life experience, though names and details have been changed in order to maintain confidentiality.

Case study 14.1
Model case of loneliness

> Mr Taylor is a 62-year-old man who was diagnosed with small-cell carcinoma of the lung in January 2002. During his ongoing courses of radiotherapy treatment, Mr Taylor lost his wife of 40 years, who had been troubled with angina for some time. Initially he cared for himself at home, where he was supported by the community nursing service (he and his wife have no children or close family contacts). His periods of treatment were followed by several days of respite care in the local palliative care unit. In September 2002 Mr Taylor developed tingling and sudden pain of the lower limbs, associated with generalized weakness and an inability to pass urine. An emergency computed tomography scan indicated spinal metastases and cord compression. Treatment was unable to prevent total paralysis and Mr Taylor is now confined to a wheelchair.

Case study 14.1
Model case of
loneliness—*Cont'd*

As an inpatient in the unit, Mr Taylor is receiving symptom control and psychosocial, spiritual and emotional support for his progressive condition. In sharing his experiences with members of the team, he describes the loss of his wife, his diagnosis of cancer, subsequent disability and poor prognosis as the major contributory factors for his extreme feelings of loneliness and social isolation. A quiet and very private man, he finds it difficult to mix with patients around him and has indicated his acceptance of death and release from what he sees as long-term unhappiness.

This model case study is of particular relevance to this concept analysis because it displays each of the 'defining attributes' of loneliness. For this patient, loneliness is characterized as an individualized and subjective experience, which I believe should be studied initially using phenomenological research methods to provide a description and interpretation of the experience as it is lived. It involves a person's social meaning of death, influenced by relationships with those around him and certainly included the experience of loss – of his wife, previous good health, independence, mobility and social relations.

RELATED CONCEPTS

Related concepts are those that convey similar or associated meanings with the concept under analysis (Rodgers 1989a). The related concepts as derived from the literature review include:

- Isolation
- Alienation
- Stigmatization
- Marginalization
- Separateness.

While related concepts are closely related to the analysis of loneliness, their significance at this stage is to give added clarity to the overall analysis.

Mellor (1993) focuses on the way in which death is hidden rather than forbidden in contemporary life. Individuals in modern societies shape their own identities and systems of meaning within a private sphere of social relations. In this context, impending death presents particular problems, threatening alienation and existential isolation. **Instead of being marginalized, it is argued by Clark (1993), that death should be of central significance to social research.** The aloneness individuals experience when having to cope with the death of others is perhaps even more intense when they themselves prepare for death. As a result of the reality-threatening power of death, Elias argues that modern peoples are increasingly reluctant to come into close contact with those who are dying. Since the maintenance of their self-identities is potentially undermined by the presence of death in others, it could be argued that there is a tendency for all persons now to die in situations of unparalleled isolation.

Mellor (1993) argues that 'death' and 'the dead' do not fit into modernity; they are sequestrated or secluded from contemporary societal thinking. However, Small (1997) proposes a counter claim by suggesting that 'dying' is different. There are ways in which it can and has been critiqued; for example, one can look at its medicalization or its privatization (Field et al 1997). Small argues that, as with modernism, we have only a partially developed approach to the overall complexity of death, dying and the dead (Small 1997). **In a society that promotes the healthy human body, in an analysis of consumer culture, gender, sexuality, health and illness, it is no surprise to find that pain, suffering and death are unwelcome intrusions in the midst of a happy life.** We live in a society characterized by 'death avoidance', and by being dominated by a survival mode we have decided that dying is what other people do (Field et al 1997).

Lawton (1998) augments this argument by providing a very emotive and thought-provoking analysis of the sequestration of the unbounded body and 'dirty dying'. In exploring the marginalization of patients within the physical space of palliative care settings, she examines some examples of why an apparent intolerance of the disintegrating, decaying body appears to have become such a marked feature of the contemporary West. Dying patients may experience a total loss of 'selfhood' and social identity once their bodies became severely and irreversibly unbounded, often as a result of such complications as uncontrolled vomiting, diarrhoea, fungating tumours and the development of gross oedema. They may withdraw, disengage or 'switch themselves off' from society.

An increasing amount of literature is focusing on the stigmatization and marginalization associated with acquired immunodeficiency syndrome (AIDS; Alonzo & Reynolds 1995, Cutcliffe 1995, Green 1995, Green & Platt 1997). Goffman (1969) has described how stigmatized persons incorporate standards from the wider society and in the process discredit themselves. Self-hatred and shame develop from internalizing negative values. The discrepancy between what is expected in a normal individual and what is actual in a stigmatized individual, 'spoils' the social identity and isolates the stigmatized individual from self-acceptance as well as social acceptance (Alonzo & Reynolds 1995).

Some diagnoses, such as epilepsy, cancer and AIDS, can make their victims feel stigmatized and links made between individual failings (particularly sexual ones), social marginality and moral inadequacy are associated with cholera, typhoid, tuberculosis and cancer (Goffman 1969). AIDS is a particularly threatening, stigmatizing illness because the patient with AIDS faces not only death but also death with a 'spoiled identity'. The interpersonal process of dying is no longer one in which personal bonds are made whole and solidified (Siminoff et al 1991); rather the stigma associated with AIDS places an almost insurmountable barrier between the patient and their relatives and friends. In this position these people often develop a sense of 'separateness'. Feelings of loneliness, isolation, alienation, stigmatization and marginalization often lead the person to developing an overriding preoccupation with AIDS, which results in communication only occurring with others who have this illness.

ANTECEDENTS

Antecedents are those events that precede the occurrence of the concept. Antecedence is not synonymous with causality. An antecedent may contribute to the occurrence of the concept, it may be associated with its occurrence, or it may need to be present for the concept to be present. Identifying antecedents may help further refine the defining attributes of the concept of interest. McKenna (1997) states that this step is useful in that it gives an indication of the purpose of the analysis and the clinical area in which the concept is normally used.

Research has demonstrated that loneliness has a high correlation with factors such as living alone, widowhood, singleness, early loss and poor health (Lopata 1969, Seabrook 1973, Townsend & Turnstall 1973, Weiss 1973, Havinghurst 1978, Hunt 1978, Power 1979). Although several writers have shown that loneliness increases with age, Tornstam (1981) demonstrated that, when the above factors are controlled, age is not significant. **It is not that ageing causes loneliness but rather that old people are more likely to experience situations/factors that may cause loneliness at any age, e.g. bereavement, living alone, lack of friends or ill-health.** A change in a person's situation may be the most obvious antecedent for loneliness, for example loss of a loved one or succumbing to a chronic and progressive illness. Another antecedent could be a person's attitude to illness, which arguably depends on childhood experiences reinforced and strengthened throughout adult years. Fromm-Reichmann (1959, p. 128) points out that: 'This frightened secretiveness and lack of communication about loneliness seems to increase its threat for the lonely ones, even in retrospect, it produces the sad conviction that nobody else has experienced or ever will sense what they are experiencing or have experienced'. Therefore, lack of communication and awareness may also be antecedents of loneliness.

The impersonal phenomenon of death is a final antecedent of loneliness. In modern society, less attention is being directed to clarifying the interrelated pattern of dying within the context of meaningful life experiences (Jones 1992). Dying is often treated as an object of scientific detachment. No longer a subjective experience of life, death has become an impersonal medical problem; however the hospice philosophy and developments in palliative care are addressing this situation by providing a charismatic alternative to the institutionalized picture of death in the UK (Corner & Dunlop 1997). Also by adopting what Good et al (1981) term 'a meaning-centred approach' to understanding practice, palliative care providers seek to access patients' interpretations of their illness in assisting them to construct new understanding of their situation. Kleinman (1988) used this approach in the context of patients' with chronic pain to develop a new model of practice in which the patient's narrative of the illness experience is used therapeutically to elicit the meaning and significance of symptoms, and the consequences of illness to the patient's personal and social world. Corner & Dunlop (1997) suggest that it should therefore be possible to construct a model for palliative care that could take these issues into account and could provide the basis for innovations in care.

CONSEQUENCES

Consequences are those events or outcomes that happen after the occurrence of the concept. It is understandable that often the consequences of loneliness are negative in nature. Decreased quality of life, possible withdrawal and social isolation could be consequences of loneliness. Even when openness towards death is present, the dying person commonly experiences isolation as they approach the terminal phase of life. As a result, many dying patients may spend their final days and hours experiencing great loneliness. Patients may also feel that they are already 'as good as dead', that they have died socially in the minds of others (Charmaz 1980). In spite of this negative interpretation attached to the consequences of loneliness, there may be positive outcomes as well. When patients are ready to talk, many will communicate and share their experience of loneliness, sometimes verbally, sometimes through gestures or other non-verbal communication.

EMPIRICAL REFERENTS

Empirical referents provide a means of measuring the defining attributes and are the events that demonstrate the existence of the concept (Walker & Avant 1995). Given that the concept of loneliness has been defined as being both vague (Seabrook 1973) and subjective (Younger 1995), and that it defies description (Fromm-Reichmann 1959), it would be extremely difficult to operationalize it. Arguably the best way to acquire further knowledge about this concept would be to undertake a phenomenological study. This would form the foundation for the commencement of a programme of research-based concept development that would lead to theory generation and the provision of patient-centred care. The identification of areas for further study will now be considered in the concluding section.

RECOMMENDATIONS FOR FUTURE STUDY AND CONCLUSIONS

Dying is treated as a procedural problem in nursing practice, through the application of nursing diagnosis and nursing process. Dying is rarely perceived as part of the experience of living, or characterized by the meanings assigned by the individual to the event (Jones 1992). Research into dying rarely explores dying as a 'living' reality that needs to be organized like any other by the dying person as a social being. Studies do not often describe dying, and the loneliness experienced as a result of dying, as a set of organized experiences at least partly directed by the dying person. Charmaz (1980) suggests that there are strong indications that dying persons themselves play a critical and active part in the social management of the dying process. As the shift from acute to chronic types of illness increases with better treatments, it can be expected that this role of the dying will become increasingly important (Kellehear 1990).

The challenge for the nursing discipline will be the construction of meaning that will help to explain the subjective and individual experience of loneliness in dying patients. Only when research is grounded in the lonely person's living reality will the long-term goal of expanding nursing's knowledge base be achieved.

The evidence base of nursing research contains few studies on loneliness as experienced by dying patients, despite the fact that nurses sometimes discuss these feelings of loneliness, aloneness and social isolation with patients. A programme of concept development through multiprofessional research should therefore be planned that emphasizes the experience of loneliness and the development of specific clinical assessment tools. Perhaps nurses need to reconsider their approach to caring for the psychosocial needs of patients, focus more on assessing each individualized experience and aim to plan care to reduce the negative impact of loneliness. Strategies to support this may include thorough patient assessment with open and sensitive communication, increased use of day care facilities, individual and therapeutic group counselling sessions, social support and various complementary therapies, e.g. pet therapy. In providing a holistic approach to care, healthcare professionals need to pay more attention to 'how they see a person'. This could be the first step towards addressing this important quality-of-life issue.

REFERENCES

Alonzo AA, Reynolds NR 1995 Stigma, HIV and AIDS: an exploration and elaboration of a stigma trajectory. Social Science and Medicine 41: 301–315

Andersson L 1998 Loneliness research and interventions: a review of the literature. Aging and Mental Health 2: 264–274

Armstrong T 2003 Symptoms experience: a concept analysis. Oncology Nursing Forum 30: 601–606

Berblinger KW 1968 A psychiatrist looks at loneliness. Psychosomatics 9: 96–102

Beyea SC 1990 Concept analysis of feeling: a human response pattern. Nursing Diagnosis 1: 97–101

Bolmsjo I 2000 Existential issues in palliative care – interviews with cancer patients. Journal of Palliative Care 16: 20–22

Charmaz K 1980 The social reality of death. Addison Wesley, Reading

Chinn P, Kramer MK 1995 Theory and nursing: a systematic approach, 4th edn. CV Mosby, St Louis, MO

Clark D 1993 The sociology of death: theory, culture, practice. Blackwell, Oxford

Cocker KL, Bell DR, Kidman A 1994 Cognitive behavioural therapy with advanced cancer patients. Psycho-oncology 3(2): 233–237

Cody WK 1997 What is nursing science? Nursing Science Quarterly 10: 12–13

Corner J, Dunlop R 1997 New approaches to care. In: Clark D, Hockley J, Ahmedzai S (eds) New themes in palliative care. Open University Press, Buckingham, pp. 288–294

Cutcliffe JR (1995) How do nurses inspire and instil hope in terminally ill HIV clients? Journal of Advanced Nursing 22: 888–895

Davis G 1992 The meaning of pain management: a concept analysis. Advances in Nursing Science 15: 77–86

Davis C, Sheldon F 1997 Therapeutic innovations. In: Clark D, Hockley J, Ahmedzai S (eds) New themes in palliative care. Open University Press, Buckingham, pp. 223–238

Dobratz M 2002 The pattern of the becoming-self in death and dying. Nursing Science Quarterly 15: 137–142

Donaldson J, Watson R 1996 Loneliness in elderly people: an important area for nursing research. Journal of Advanced Nursing 24: 952–959

Elias N 1985 The loneliness of the dying. Basil Blackwell, Oxford

Ernst E 2001 Complementary therapies in palliative cancer care. Cancer 91: 2181–2185

Faulkner A, Maguire P 1994 Talking to cancer patients and their families. Oxford University Press, Oxford

Field D, Hockey J, Small N 1997 Death, gender and ethnicity. Routledge, London

Fromm-Reichmann F 1959 On loneliness. In: Bullard DM (ed) Psychoanalysis and psychotherapy. University of Chicago, Chicago, IL, pp. 326–336

Goffman E 1969 Stigma: notes on the management of spoiled identity. Penguin, Harmondsworth

Good BJ, Delvicchio S, Good MJ 1981 The meaning of symptoms as a cultural hermeneutic model for clinical practice. In: Eisenberg I, Kleinman A (eds) The relevance of social science for medicine. Reidal, Boston, MA

Green G 1995 Attitudes towards people with HIV. Social Science and Medicine 41: 557–568

Green G, Platt S 1997 Fear and loathing in health care settings reported by people with HIV. Sociology of Health and Illness 19: 70–92

Havinghurst R 1978 Aging in Western society. In: Hobman D (ed) The social challenge of ageing. Croom-Helm, London, pp. 15–44

Hinshaw AS 1989 Nursing science: the challenge to develop knowledge. Nursing Science Quarterly 2: 162–171

Hunt A 1978 The elderly at home: a study of people aged 65 and over living in the community in England in 1976. Social Survey Division, Office of Population and Census Surveys, London

Jacob SR 1993 An analysis of the concept of grief. Journal of Advanced Nursing 18: 1787–1794

Jones SA 1992 Personal unity in dying: alternative conceptions of the meaning of health. Journal of Advanced Nursing 18: 89–94

Kellehear A 1990 Dying of cancer: the final year of life. Harwood Academic, Reading

Kemp V 1985 Concept analysis as a strategy for promoting critical thinking. Journal of Nursing Education 24: 282–284

Kleinman A 1988 The illness narratives: suffering, healing and the human condition. Basic Books, New York

Kurtz I 1982 Loneliness. Basil Blackwell, Oxford

Lawton J 1998 Contemporary hospice care: the sequestration of the unbounded body and dirty dying. Sociology of Health and Illness 20: 121–43

Lopata H 1969 Loneliness: forms and components. Social Problems 17: 248–262

McKenna H 1997 Nursing theories and models. Routledge, London

Mason DJ, Backer BA, Georges CA 1991 Towards a feminist model for the political empowerment of nurses. Image – Journal of Nursing Scholarship 23: 72–77

Mellor P 1993 Death in high modernity: the contemporary presence and absence of death. In: Field D, Hockley J, Small N (eds) Death, gender and ethnicity. Routledge, London

Moody LE 1990 Advancing nursing science through research, vol 1. Sage, Newbury Park, CA

Morse JM 1995 Exploring the theoretical basis of nursing using advanced techniques of concept analysis. Advances in Nursing Science 19: 31–46

Mort F 1993 Dangerous sexualities. In: Clark D (ed) The sociology of death. Blackwell Science, Oxford

Moustakas CE 1961 Loneliness. Prentice-Hall, Englewood Cliffs, NJ

Norris CM 1970 Proceedings from the second annual nursing theory conference. University of Kansas, Lawrence, KS

O'Leary E, Nieuwstraten I 2001 Emerging psychological issues in talking about death and dying: a discourse analytic study. International Journal for the Advancement of Counselling 23: 179–199

Oxford English Dictionary 1993 Oxford English Dictionary, 2nd edn. Clarendon Press, Oxford

Power B 1979 Old and alone in Ireland. St Vincent de Paul, Dublin

Robinson DS, McKenna HP 1998 Loss: an analysis of a concept of particular interest to nursing. Journal of Advanced Nursing 27: 779–784

Rodgers BL 1989a Concepts, analysis and the development of nursing knowledge: the evolutionary cycle. Journal of Advanced Nursing 23: 305–313

Rodgers BL 1989b Loneliness. Easing the pain of the hospitalized elderly. Journal of Gerontological Nursing 15: 16–21

Rodgers BL 1994 Concepts, analysis and the development of nursing knowledge. In: Smith JP (ed) Models, theories and concepts. Blackwell, Oxford

Seale C, Addington-Hall J 1995 Dying at the best time. Social Science and Medicine 40: 589–95

Seabrook J 1973 Loneliness. Maurice Temple Smith, London

Siminoff LI, Erien JA, Lidz CW 1991 Stigma, AIDS and quality of nursing care: state of the science. Journal of Advanced Nursing 16: 262–269

Slevin E 1995 A concept analysis of and proposed new term for, challenging behaviour. Journal of Advanced Nursing 21: 928–34

Small N 1997 Death and difference. In: Field D, Hockley J, Small N (eds) Death, gender and ethnicity. Routledge, London

Smith EE, Medin DL 1981 Categories and concepts. Harvard University Press, Cambridge, MA

Thomas J, Retsas A 1999 Transacting self-preservation: a grounded theory of the spiritual dimensions of people with terminal cancer. International Journal of Nursing Studies 36: 191–201

Tornstam L 1981 Daily problems in various ages. Paper presented to X11th International Congress of Gerontology, Hamburg

Townsend P, Turnstall S 1973 Sociological explanations of the lonely. In: Townsend P (ed) The social minority. Allen Lane, London, pp. 257–263

Walker LO, Avant KC 1995 Strategies for theory construction in nursing, 3rd edn. Appleton & Lange, Norwalk, CT

Weiss RS 1973 Loneliness: the experience of emotional and social isolation. MIT Press, Cambridge, MA

Wenger C 1983 Loneliness: a problem of measurement. In: Jerrome D (ed) Aging in modern society. Croom Helm, London, pp. 145–165

Witzleben HD 1968 On loneliness. Psychiatry 21: 31–43

Wilkinson S, Aldridge J, Salmon I et al 1999 An evaluation of aromatherapy massage in palliative care. Palliative Medicine 13: 409–417

Wright K, Flemons D 2002 Dying to know: qualitative research with terminally ill persons and their families. Death Studies 26: 255–271

Younger JB 1995 The alienation of the sufferer. Advances in Nursing Science 17: 53–72

Zack MV 1995 Loneliness: a concept relevant to the care of dying persons. Nursing Clinics of North America 20: 403–14

A concept analysis of shame

Mary Haase and Lanny Magnussen

EDITORIAL

As stated in the previous editorial, through the course of writing this book and as a result of thinking about nursing concepts over the last decade and more, it strikes the editors that there are certain concepts that are 'difficult' to talk about. That is not to imply that these are tacit concepts: concepts that exist beyond our ability to express them in words. Moreover, they are concepts that, for a range of reasons, nurses appear to be uncomfortable with. Perhaps by its very nature shame is one such concept. It is not without a great deal of discomfort that we, as practitioners, explore ways in which patients and nurses may be experiencing shame; how we may be contributing to a sense of shame; and what we might do by way of interventions to alleviate this sense of shame. Accordingly, it may come as little surprise that the literature, particularly the nursing literature, is hardly replete with references to shame and the healing of shame. But is encouraging, nonetheless, that some literature exists. Mary and Lanny remind us in their chapter that shame is pervasive, it is common and it is frequently encountered in healthcare settings, particularly but not exclusively within mental healthcare settings. However, despite the pervasive and sometimes imperceptible nature of shame, Mary and Lanny also remind us that there is a large amount we can do as practitioners to help alleviate and combat the patient's sense of shame.

Interestingly, shame within healthcare settings is by no means exclusive to patients and there is a great deal of research that needs to be undertaken to examine experiences of shame in nurses. The classic work of Menzies comes to mind and the ways in which nurses dealt with their sense of shame some 40+ years ago. While much has changed in healthcare over this time, the capacity for nurses to feel shame has not necessarily diminished, indeed, with an increasingly litigious undercurrent to much of health care, an argument could be made that the capacity for shame in nurses within health care has increased.

There are some additional and as yet hitherto unanswered questions about the nature of shame, particularly its compound effects. For example, does previously unresolved shame make one's present shame more difficult to deal with? Is the nurse who is experiencing an unresolved sense of shame likely to be less effective than her 'shameless' colleague? Does one need to attend to one's own shame issues before one can engage and help with another person's shame? The parallels here with the notion of 'the wounded healer' are not lost on the editors, and there may be a great deal we can learn about dealing with shame by scrutinizing this body of work. What is clear is that healthcare organizations have both a professional and moral obligation to their employees; one that includes findings ways to help nurses deal with and/or cope with any unresolved shame. Furthermore, it is incumbent upon these organizations to minimize any sense of unnecessary shame that they foster in or bestow upon their nurses.

INTRODUCTION

> *It is shame or pride which reveals to me the other's look and myself at the end of that look. It is shame or pride which makes me live, not know the situation of being looked at.*
>
> *Sartre 1956*

Concept analysis can be defined as the examination of the attributes or characteristics of a concept (Walker & Avant 1995). It is through careful examination of the concept that the attributes or characteristics are unveiled and a deeper more meaningful description of the concept is revealed. Yet concept analysis does not prescribe a permanent definition of a concept; rather, a concept analysis provides a tentative suggestion (Walker & Avant 1995). The meaning of a concept may change over time or with another's experience. Having acknowledged the possibility of the changing meaning of a concept, this chapter presents a concept analysis of shame as it is understood at this point in time. The meanings of shame should be clearer once you have read and thought about this concept analysis. In this chapter the approach and procedure for conducting a concept analysis suggested by Walker and Avant (1995) will be used as a framework, although not strictly adhered to.

SELECT A CONCEPT

Possibly the most difficult step of a concept analysis is the selection of the concept to be examined. Walker and Avant (1995) suggest that this should be done with care and that a concept of deep interest should be selected. The process of conducting a concept analysis should not drag the researcher down but rather excite and enlighten. Accordingly, we have selected the concept of shame. Shame is a concept that has not been well defined by the nursing discipline, despite the fact that shame influences a nurse's activities daily (Grainger 1991, Zupancic & Kreidler 1998). Shame may be experienced many times in a day; the ability to manage our reaction to shame often disguises or minimizes the impact of the shame experience both for the one experiencing it and the observer. Although nurses (and other healthcare practitioners) experience it, they seldom have meaningful conversation about the experience of shame. Perhaps we often lack the ability and skills to talk about it. However, the disorganizing tendencies of shame may well put patients at risk while we respond to our experience of shame.

Thus, the aim of this analysis of shame is to assist the reader to gain a deeper understanding of the concept. We hope to unveil the attributes and characteristics of shame, making the concept clearer and more visible. This unveiling will lead nurses (and other practitioners) to learn about shame and how it influences what we feel, what we do, what we say and even who we are. Most importantly, it will improve our ability to manage disorganizing emotion so it does not negatively impact how we deliver nursing care to/with our patients. Shame can lurk in the background of all interactions and can quickly become the dominant emotion. Ignoring the impact of shame in healing relationships can, and often does, destroy or hinder the therapeutic alliance between nurse and patient. Furthermore, the connection between team members and the resultant impact on the quality of care provided is powerfully shaped by the individual and team's ability to manage shame affect.

IDENTIFY USES OF THE CONCEPT

In this step of the concept analysis, as many uses of the concept as can be found are identified. We used dictionaries, thesauruses, literature and interviews with those who have experienced shame. Commonly, shame is described as a phenomenon covering a continuum that starts as a slight blush of modesty and ends in a crushing experience of being unfit for human contact. The experience of shame involves a biological dimension, in addition to having social and cultural determinants. Studying shame is confounded by the multiple factors that are linked to the shame experience. The word shame comes from the Old English *sceamu*, akin to Old High German *scama*, 'shame', meaning feeling of disgrace; state of disgrace; circumstances causing disgrace; modest feeling (Hoad 1986). Macdonald (1988, p. 142) writes that 'the word shame is in fact thought to derive from an Indo-European word meaning hide'.

Shame is probably from the root meaning 'to cover' according to the *New Webster Encyclopedic Dictionary* (Thatcher & McQueen 1984).

Shame is defined in the *Concise Oxford Dictionary* (Fowler & Fowler 1958) as:

1. Feeling of humiliation excited by consciousness of guilt or shortcoming, of having made oneself appear ridiculous, or of having offended against propriety, modesty, or decency
2. Restraint imposed by desire to avoid humiliation
3. State of disgrace, ignominy, or discredit.

Shame is defined in the *Oxford Dictionary* (Thompson 1995) as a noun:

1. A feeling of distress or humiliation caused by consciousness of the guilt or folly of oneself or an associate
2. A capacity for experiencing this feeling, esp. as imposing a restraint on behaviour (has no sense of shame)
3. A state of disgrace, discredit, or intense regret

4a. A person or thing that brings disgrace
4b. A thing or action that is wrong or regrettable.

As a verb:

1. To bring shame on, make ashamed, put to shame
2. Force by shame (was shamed into confessing).

And also:

- For shame! (a reproof to a person for not showing shame)
- Put to shame (disgrace or humiliate by revealing superior qualities)
- Shame on you! (You should be ashamed)
- What a shame! (How unfortunate).

In the *New Webster Encyclopedic Dictionary* (Thatcher & McQueen 1984) the word shame is defined as a painful sensation excited by the exposure of that which nature or modesty prompts us to conceal, or by a consciousness of guilt, or of having done something which injures reputation; the cause or reason of shame; reproach; disgrace; contempt. Related words include shamed, ashamed, shamefaced, shamefully, shamefulness, shameless, shamelessly and shamelessness. These related words describe how and when shame is experienced. Shame has been defined by many, yet controversy about the definition still exists (Tomkins 1963, Lewis 1971, Tangney &

Dearing 2002, Nathanson 1992). Are guilt, humiliation and embarrassment merely synonyms for shame? Or is each of the words uniquely distinct?

An extensive review of the literature revealed that shame is a relatively new area of interest in the healthcare literature. The concept has been examined from points of view that include Eastern and Western religion, psychoanalytic theory, affect theory, affect–cognitive theory, cognitive–behavioural theory, developmental theory, transpersonal theory, developmental psychology and social psychology. The point of view promoted by Nathanson (1992) is that shame affect interrupts the experience of interest or joy. His rather dense theory builds on the original work of Tomkins (1963). Tomkins suggests that the role of shame is to promote survival by providing a stimulus powerful enough to interrupt the effect of interest/excitement or enjoyment/joy. Interruption of these rewarding effects occurs when continuing the behaviour may be potentially damaging to an important relationship or to the self. Stosny (1995) writes about how shame can reinforce anti-social behaviour in individuals who are resistant to the experience of shame.

Nathanson (1992) offered a model that explained what he referred to as the cognitive phases of shame, as well as a structure to examine common defensive reactions to anticipated and actual shame – what he called the compass of shame. These cognitive phases of shame follow the developmental path of children. The successful negotiation of all phases results in a shame-resistant but socially responsive adult. Nathanson makes the case that the most potent antidote to shame is healthy pride.

Other prominent writers who have been exploring the many dimensions of shame are Tangney and Dearing (2002), who further developed and tested the work of Lewis (1971). Their thesis is that the experience of shame is about the diminishment of self, without the ability or opportunity to repair or change the defective characteristics. **It is the individual's sense of self that is under attack, not simply their behaviour. Tangney and Dearing provide a definition that helps us differentiate between shame and guilt, which are commonly used interchangeably in the literature.** The difference is 'I did a horrible thing' (guilt) and 'I am horrible' (shame). Shame is the effect of connection/disconnection, providing powerful and immediate emotional information to all participants.

Freud studied shame but only as it related to his focus on anxiety and guilt (Zupancic & Kreidler 1998). He thought of shame as a social moderator that opposed the pleasure principle. Erickson (1950) identified the second stage of psychosocial development as the critical task of learning autonomy versus shame and doubt. If a child at this stage did not succeed at the developmental task of autonomy then they would be plagued with experiences of shame and doubt. Kohut and Fairbairn suggest that when the child's exhibitionist demands are not responded to with admiration, approval, or empathic understanding by the primary caregivers, the child experiences a narcissistic injury (Kohut & Fairbairn 1971) This early non-acceptance is experienced by the child as shame and results in instinctual shame – the shame of being seen. The resulting accumulation of shameful memories is experienced repeatedly when the adult is aware of being seen. When adults have not developed adequate character adjustments to the exposure of self they will experience an outbreak of shame. Dysfunctional reactions can include anger, fear, depression, obsessive–compulsive behaviours, self-harm behaviours, even suicide, and violence against others (Jacobson & Gottman 1998).

Nathanson (1997) and Tomkins (1963) state that shame is one of nine innate effects. Nathanson believes an affect is primal and that shame may serve an evolutionary function by protecting individuals from becoming too excited over potentially harmful situations. Beck et al (1985, p. 156) describe shame as 'an affect related to a person's conception of his public image at the time that he is being observed or believes he is being observed'.

Tangney (2002) describes shame as a member of the family of self-conscious emotions. Other members of the family are guilt, embarrassment and pride. Feelings of shame are unwelcome and often difficult to manage. Shame generally results following the exposure and consequent disapproval, by the other, of a significant incorrectness or personal shortcoming. During the shame experience, we become intensely aroused and acutely aware of the scrutiny of the other (Lewis 1986). Beck et al (1985) state that if individuals engage in a shameful activity in private they will not feel shame. This belief is supported by Hahn (2001). The modulating factor in shame is the scrutiny or perceived scrutiny of the other.

Feelings of shame challenge the internal belief that one is decent, good and competent (Street & Arias 2001). Shame causes us to feel less of a human being. It is as if the capability of rational thought leaves us. Our eyes avoid contact with the other, our head drops forward and our body turns inward. We may experience feelings of self-loathing, anger and disgust. We find ourselves wanting to just disappear from sight, to cover up and become invisible to others. We want to run or hide, not wanting to be found out.

Our perception of the scrutiny of the other may be totally skewed but if we believe our perception then we will experience shame. The other does not need to be known to us: they may be a total stranger. According to Gilbert (1998), anxiety is a central element in the experience of shame, but Beck, et al (1985) have a different opinion. They note that, while anxiety typically occurs before a person enters a stressful situation and ends when the situation is over, shame starts with a person's reaction to scrutiny and feelings of shame may last long after the experience has ended. Leaving the situation does not mean an end to the feelings of shame. Anticipatory shame may be experienced as anxiety and often develops into depression if there is not adequate relief from the experience (Nathanson 1992).

Researchers of shame have found that anger is sometimes a response to shame but the anger can be activated so quickly that a person may lack conscious awareness of the experience of shame (Gilbert 1998). When a person is shamed they may react with anger to save face. This is not to say that all anger is related to shame – sometimes a person may just be frustrated. In Tomkins' (1963) model of affect, anger is stimulated when there is a higher than optimal level of stimulation.

Many people use the words guilt and shame interchangeably, but Tangney (2001, 2002) clearly separates the two. Guilt and shame are both reactions involving a negative evaluation of self. Guilt is the disapproving evaluation of one's behaviour but shame is the negative evaluation of one's entire self (Lewis 1971, Tangney 2001, 2002, Street & Arias 2001). Guilt expresses the thought, 'I have made a mistake!' while shame cries out, 'I am a mistake!' (Albers 2000). People who experience guilt often feel compelled to confess or make amends for their behaviour to the other person. Shame experiences make a person feel worthless and powerless and make them want to escape or hide.

Humiliation and shame are also often used interchangeably but Miller (1993, p. 145) notes the differences.

> *... humiliation is the emotional experience of being caught inappropriately crossing group boundaries into territory one has no business being in. If shame is the consequence of not living up to what one ought to, then humiliation is the consequence of trying to live up to what one has no right to.*

Miller (1993) states that to be humiliated is to be brought down in some manner. Humiliation is an act done to one person by another. Shame is a reflection of one's self by the self. Shame is the person's interpretation of the action of another. It is possible to experience shame and humiliation at the same time.

One way of handling feelings of shame is keeping it a secret. If you are able to cover your shame by hiding your bodily reactions and not telling the secret, no one will know. It will be your secret.

In religious circles shame and sin have been associated for hundreds of years. Feelings of shame were relieved through confession and prayer. It also seems that a display of shame results in less harsh attention from others. We know that the experience of shame causes us to turn away from the other, thus making disclosure of feelings of shame doubtful. We try to hide our shame. **We are ashamed of our shame. How then can shame be healed? Gilbert (1998, p. 25) writes that the 'repair of shame may involve forgiveness of self and belief in the forgiveness of others'. The research on forgiveness is just beginning to be studied and developed (Konstam et al 2001).**

Kaufman (1992, p. 5) very neatly sums up the effects of shame on an individual and gives some direction for beginning to heal the individual who has experienced shame:

> *Because shame is central to conscience, indignity, identity, and disturbances in self-functioning, this affect is the source of low self-esteem, poor self-concept or body image, self-doubt and insecurity, and diminished self-confidence. Shame is the affect that is the source of feelings of inferiority. The inner experience of shame is like a sickness within the self, a sickness of the soul. If we are to understand and eventually heal what ails the self, then we must begin with shame.*

Kaufman suggests group therapy as an effective method for dealing with shame. He also suggests symptom management, repatterning of cognitive distortion and teaching of self-care strategies, but gives no indication of how to proceed with these strategies.

What becomes apparent is that there is a degree of consistency in the literature that focuses on shame, the experience of shame is disorganizing, demoralizing, often comes without warning and can bring whatever you were doing to a complete halt, if only momentarily.

DETERMINE DEFINING ATTRIBUTES

Once the many instances of a concept have been found the next task is to read through them and make note of the characteristics that repeat. It is these characteristics that come to be known as the defining attributes of the concept. In Walker and Avant's (1995) view, the defining attributes differentiate one concept from another; they clearly describe the concept under review.

Not all concepts have a behavioural component, but the concept of shame does. When someone is shamed or experiences shame their head drops, eyes avert, and they seem to shrink in on themselves. A similar response can also be seen animals. A shamed dog drops his head and tail, averts his eyes and cowers. In defeat there is shame: the defeated slink away, not daring to look up, hoping to become invisible until the experience passes.

Central to the differentiation of shame from the other self-conscious emotions is that repair or redemption is not possible. A particular experience is defined as shame by the person having the experience. Tangney's research was not able to distil out a clear set of experiences that would produce shame in anyone exposed to those experiences. We conclude, then, that once the brief affect and action tendency phase of shame stimulation pass the subsequent events can be under the control of the individual. **It is how the individual interprets and then responds to the event that decides whether it is shame or one of the other self-conscious emotions. We further propose that, with adequate recondition/learning, the majority of us can undo the harmful effects of early shame.**

DEVELOP MODEL CASES(S)

A model case holds all the defining attributes of the concept and no attributes of any other concept. It is a pure example of the concept under study. There is no doubt that the case is a true example. A model case for shame follows.

Case study 15.1
A model case for shame

> Jane is excited about the excellent assessment and care she has pro-
> vided her patient. She shares her findings with her colleague. Her col-
> league responds, 'I expected better of you. It is clear to me that Mrs Jones
> was having a hypoglycaemic reaction, not an anxiety attack. How could you
> mix up the symptoms?' Jane's chin drops to her chest, she looks away from
> her colleague, her head spins with confusion as she tries to assimilate what
> is being said to her. As her stomach churns, she wishes she could sink into
> the floor. She thinks, 'I am so stupid!'

CONSTRUCT ADDITIONAL CASES

Now the model case has been constructed the next step is to construct additional cases. These cases are constructed to show what the concept is not and to promote further understanding of the concept. Walker and Avant (1995) suggest five additional cases, borderline, related, invented, contrary and illegitimate. Constructing the additional cases enables the researcher to ensure that there are no overlapping attributes and no conflicting defining attributes.

BORDERLINE

A borderline case contains some of the critical attributes but not all of them. In some cases they may contain most or all of the attributes but there may be a difference in one of the attributes. It is these small differences that further help to define the concept in question.

In a borderline case Jane listens to the feedback from the colleague and assesses the new information against her findings. Although she feels shame it is short-lived and she moves into action to examine the care the patient required. She also feels confident in her nursing skills and acknowledges that even the most skilled nurse can miss relevant information in an assessment. Jane is also puzzled at the disrespectful elements in her colleague's feedback. She decides to wait a while and then to approach the colleague to see if she can re-establish comfort and ease in the relationship.

If she found she was not accurate in her assessment, Jane would revise her care plan, discuss it with the doctor and the patient then begin the new treatment. This is different from a shame response because Jane attempts to repair the relationship, does not feel diminished or flawed as a person or a nurse and she does not react out of old responses learned in childhood.

RELATED

Related cases are related to the concept but do not contain the critical attributes. Related cases help to clarify all the concepts that surround the concept under review. In the case of shame, related concepts are guilt, embarrassment, humiliation and perhaps even anger.

Jane shows her assessment to her colleague, who then asks if she can present the assessment in grand rounds later that day. At the grand rounds, Jane's case is held up as an example of incompetent nursing. Jane is asked to explain how she so badly missed the obvious symptoms of hypoglycaemia and whether she feels she should be allowed to continue to practise given her pathetic assessment skills. This public humiliation is much more than the simple interruption of positive affect, it continues on in an attempt to destroy Jane's credibility as a nurse.

An example of guilt would be if Jane had not followed the procedure for a complete assessment because the ward was very busy. She relied on her initial impressions and had not waited for the lab results to come back before starting the nursing care. She then ignored new information from the patient and convinced herself that she was doing a wonderful job. When her assessment was reviewed she knew she had been premature in her assessment. She still has confidence in her skills and is not diminished in the eyes of her colleagues. She promises herself always to complete the assessment before committing to a care plan.

INVENTED

Invented cases are constructed using ideas that do not exist within our own experience. In the invented case all Jane's thoughts and feelings about this patient, as well as her fears and doubts about herself, are projected on to a huge screen in the main lobby of the hospital for everyone to see. When Jane realizes that everyone has seen this numerous times and her flaws and her most painful secrets are exposed, she is flooded with shame.

CONTRARY

A contrary case is clearly not an example of the concept. A contrary case would be when Jane's colleagues see her work and say 'Well done – see you tomorrow'. Their complements are not so glowing as to put Jane above the crowd and invite jealousy, yet they accurately reflect a job well done and it is appreciated by the team.

ILLEGITIMATE

An illegitimate case shows the concept used improperly. It is not always included in a concept analysis. An illegitimate case would occur if Jane's error was pointed out in a respectful way and she then corrected the treatment plan to reflect the new information. Someone observing the interaction felt, however, that Jane had been shamed because the error had been pointed out to her. They drew this conclusion because Jane blushed when the conversation began and stammered a bit when she began talking about the assessment process she used. Because the colleague bringing the error to her attention was a man, the observer felt that he used his superior size and strength to intimidate Jane and that this is further proof of the toxic heritage of the patriarch. The observer's conclusion is that if any man speaks to a woman he will shame her because of the systemic power imbalance.

IDENTIFY ANTECEDENTS AND CONSEQUENCES

Antecedents are the events that come before the occurrence of the concept. An antecedent cannot also be an attribute of the concept. Consequences are the events that come about as a result of the occurrence of the concept. In other words, antecedents lead up to the concept and consequences follow it.

ANTECEDENTS

Any observant parent can tell you about the infant's reaction when the mother suddenly breaks away when they are participating in that intensely intimate mutual gaze that is the essential to the bonding process. Suddenly the infant responds with a loss of coordination, a dropped head, perhaps crying or whimpering, and flushing. This is the innate response to an interruption of a highly valued activity. It is shame prior to the influences of learning and living in a social world. The particular biology of the child interacts with the environment to produce the unique and intensely complex set of rules that becomes the shame experience of the adult.

Tangney's (2001, 2002) research confirmed the powerful role that experience has in shaping the response. She was unable to find any consistency in which experiences would produce shame, humiliation or guilt in her study sample. The role of appraisal influences our response to the stimuli to the extent that what is devastation for one is experienced as a social hiccup for another. The conditions of preperception are the unique mediators that dampen or amplify the shame experience.

For shame to occur the person must first be engaged in an activity that is of interest, even exciting, to them. As they are participating in the activity they experience a series of small victories or conclusions that release the neural density that accompanies concentration and effort. This release is the experience of joy. The waves of engagement completion and joy continue until the person shifts their attention to something else or the activity comes to its natural end, such as finishing 18 holes of golf. When excitement or joy ends abruptly, shame is felt. With the shame there are immediate changes in the person's behaviour. The head falls forward, the eyes avert and the person shrinks into him/herself.

CONSEQUENCES

After the shame experience we continue on with what comes next. Which pole of the compass of shame we use influences our response. Our response options are mostly narrow as we repeat our own history. A novel response to shame is a noteworthy event – it is the climatic moment in the movie where the antihero pulls himself up by his bootstraps and does the opposite of what his usual response is. Sadly, that is mostly the other pole of the compass of shame. A truly novel response would be to face and learn from what in the past has crushed us under our own shame response.

CONCLUSION

Shame is relatively new to nursing and we feel it is important to examine the impact shame responses have on each nurse's practice. There is strong evidence that the disorganizing features of shame reduce the nurse's ability to access complex information, to be creative in problem-solving and to act quickly in a coordinated, purposeful way. This may mean that our patients do not receive the best possible care. The defining attributes of the concept of shame are also useful in relating to the emerging study of workplace bullying and horizontal violence. Understanding the concept of shame as it relates to nursing will bring a greater understanding of how shame influences a nurse's work life. This understanding of shame will pave the way to developing skills to change our behaviours toward each other, understanding why we treat each other the way we do, and to improving nursing care.

REFERENCES

Albers RH 2000 Shame and the conspiracy of silence. Journal of Ministry in Addiction and Recovery 7: 51–68

Beck AT, Emery G, Greenberg RL 1985 Anxiety disorders and phobias. Basic Books, New York

Erickson E 1950 Childhood and society. Norton, New York

Fowler HW, Fowler FG (eds) 1958 The concise Oxford dictionary, 4th edn. Clarendon Press, Oxford

Gilbert P 1998 What is shame? Some core issues and controversies. In: Gilbert P, Andrews B (eds) Shame: interpersonal behaviour, psychopathology, and culture. Oxford University Press, Oxford

Grainger RD 1991 Guilt and shame. American Journal of Nursing 12: 348–356

Hahn WK 2001 The experience of shame in psychotherapy supervision. Psychotherapy 38: 272–282

Hoad TF 1986 The concise Oxford dictionary of English etymology. Oxford University Press, Oxford

Jacobson N, Gottman J 1998 When men batter women. Simon & Schuster, New York

Kaufman G 1992 The psychology of shame, 2nd edn. Springer, New York

Kohut H, Fairbairn J 1971 The analysis of the self. International University Press, New York

Konstam V, Chernoff M, Deveney S 2001 Toward forgiveness: the role of shame, guilt, anger, and empathy. Counseling and Values 46: 26–39

Lewis HB 1971 Shame and guilt in neurosis. International Universities Press, New York

Lewis HB 1986 The role of shame in depression. In: Rutter M, Izard CE, Read PB (eds) Depression in young people: developmental and clinical perspectives. Guilford Press, New York

Macdonald J 1988 Disclosing shame. In: Gilbert P, Andrews B (eds) Shame: interpersonal behavior, psychopathology, and culture. Oxford University Press, Oxford, pp. 141–157

Miller WE 1993 Humiliation. Cornell University, New York

Nathanson DL 1992 Shame and pride: affect, sex, and the birth of the self. WW Norton, New York

Nathanson DL 1997 Shame and the affect theory of Silvan Tomkins. In: Lansky MR, Morrison AP (eds) The widening scope of shame. Analytic, New York, pp. 107–138

Sartre JP 1956 Being and nothingness: a phenomenological essay on ontology. Washington Square, New York

Stosny S 1995 The powerful self. Compassion Alliance, Gaithersburg, MD

Street AE, Arias I 2001 Psychological abuse and posttraumatic stress disorder in battered women: examining the roles of shame and guilt. Violence and Victims 16: 65–77

Tangney JP 2001 Constructive and destructive aspects of shame and guilt. In: Bohart AC, Stipkek DJ (eds) Constructive and destructive behavior: implications for family, school, and society. American Psychological Association, Washington, DC, pp. 127–145

Tangney JP 2002 Perfectionism and the self-conscious emotions: shame, guilt, embarrassment, and pride. In: Flett GL, Hewitt PL (eds) Perfectionism: theory, research, and treatment. American Psychological Association, Washington, DC, pp. 199–215

Tangney JP, Dearing RL 2002 Shame and guilt. Guilford Press, New York

Thatcher VS, McQueen A (eds) 1984 The new Webster encyclopedic dictionary of the English language. Avenel, New York

Thompson D (ed) 1995 The concise Oxford dictionary, 9th edn. Clarendon Press, Oxford

Tomkins S 1963 Affect, imagery, consciousness: the negative affects. Springer, New York

Walker LO, Avant KC 1995 Strategies for theory construction in nursing. Appleton & Lange, Norwalk, CT

Zupancic M, Kreidler MC 1998 Shame and the fear of feeling. Perspectives in Psychiatric Care 34: 29–34

Towards a praxis theory of suffering

Janice M. Morse

EDITORIAL

Relieving or attempting to alleviate a patient's suffering strikes the editors as being another of these concepts that might be regarded as a core element of nursing practice. Further, few credible nursing scholars would dispute that, if a patient is suffering, then it is the nurse's responsibility and duty to attempt to alleviate this. Assuaging this suffering, as Jan points out in her chapter, is by no means limited to the historical, myopic preoccupation with physical suffering – most often suffering in the form of pain. This is not to belittle the importance of pain relief as a crucial aspect of some nursing practice, but suffering transcends unidimensional aspects of the person and it is the responsibility of the nurse to be aware of this.

Jan's chapter further reminds us of another important, if not crucial aspect of practice and that is the need sometimes to leave well alone! As stated in a previous editorial, there is a time for consciousness-raising and there is a time for leaving well alone. It is immensely encouraging to see that the findings of Jan's research add support to this position but it is a position that does not often occur naturally in nursing. One common dynamic that relates to and influences this argument is that nurses often 'feel the need to be doing'. There is a sense that, if they are not busy, if they are not engaged in overt, highly visible interventions, then they are somehow doing wrong, somehow not doing their job properly. Similarly, there is a sense that if they are not engaging in 'active' attempts to make it better (e.g. to relieve or alleviate a person's suffering) then they are being negligent or remiss. When combined, these perceptions, while having perhaps a sound moral underpinning, may well be counterproductive from the point of view of the patient's well-being and recovery. It is a difficult lesson for many nurses to learn but sometimes the hardest thing to do is nothing!!

INTRODUCTION

Understanding the experience of suffering and knowing how to assist those who are suffering are important goals. Yet, despite the vast amount of literature on suffering, little research has been conduced from a behavioural–experiential perspective. In short, although many have conducted interviews and written about the plight of the sufferer (Starck & McGovern 1992) and the ethical–moral implications of suffering (Rawlinson 1986), few have conducted research that observed those who were suffering. Similarly, few have linked sufferers' emotional responses with their behaviours – and the responses of others to the sufferer – over the course of the suffering. Until such research is conducted, we cannot fully understand the behavioural cues of the sufferer and how best to assist those who are suffering.

Nurses are the caretakers of suffering (Morse et al 1996). Understanding suffering, and the responses and needs of those who are suffering, rests squarely on the shoulders of nurses, and easing and alleviating suffering can be considered to be at the heart of nursing (Eriksson 1997, Rodgers & Cowles 1997). Nurses are at the bedside throughout the course of illness and they are often the only support for those suffering, both patients and their families (Travelbee 1971, Kahn & Steeves 1994). Although nursing has given voice to patients' stories of suffering (Gregory & Russell 1999), the literature does not contain an accurate behavioural description of suffering. Links between these stories and patients' behavioural responses are lacking. More seriously, there is no connection between these stories of suffering, behavioural cues and the responses of caregivers. Nursing texts contain recommendations for interacting with the sufferer that are not research-based, and they promote caregiver responses, such as empathy, that are possibly inaccurate and may even be harmful (Morse et al 1992a). There is an urgent need to explore suffering from a number of research perspectives, examine suffering within the clinical context and evaluate nurses' interactions with patients who are suffering.

LITERATURE REVIEW

Medicine has played a dominant role in examining suffering, considering suffering to be inextricably linked to pain (Scarry 1985, Chapman & Gavrin 1999) and other unpleasant symptoms, such as nausea and vomiting (Roy 1998). From this perspective, suffering is a behavioural/emotional pain response. **The primary effort in medical research on suffering, therefore, has been to alleviate pain.** Cassell (1991) notes that this perspective of suffering is simplistic: to remove pain is to remove suffering. For many decades, social scientists have noted that suffering also occurs in response to the meaning of the symptoms to the sufferer (see, for instance, the classic work of Zborowski 1969). Despite this, medicine has been slow to recognize that suffering goes beyond the physical (Cassell 1991). Cassell defines suffering in physical terms but states that it results in an emotional response of the whole person. He writes 'suffering occurs when an impending destruction of the person is perceived; it continues until the threat of destruction has passed or until the integrity of the person can be restored in some other manner' (Cassell 1991, p. 33).

The final major perspective on suffering is the ethical and theological-moral perspective, which considers the purpose of suffering and its redemptive qualities. The ethical perspective considers the relationship between treatment and the value of suffering in human life (Cassell 1992). It also considers the moral responsibility of preventing and relieving suffering (Gadow 1991), and the problem of causing suffering in the process of providing treatments. These and other authors explore the process of suffering and the transformative processes that occur when the meaning of suffering is realized and suffering is relinquished (Watson 1986, Steeves & Kahn 1987).

Kleinman's (1988) early work explored the cultural representations of suffering within an ecological framework and cultural variations in normative behavioural responses. With Veena Da, Margaret Lock and others, he later developed the notion of *social suffering*; in other words, the suffering resulting from 'political, economical, and institutional power' and reciprocally 'how these forms of power themselves influence responses of social problems' (Kleinman 1988, p. ix). Such human suffering occurs as a result of war (Frankl 1992, Asad 1997), famine (Frankl 1992, Asad 1997, Kleinman 1997) or violence (Young 1997) and occurs at the societal (national/population) level (Daniel 1997) within ethnic/cultural groups (Schwarcz 1997).

Suffering has been linked with nurses' imperative to care (Eriksson 1992). The suffering of caregivers resulting from viewing or assisting those who are suffering has been a professional concern for many decades, and it is often linked to burnout. However, inherent in the process of providing care is the sharing of the suffering experience (Kreidler 1984) and the moral obligation to speak of this suffering (Kahn & Steeves 1994). Recent caring theorists expanded beyond empathy to discussions of authenticity (Daniel 1998) or genuineness, which Ray (1997 p. 115) defines as 'unconcealment of affect to self and others.'

Our previous research (Morse et al 1997) indicated that such genuineness may not always be present – nurses apparently either 'matched' or 'countered' the patient's affect depending on their perception of the patient's needs. The interaction is apparently patient-led, with nurses taking their cues from the patient. In order to provide optimally effective care, there is an urgent need to explore this phenomenon further.

Despite the vast amount of research into suffering, enquiry into the nature of suffering has rarely been approached, considering it as an emotional response and using a behavioural-experiential approach. Suffering has been viewed as a response to losses – the loss of a pain-free existence (Chapman & Gavrin 1999), the loss of health (Jones 1999), the loss of dignity, the loss of movement, the loss of an anticipated future, the loss of another, the loss of self (Charmaz 1983, DeBellis et al 1986, Morse & Johnson 1991).

What is suffering? Many synonyms illustrate the affective nature of suffering: discomfort, anguish, distress, torment, pain, heartache, misery, anxiety and affliction. Interestingly, 'endure' is not listed under suffering, but under 'endure' we find support, survive, brave, hold out against, withstand and suffer. From our interviews, laypeople speak about 'enduringandsuffering' under the rubric of suffering, as though both concepts were one word (and therefore one concept) or different manifestations of one concept (i.e. two parts or states within one concept), or two separate but inextricably linked concepts (enduring-and-suffering.) The perceived relationship between enduring and suffering has important ramifications for exploring suffering, because it determines *how* the studies are conducted methodologically, how the resulting theory is conceived and diagrammed, and ultimately how therapeutic interactions and therapeutic outcomes are established for those who are suffering.

It also raises significant research questions. For instance, if suffering and enduring are separate states, can a person emerge from enduring without releasing emotions? And is it possible to experience emotional release and resolve suffering without at some point enduring? It is also important to note that some researchers consider enduring to be an integral part of suffering but have not labelled it 'enduring'. For example, Frankl (1992) writes about keeping suffering privately contained; Reich (1987, 1989) has a stage labelled 'mute suffering'. Is 'mute suffering' another label for enduring? The literature is certainly conceptually confusing.

In this research program, we are exploring suffering using narrative accounts or stories of suffering and linking these with behavioural observations of those who are suffering. Our research program is divided up into discrete research projects, each exploring various aspects of suffering. The research began as an 8-year National Institutes of Health (NIH) grant delineating comfort for the improvement of nursing care. Then we realized that we could not understand comforting unless we first understood what was being comforted. We interviewed trauma and burns patients, and patients with chronic conditions, and observed (including videotaping) in the trauma (Accident and Emergency) room. We continued to study enduring and suffering directly with a 3-year grant from the Medical Research Council of Canada (MRC), exploring suffering in oncology and palliative care populations. (A number of projects were funded by these grants. Please refer to the original publications for methodological details.)

We developed a model of suffering that consisted of two states: enduring and suffering (Morse & Carter 1995, 1996). This model has been revised considerably as our understanding of the second phase (releasing) has developed: we relabelled this suffering as *emotional suffering*, identified the consequences of failing to endure, identified escapes from enduring and emotional suffering and finally described the relationship between states of enduring or emotional suffering and caregiver response. This chapter represents the revised and expanded theory.

A PRAXIS THEORY OF SUFFERING

We identified two broad and divergent stages of suffering: emotional suppression or *enduring* and *emotional suffering* (Morse & Carter 1996) These states are not only distinct but also diametrically opposite; each demands that the person be treated in a distinctly different way.

ENDURING

Enduring occurs as a response to a threat to integrity of self. It results in a shutting down of emotional responses while the person 'comes to grips' with a situation. Enduring is the blocking of the emotional response: emotions are suppressed, squelched, sealed off. Enduring is a strategy that enables the person to 'go through the motions', doing what must be done. It is therefore a natural and necessary behaviour that permits the person to continue day-to-day functioning, but the internalizing of emotions does not bring about relief (Morse & Carter 1996). The individual *must* experience an emotional release *if* healing (i.e. healing that is not of the physical body) is to occur (Moulyn 1982).

Enduring occurs at various levels of intensity, depending on the severity of the threat (Morse & Carter 1996). In its most extreme form, the person appears emotionless, with a mask-like expression. The person has an erect posture, with shoulders back and head up, and mechanical, 'chunky' movements. Walking is characterized by a robot-like gait, swaying from side to side. There is little facial expression and little movement of the mouth and lips when speaking; the person speaks in an expressionless monotone, using short sentences and sighing often. The eyes appear dull and unfocused, the person shows little interest in life (Morse & Carter 1996) and appears vague. In its most severe form, emotional suppression disconnects the person from life, such that later he or she may have no memory of the funeral or stressful event.

Persons who are enduring focus on the present, and it is this focus that enables them to keep going, minute by minute. By focusing on the present, one blocks out the past and the future. If whatever is being endured is a physical threat, then individuals develop strategies for physically holding on to the present, such as counting something, breathing in and out or watching the clock (Morse & Carter 1996).

ESCAPES FROM ENDURING

The suppressed energy must go somewhere, and persons who are enduring often erupt emotionally, expressing anger at some trivial and tangential concern ('displacement comments'). For example, we see relatives in the trauma room furious with staff over some minor matter. These emotional outbursts provide an escape for pent-up energy and escape from that which is being endured; they are usually episodes of short duration, with the person quickly returning to enduring (Dewar &

Morse 1995). Escapes used are 'mind-absenting' behaviours that require purposeful concentration; tasks that distract and remove one's mind from what is being suffered (e.g. doing puzzles); concentrated cognitive work; hard physical exercise; or laughing hysterically. In its most extreme form, participants tell us that they count – they count the tiles on the ceiling or the leaves on the tree (Morse & Carter 1996).

We argue that enduring behaviours are instinctive and helpful because they are a normal response that enables preserving of the self. According to the context and circumstances, we have identified three types of enduring (Morse & Carter 1996):

- *Enduring to survive* occurs in instances of serious physiological threat. It enables the person to focus on vital physiological functions, such as breathing, in order to control intractable pain, to focus on the self. It enables the trauma patient to remain in control, not to fight caregivers, so that care is provided more quickly and efficiently, and not to scream. It conserves the patient's energy and enables the provision of safe care.
- *Enduring to live* occurs in untenable life situations. It enables the person to focus on getting through each moment and thus getting through day by day, thereby getting through the untenable situation.
- *Enduring to die* occurs at the end of life. It enables the person to prioritize, conserve energy, maintain control and remain focused on the present in order to bear the unbearable. Although enduring requires energy, it requires much less energy than emotional releasing. As the person's condition deteriorates, fatigue overwhelms them and the person slips from enduring and relinquishes themselves to death.

EMOTIONAL SUFFERING

On the other hand, emotional suffering is a very distressed state in which emotions are released. (Previously (Morse & Carter 1995, 1996) we labelled this state as suffering, but it was confusing to label the model 'suffering' as well as having one of the states within the model with the same label. We have revised the model to call this 'emotional suffering'.) The person who is emotionally suffering is filled with sadness. The person may cry, sob, moan or weep constantly. The person talks to whomever will listen, repeating the story of the loss over and over, as if to convince themselves that the 'nightmare' is real. ('When I tell you it makes it true.') The person's posture is stooped, with head down and looking as if he or she is 'falling apart'. The face is lined and the facial expression is described as 'drooping'.

When one is emotionally suffering, one can recognize the meaning or significance to one's life of whatever is lost; there is recognition too that the future is changed and irrevocably altered. Gradually, when one has 'suffered enough', hope begins to seep in (Morse & Doberneck 1995, Morse & Penrod 1999) and possible alternative futures are envisioned, realistic goals are established and strategies to work towards achieving these goals are made. **It is the work of hope that brings the person from despair to the reformulated self. Once suffering has been worked through, people report that they revalue their lives; they live more deeply.**

ESCAPES FROM EMOTIONAL SUFFERING

Escapes from releasing are 'mind-numbing' strategies. The person may sleep, drink or eat excessively or try to remove themselves from the situation by mindlessly watching television. Note that the physical escapes used when enduring are actions that use excessive energy; emotional suffering itself uses energy. Those who have emotionally suffered report feeling drained. Therefore escapes from emotional suffering tend to conserve physical energy (Morse & Carter 1996).

THE TRAJECTORY OF SUFFERING

When a catastrophe occurs, the initial response of the individual is shock. The person's senses are acute, they are trying to absorb and make sense of what is happening. If it is an accident, then the person 'checks himself out' to see if his body is intact and how seriously it is injured. The immediate response may be denial, 'No, NO!' There may be a failure to endure, manifest as a loss of control or screaming. As soon as the person recognizes what has happened and recognizes that he must function in order to survive or get through the situation, then 'the person pulls himself together' and begins to endure.

FAILURE TO ENDURE

Through our observations of patients receiving trauma care, we identified six behavioural states. With the first four (unconscious, relaxed/normal, scared, afraid) some degree of relinquishment for care and enduring was evident. The last two (terrified and out of control) may be classified as *a failure to enter enduring*.

Nurses' comforting actions, using the *Comfort Talk Register* (Proctor et al 1996), and eye contact and touch (Morse & Proctor 1998) with patients who are terrified, facilitates the patient's ability to hold on, prevents the loss of control and moves the patient towards enduring. Comforting strategies are not attempted with those who have lost control. Loss of control is a dangerous state for trauma patients; they are screaming and unable to hear or hold still, may fight caregivers, are restrained and are usually pharmaceutically paralysed as soon as possible so that care may proceed.

ENTERING EMOTIONAL SUFFERING

Those who are enduring do not move from enduring to emotional suffering until they are tentatively ready to accept their loss. People may move slightly beyond enduring and 'taste' emotional suffering, then sense the possibility of psychologically disintegrating and instantly move back into enduring. They may also flip back and forth between enduring and emotional suffering according to energy level, context and available supports. In this way, progression through the model is not a linear movement from enduring to suffering. The person may move back and forth quickly between enduring and emotional suffering, and emotional suffering may suddenly, and at any time, overwhelm a person who is enduring. Furthermore, within each state, the emotional levels change in intensity. Sometimes, when enduring, it may take a great deal of energy to contain the emotion; at other times the emotional suppression will occur without the sufferer being aware of it. Sometimes, when emotionally suffering, the sadness will be intense; at other times it will be manifest as an all-encompassing sadness resembling depression.

Individuals move back into enduring in two ways. First, the taste of releasing, with its overwhelming emotions, may cause the person to fear loss of control, fear they may disintegrate and fear not being able to regain control. Second, emotional suffering requires energy: after a period of sobbing the individual is depleted of energy and it is this depletion that enables the person to move back into enduring.

What moves individuals from one state to another, from enduring to emotional suffering and vice versa? We have identified two factors:

- Cultural and behavioural norms and context, contributing to the individual's ability to withstand the loss
- Levels of understanding/acceptance about the event that is causing the response.

First, whether one endures or emotionally suffers is a process of *appropriate behavioural norms*. For example, one may endure in public and emotionally suffer in private; one may express emotional suffering in front of some family members and hide emotional suffering from others. Family members suffering in the waiting room may 'pull themselves together' as they walk around the patient's room, ceasing to exhibit suffering quenching their emotions. They endure as they enter the patient's room for to reveal the extent of the suffering by revealing emotional suffering is to reveal the seriousness of the anticipated loss, which might place a burden on the patient. It is paradoxical that at the same time patients are concealing their emotions from the family by enduring for the same reasons and, sometimes with a great effort, suppressing their emotions and returning to enduring. This enduring behaviour sometimes causes much distress to caregivers, who have been taught that crying is normal and who therefore try to encourage emotional releasing, particularly in families in which someone is dying. Thus, first it is the *appropriate situation* and context that, in part, determines whether or not a person endures or releases emotions.

Second, as previously mentioned, it is *recognition* that the event has happened that moves people into enduring, *acknowledgement* that it really occurred moves them into emotional releasing and *acceptance* of the lost past and the altered future that moves them beyond suffering. Once the loss is accepted, hope seeps in; it is the work of hope that enables the person to move on to the reformulated future. **We argue that suffering is a necessary means to recovery. In other words, emotional suffering is a healing agent (Moulyn 1982).**

OUTCOME OF SUFFERING

People who have suffered reconstitute their lives and they describe themselves as becoming richer for the experience of suffering. They have an urge to 'give back', to help those who are suffering get through the experience. They volunteer to help with support groups and become involved in the lives of those who are suffering, and they are prepared to speak publicly about their experience, their loss and their own suffering (Morse & Carter 1996).

To reiterate, the process is not linear. Note that enduring and releasing in Figure 16.1 are drawn with shaky circles, indicating that the nature and intensity of the experience vary over time, sometimes from minute to minute, sometimes more slowly. People switch back and forth between enduring and emotional releasing, using the escapes when they can no longer endure or tolerate releasing.

THE ROLE OF SUFFERING

We live within a social world of mutuality – of interaction, of dependence, of community. As such, behavioural cues of suffering communicate distress. From this perspective, we consider suffering behaviours, such as the signs of overt distress of

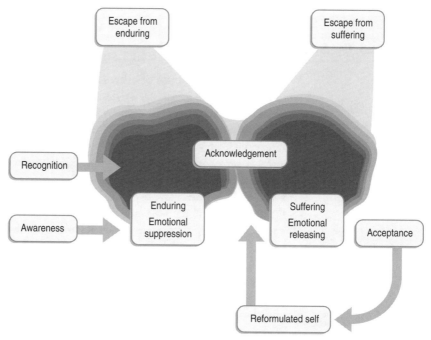

Figure 16.1 Model of suffering

emotional releasing (e.g. weeping, sighing, stooped posture, verbal expressions of distress, and so forth), *as signals that motivate others* to comfort those who are suffering (Morse et al 1992b). Enduring is a natural response that enables the individual to function. Enduring gives signals to others that imply dignity, capability, strength and coping. It sends a message: 'Don't touch me – I'm fine, thank you'. When enduring, individuals have an erect posture; their arms lie impassively at their sides or they may be crossed as though they are 'literally' holding themselves together.

Family groups who are enduring stand apart. When one person is more distressed than others, family members may stand on either side of the one who is most enduring. There are spaces, gaps between each individual. They do not touch, maintain eye contact, or talk to the person who is enduring; they may 'talk for' him or her when approached by others.

When sufferers are releasing suffering, their posture is stooped; the extreme is to collapse on the floor. Those observing the sufferer to some extent share the emotional response or are moved to compassion, compelled to console, commiserate, sympathize and pity. People step forward to touch, support, hold or hug, give reassurances and so forth. They may encapsulate the sufferer with their body, as if to hold the sufferer together. This response in others to alleviate suffering is probably innate, although we recognize that those with certain relationships to the sufferer or with certain roles or professional preparation have priority access to comfort the sufferer. That is, one is less likely to offer comfort to a stranger than to a family member or a friend, but comforting a stranger is not taboo if the signals of distress are acute or the circumstances are extraordinary.

PARADOXES OF SUFFERING BEHAVIOUR

Because of the response of others to suffering (i.e. suffering signals distress, which motivates others to assist), we describe emotional suffering as an external or public state. The nature of the distress and the type of behavioural signals present communicate the severity of the distress and place the responsibility onto others to intervene, to try to alleviate the distress by comforting, by *'being there'* for the sufferer. *A paradox* occurs because emotional suffering is a state that is communicated, can be instinctively evaluated and motivates others to alleviate distress. It can also result in the distress of the other. Such is the basis of empathic response. Further, the sufferer is aware that, *if* the reason for the suffering was caused by another, *if* it will distress the other person to see the suffering, *if* the very act of seeing the suffering will make the other suffer as well or *if* the suffering is considered a sign of personal weakness, inappropriate in the context, then the emotional release of suffering will be concealed. The paradox is that, whereas its public nature enables others to assist in alleviating the suffering, its public nature demands that emotional suffering be a private behaviour. In our data, we have records of sufferers concealing their suffering, crying in secluded places (in a car on the way home from work (Wilson & Morse 1991)), by retreating to the bathroom or by simply turning away from others. Some people prefer to be consoled by counsellors and clergy rather than by family members and close friends in order to remove the responsibility and the burden of comforting from others who may also be suffering. The person may also conceal the suffering by moving from emotional releasing to enduring.

ENDURING BEHAVIOURS

The suppression of emotions in the person who is enduring demands a distant respect from others. This makes enduring a private state in which the person's emotions are concealed. The upright posture and controlled emotions do not invite others to console – quite the converse. Those who are enduring send a signal to others not to touch or hug, not to console or to comfort; rather, the message ranges from 'Leave me alone' to 'Stand back, I'm OK'. The suppression of emotions and the focus on the present enable the enduring person to 'get through' the immediate untenable situation beyond comprehension: the funeral, the medical treatments, and so forth. It enables them to continue to care for children rather than to 'fall apart', emotionally disintegrate and be unable to function in day-to-day events. However, it is interesting to note that, although enduring people consider themselves to be functioning quite well, in retrospect they may rate their level of functioning as poor. Because emotions are suppressed and not communicated to others, we have classified enduring as a private state. Again, note an interesting paradox: the encapsulating or blocking of the emotions when enduring (hence making it a private state) enables *public behaviour/public functioning*.

Returning to Figure 16.1, note that individuals may move back and forth between enduring and emotional releasing. It is also important to note that both concepts vary in intensity depending on what is being endured, the distractions present and the overall context. As their state alters, so do the others' styles of interaction with those who are suffering. From silent support and being there when they are enduring to moving in and comforting when they are releasing.

THE SYNCHRONY OF SUFFERING

Day-to-day events demand that responsibilities be met, children be cared for and one spouse 'be there' for another. Thus, one spouse may endure to 'keep things going' while the other suffers; some time later they may switch these roles. In this way there is a certain synchronicity or pacing of enduring and suffering states that depends upon the responses of others and on context. As previously mentioned, people may suffer in the family waiting room, walk down the corridor to visit the relatives, pull themselves together, move to enduring and enter the room concealing emotional distress from the sick person. Later, when leaving the room, they may 'break down' and return to the waiting room to suffer. Therefore, whether one endures or suffers depends upon the context and the support available.

IMPLICATIONS

I have previously made the argument that 'nurses are the caretakers of suffering' (Morse et al 1996). This means that the primary responsibility for the care, and the comforting, of those who are suffering is the professional responsibility of nursing and rests squarely on the shoulders of nurses. From the above, what can we ascertain that will help nurses achieve this goal?

First and foremost, we see that *care must be patient-led* (or *sufferer-led*). Nurses are experts at reading the non-verbal behavioural cues of patients. Perhaps it is experience, intuition or simply a part of human interaction that enables this 'reading' of the patient. **Nevertheless, being able to recognize the behavioural patterns that patients exhibit as they suffer – and use them to guide therapeutic interventions – is an advanced nursing skill.** Nurses must be able to recognize and articulate behaviours related to suffering, to differentiate between those who are enduring and those who are emotionally releasing and to recognize that they need to be treated differently.

Those who are *enduring* should have their enduring behaviours supported. They should not be touched. Verbal statements should be used that support their enduring; for example, 'You are holding up well' is appropriate. Being with the person in silence – not saying anything – is also helpful, although it may appear that the person is unaware of your presence. Support must be present-focused, making no reference to the future ramifications of the event.

When persons are enduring, empathy should *not* be used. These people are 'emotionally available' as they attempt to come to grips with their situation. Empathic statements, consolation, commiseration, condolences and expressions of sympathy and pity 'break through' the enduring, so that the person will move unwillingly to emotional releasing. We call empathic expressions that are unanticipated and cause the individual to 'break down' *side-swiping* and nurses must recognize that helping a patient to cry or face the reality of the situation is not necessarily therapeutic (Morse et al 1992b). The value we place on tears as a therapeutic sign – a notion perhaps adopted from counselling – must be re-examined, for releasing may not be appropriate during a crisis. Individuals intuitively sense that during a crisis they must be 'strong' or they will not be able to support others and do what needs to be done. Empathic statements and the use of touch with those who are enduring give them something else to resist if they are going to maintain control – another thing to resist and to be endured. Thus, empathy, when used with persons who are enduring, is not helpful and may even be harmful (Morse et al 1992a).

On the other hand, when people are *emotionally suffering,* others encase them with an embrace, as if to give them a new body boundary, a support on which to lean. Touch is firm. These people are held and stroked, and the voices of caregivers console. When emotionally suffering, sufferers need to talk; listening is important and empathy is appropriate. If they seek reassurances, these must be realistic ('I'll be here for you' rather than 'Things will work out'.) These people do not cry constantly – sobbing comes and goes, increasing and decreasing in intensity – but they may continue to cry easily. Assistance with daily tasks, comfort food and emotional warmth are important at this time.

DISCUSSION

Nursing is beginning to recognize the significance of suffering in the provision of care, and expanding its conceptualization of suffering. However, much of our research on suffering still focuses on pain (Paulson et al 1999) and other unpleasant symptoms (van Post & Eriksson 1998). There is a failure to recognize that not all pain, in particular chronic pain, the immediate pain of trauma or transient (but sometimes severe) procedural pain, can be eliminated; neither is it appropriate always to anaesthetize these patients. **Apart from the natural childbirth movement, which actively resists analgesics and replaced them with coping strategies, we have done little to investigate ways to enhance enduring or foster stoicism, preferring instead to use restraints of one type or another, including simply holding patients down.** There is an urgent need to investigate non-pharmaceutical measures to enhance patients' abilities to endure, such as the *Comfort Talk Registry* (Proctor et al 1996), patterns of touch and the most effective and kindest ways to conduct distressing procedures such as a nasogastric tube insertion (Penrod et al 1999, Morse et al 2000).

While the focus on clinical pain continues, some authors are beginning to recognize enduring as a legitimate coping style (Nannis et al 1997) or an aspect of hardiness (Craft 1999), more often associated with psychosocial distress (such as homelessness (Montgomery 1994) or imprisonment (Keavney & Zausszniewski 1999)) and catastrophes (such as tornadoes (Goldeski 1997) or war (Summerfield 1999)). Nurse-authors are beginning to attend to suffering as the basis of patient needs (Fagerstrom et al 1998, Eifred 1998), caring (Eriksson 1992), and comforting (Morse 1992), to interpret and follow patient cues in our efforts to provide patient-centred care (Morse & Proctor 1998). Nevertheless, we still have an immense amount of research to do in learning to understand the behavioural cues of enduring and emotional releasing. Researchers continue to prefer to rely on the perspectives of professionals and patient reports of their needs and the nurse–patient relationship, rather than using technologies and observation methods that will enable the actual identification of cues. We still have an immense amount to learn about appropriate methods of comforting those who are suffering.

This chapter is reproduced, with kind permission from Lippincott Williams & Wilkins, from a paper that first appeared in *Advances in Nursing Science* – Morse JM 2001 Towards a praxis theory of suffering. Advances in Nursing Science 24(1): 47–59.

REFERENCES

Asad T 1997 On torture, or cruel, inhuman and degrading treatment. In: Kleinman A, Das V, Lock M (eds) Social suffering. University of California Press, Berkley, CA, pp. 285–308

Cassell E 1991 The nature of suffering and the goals of medicine. Oxford University Press, New York

Cassell E 1992 The nature of suffering: physical, psychological, social and spiritual aspects. In: Starck PL, McGovern JP (eds) The hidden dimension of illness: human suffering volume. National League for Nursing Press, New York, pp. 291–303

Chapman RC, Gavrin J 1999 Suffering: the contributions of persistent pain. Lancet 353: 2233–2237

Charmaz K 1983 Loss of self: a fundamental form of suffering in the chronically ill. Sociology of Health and Illness 5: 168–195

Craft CA 1999 A conceptual model of feminine hardiness. Holistic Nursing Practice 13: 25–34

Daniel EV 1997 Suffering nation and alienation. In: Kleinman A, Das V, Lock M (eds) Social suffering. University of California Press, Berkley, CA, pp. 309–358

Daniel LE 1998 Vulnerability as a key to authenticity. Image – the Journal of Nursing Scholarship 30: 191–192

DeBellis R, Marcus E, Kutscher AH et al 1986 Suffering: psychological and social aspects in loss grief, grief and care. Haworth Press, New York

Dewar AL, Morse JM 1995 Unbearable incidents: failure to endure the experience of illness. Journal of Advanced Nursing 22: 957–964

Eifred S 1998 Helping patients find meaning: a caring response to suffering. International Journal of Human Caring 2: 33–39

Eriksson K 1992 The alleviation of suffering: the idea of caring. Scandinavian Journal of Caring Sciences 6: 119–123

Eriksson K 1997 Understanding the world of the patient, the suffering human being: the new clinical paradigm from nursing to caring. Advanced Practice Nursing Quarterly 3: 8–13

Fagerstrom L, Eriksson K, Engberg IB 1998 The patients' perceived caring needs as a messenger of suffering. Journal of Advanced Nursing 28: 978–987

Frankl V 1992 Man's search for meaning, 4th edn. Beacon Press, Boston, MA

Gadow G 1991 Suffering and interpersonal meaning. Journal of Clinical Ethics 2: 103–112

Goldeski LS 1997 Tornado disasters and stress responses. Journal of the Kentucky Medical Association 95: 73–89

Gregory DM, Russell C 1999 Stories on life and suffering. Carelton University Press, Montreal

Jones A 1999 'Listen, listen, trust your own strange voice.' Psychoanalytically informed conversations with a women suffering serious illness. Journal of Advanced Nursing 24: 826–831

Kahn DL, Steeves RH 1994 Witnesses to suffering: nursing knowledge, voice and vision. Nursing Outlook 42: 260–264

Keavney ME, Zausszniewski JA 1999 Life events and psychological well-being in women sentenced to prison. Issues in Mental Health Nursing 20: 73–89

Kleinman A 1988 The illness narratives: suffering, healing and the human condition. Basic Books, New York

Kleinman A, Das V, Lock M (eds) 1997 Social suffering. University of California Press, Berkley, CA

Kreidler M 1984 Meaning in suffering. International Nursing Review 31: 174–176

Montgomery C 1994 Swimming upstream: the strengths of women who survive homelessness. Advances in Nursing Science 16: 34–45

Morse JM 1992 Comfort: the refocusing of nursing care. Clinical Nursing Research 1: 91–113

Morse JM, Carter B 1995 Strategies of enduring and the suffering of loss: modes of comfort used by a resilient survivor. Holistic Nursing Practice 9: 33–58

Morse JM, Carter B 1996 The essence of enduring and the suffering of loss: the reformulation of self. Scholarly Inquiry for Nursing Practice 10: 43–60

Morse JM, Doberneck BM 1995 Delineating the concept of hope. Image – the Journal of Nursing Scholarship 27: 277–285

Morse JM, Johnson JL (eds) 1991 The illness experience: dimensions of suffering. Sage, Newbury Park, CA

Morse JM, Penrod J 1999 Linking concepts of enduring, suffering and hope. Image – the Journal of Nursing Scholarship 31: 145–150

Morse JM, Proctor A 1998 Maintaining patient endurance: the comfort work of trauma nurses. Clinical Nursing Research 7: 250–274

Morse JM, Anderson G, Bottoroff J et al 1992a Exploring empathy: a conceptual fit for nursing practice? Image – the Journal of Nursing Scholarship 24: 274–280

Morse JM, Anderson G, Bottoroff J et al 1992b Beyond empathy: expanding expressions of caring. Journal of Advanced Nursing 17: 809–821

Morse JM, Whittaker H, Tason M 1996 The caretakers of suffering. In: Chesworth J (ed) Transpersonal healing: essays on the ecology of health. Sage, Newbury Park, CA, pp. 91–104

Morse JM, Havens GA, Wilson S 1997 The comforting interaction: developing a model of nurse–patient relationship. Scholarly Inquiry for Nursing Practice 11: 321–343

Morse JM, Penrod J, Kassab C et al 2000 Evaluating the efficacy and effectiveness of approaches to nasogastric tube insertion during trauma care. American Journal of Critical Care 9: 325–333

Moulyn A 1982 The meaning of suffering: an interpretation of human existence from the viewpoint of time. Greenport Press, Westport, CT

Nannis ED, Patterson TL, Semple SJ 1997 Coping with HIVV disease among seropositive women: psychosocial correlates. Women and Health 25: 1–22

Paulson M, Danielson E, Norberg A 1999 Nurses' and physicians' narratives about long-term and non-malignant pain among men. Journal of Advanced Nursing 30: 983–989

Penrod J, Morse JM, Wilson S 1999 Comforting strategies used during nasogastric tube insertion. Journal of Clinical Nursing 8: 31–38

Proctor A, Morse JM, Khonsari ES 1996 Sounds of comfort in the trauma centre: how nurses talk to patients in pain. Social Science and Medicine 42: 1669–1680

Rawlinson MC 1986 The sense of suffering. Journal of Medical Philosophy 11: 39–62

Ray MA 1997 The ethical theory of existential authenticity: the lived experiences of the art of caring in nursing administration. Canadian Journal of Nursing Research 29: 111–126

Reich WT 1987 Models of pain and suffering: foundations for an ethic of compassion. Acta Neurochirurgica 38(Suppl): 117–122

Reich WT 1989 Speaking of suffering: a moral account of suffering. Soundings 72: 83–108

Rodgers BL, Cowles KV 1997 A conceptual foundation for human suffering in nursing care and research. Journal of Advanced Nursing 25: 1048–1052

Roy DJ 1998 The relief of pain and suffering: ethical principles and imperatives. Journal of Palliative Care 14: 3–5

Scarry E 1985 The body in pain. Oxford University Press, New York

Schwarcz V 1997 The pain of sorrow: public uses of personal grief in modern China. In: Kleinman A, Das V, Lock M (eds) Social suffering. University of California Press, Berkley, CA, pp. 47–66

Starck PL, McGovern JP 1992 The meaning of suffering. In: Starck PL, McGovern JP (eds) The hidden dimension of illness: human suffering volume. National League for Nursing Press, New York, pp. 25–42

Steeves RH, Kahn DL 1987 Experience of meaning in suffering. Image – the Journal of Nursing Scholarship 19: 114–116

Summerfield D 1999 A critique of seven assumptions behind trauma programmes in war affected areas. Social Science and Medicine 48: 1449–1462

Travelbee J 1971 Illness and suffering as human experiences. In: Interpersonal aspects of nursing. FA Davis, Philadelphia, PA

Van Post I, Eriksson K 1998 A hermeneutic textual analysis of suffering and caring in the pert-operative context. Journal of Advanced Nursing 30: 983–989

Watson JA 1986 Suffering and the quest for meaning. In: DeBellis R, Marcus E, Kutscher A et al (eds) Suffering: psychological and social aspects in loss, grief and care. Haworth Press, New York

Wilson S, Morse JM 1991 Living with a wife undergoing chemotherapy: perceptions of the husband. Image – the Journal of Nursing Scholarship 23: 78–84

Young A 1997 Suffering and the origins of traumatic memory. In: Kleinman A, Das V, Lock M (eds) Social suffering. University of California Press, Berkley, CA, pp. 245–260

Zborowski M 1969 People in pain. Jossey-Bass, San Francisco, CA

A concept analysis of nursing support

Dianne Ellis, Sue Jackson and Chris Stevenson

EDITORIAL

'Offer support' is a term that appears in nursing care planning documentation with conspicuous regularity. It is also a phrase that is bandied around nursing staff and healthcare organizations. Yet there is little consistency in the way the term is used. As Dianne, Sue and Chris remind us in their chapter, even a cursory examination of dictionaries and related literature demonstrates a range of meanings for the term 'support', ranging from: 'preventing a person from giving way, holding up' to 'corroborating a statement'. They also remind us that this support within nursing is quite clearly a holistic phenomenon and that, as a result, nurses provide physical, emotional, intellectual, social and spiritual support to patients. One might be forgiven for thinking that there would be little dissent or disagreement around the notion of providing support to patients. However, by drawing on Peplau's seminal 1952 text, the issue of providing support becomes more complex than originally thought. Peplau is adamant that what patients want is not always what they need. Accepting the cogency of Peplau's position, something of a paradox becomes evident. In the instances where the patient is not getting what they want, would they feel supported? Probably not. Yet, from the nurse's point of view, if they were attempting to give the patient what he needed, nurses are likely to feel that their actions were indeed supportive. Thus support in these situations, or a sense of support, might be something that is best determined *ex post facto*.

What becomes clear in Dianne, Sue and Chris's chapter is that the nature of support between nurses and patients is negotiated; it is likely to be unique and this gives rise to a significant practice implication – the need for specificity in care plans. What precisely do we mean when we write the term 'support' in our care plans? Accordingly, there is a need to spell out the precise nature of that support and how it will be manifest for each individual need. Perhaps writing 'provide support' is analogously non-specific and as ambiguous as writing 'provide care' or 'nurse the patient'. On a related note (the evaluation component of a care plan) measuring support is problematic. Is it limited to patient expressed senses of feeling supported (as this would rule out unconscious and uncommunicative patients)? The issue of specificity may once more inform this issue. If one is able to negotiate and identify highly specific interventions as manifestations of providing support (e.g. provide physical support to help the patient to become mobile following surgery, listen to the patient's concerns, anxiety and fears without prejudice or judgement), then the measurement of support might be expressed as an accomplishment of carrying out those interventions.

INTRODUCTION

The term 'support' is commonly used within health care, usually with very little description offered as to what is actually 'meant'. Rather, the meaning appears to be implicit. This chapter aims to provide researchers and healthcare professionals with a broader understanding of the use of the term 'nursing support'.

Concept analysis has been variously described. The chapter questions the benefits of reductionist-based approaches to concept analysis, especially as applied to the field of nursing, and more specifically in analysing nursing support. Support is multifaceted and best thought about as intricately linked to the varied context in which it is practised. Citing nursing support within the healthcare system leads to the need for a more complex analytic approach. The chapter introduces a communications theory, the coordinated management of meaning (CMM; Pearce 1976, Pearce & Cronen 1979), in order to investigate the versatile nature of nursing support.

CONCEPT ANALYSIS

Norris (1982) describes a concept as an abstraction of concrete events and Polit and Hungler (1987) as being based on observation of certain behaviours or characteristics. The *Oxford Paperback Dictionary* (Allen 1990) defines a concept as an idea, a thought or a hypothesis. George (1995) takes the view that concepts (elements/ objects) such as 'support' generate nursing theories and therefore, for some, the delineation of a concept is fundamental for the development of theory (Hardy 1974, McKenna 1997). Concept analysis holds out the possibility of arriving at a definite meaning for a concept and the definition becomes the precursor of theory development.

The developing field of concept analysis is inclusive of a number of different approaches, beginning with and elaborating on the early work by Wilson (1966). Walker and Avant (1995) have constructed an approach that originates from the logical positivism movement, which requires reduction of the term, enabling isolation of the essence of the concept. Here, the view of a concept is as constant, specific and occurring within clear and strict boundaries. Rodgers (1989) argues that the use of this process for concept analysis can be problematic. She developed an inductive, descriptive model as a means of enquiry that values the evolving nature of a concept.

Despite many differences, both Walker and Avant's and Rodgers's techniques require the investigator to highlight one model case able to reflect all the concept's critical attributes. Thus, one of the first tasks is identification of such a model case. However, with regard to nursing support this is not easy. The following section looks in more detail at the problematics of 'nursing support'.

NURSING SUPPORT

When spoken about, or enacted by nurses, support can be used as a noun to represent a bandage, splint, crutch or life-support machine. and can also signify the people (or group) that provides the support – for example support agency, support network, support staff, support systems and supporting role. The verb 'to support' refers to the practice (doing) of nursing. The *Collins Concise Dictionary* (2002) defines support as, the action of:

- preventing a person from giving way, holding up
- providing/supplying a service/something to enable someone to remain operational or to preserve life
- corroborating a statement
- bearing the cost or weight of something
- giving aid or assistance
- contributing to the value/success of something
- advocating a proposal.

An electronic search for the term 'support' on the CINAHL database (from 2000–2003) established 10393 hits and, when teamed with the word 'nursing', 1514 papers were identified that referred to some aspect of the nursing support. A closer inspection of the findings highlights the extensive usage of this term within nursing. Table 17.1 is one example of how support can be categorized.

Table 17.1

Categories of support

Category	Example
Physical support	Bodyweight support, life support, support function
Social support	Organizational support, family support, public support
Emotional support	Grief support, individual support, labour support
Psychosocial support	Psychosocial support, victim support

According to Morse et al (1996), for a concept to be regarded as mature, the characteristics of the concept need to be found recurrently within the same set of conditions. However, an exploration of the term support in relation to nursing reveals a spectrum of application. Thus, it becomes more likely that the nature of support is being determined and interpreted according to the circumstances of everyday practice, and these views would be in keeping with Rodgers' (1989) approach to concept analysis. Consequently, pinpointing one single set of features is difficult, making approaches to concept analysis that require such procedures problematic. This may be particularly difficult for abstract concepts; Chinn and Kramer (1993) support this argument suggesting, as they do, that abstract concepts are less open to such analysis.

A simple breakdown of the word support results in the discovery of other concepts, for example help/aid, safety/security, evidence and preservation, each of which could be subjected to a concept analysis in its own right. However, in practice, these other concepts tend to become isomorphic with the concept of support, and something about the whole of support is lost. Unfortunately it is perhaps 'what is lost' that is the subject of this enquiry. Similarly, a straightforward dictionary definition may be helpful but will only give a reduced explanation of the term and not a description of what it means to those giving, receiving or being involved in nursing support. It is to those 'meanings in use' that the remainder of the chapter is devoted.

THE WHOLE SYSTEM

By acknowledging that this concept has different 'meanings in use', the issue of context becomes vital. A nurse does not operate independently but as part of a healthcare system that is very complex. It is necessary to bear in mind the dynamic and detailed nature of this system, which has a large number of variables and components with a massive amount of interaction and feedback between them. The healthcare system also has people with a wide range of interests, capabilities, perceptions and stakes in the system and, because of potential coercive relationships between people in social situations, power is a further dimension for consideration (Mwaluko & Ryan 2000). This vast context of 'nursing support' eradicates any plans of using a simplistic approach, accentuating the need for the application of whole systems theory.

'Whole systems theory' has its roots in general systems theory, first mooted by von Bertalanffy (1940) and developed by Ross Ashby in the 1950s and 1960s (Ashby 1952). **To employ a 'whole systems approach' is to take the view that the properties of the concept are not intrinsic and can be understood only within the context of the larger whole, for example through contextual thinking.** This enables support to exist within the entire whole, in different ways and at different times, rather than being a definite thing that occurs at a specific time. The whole is not limited to nursing but to the complete healthcare system and beyond and it consists in an interconnection of inseparable relationships.

So, for instance, if a man is chopping down a tree with an axe, the man is not separate from the tree. Bateson (1972) argues that the tree is providing feedback all the time to the man as the man provides feedback to the tree (through the axe). Therefore, without the tree showing the man where he has cut, leaning to one side, etc., he would not know how to go on with the episode. Thus, the man does not cause the tree to fall through linear cause and effect; rather, there is a kind of circular causation.

Applying the idea of circular causation to nursing support, it becomes the product of interaction and relationships, and in turn redefines the meaning of relationships. Viewing health care as an interconnected network of concepts is to see it as a pattern and when the pattern is 'broken down' its design becomes distorted. Therefore, to fully appreciate a pattern it requires mapping out, as does the notion of support within nursing.

The whole systems approach does not seek to find a static big picture of how things are or should be. Rather, it celebrates the dynamic nature of systems and finds ways in which to both analyse and develop them (Cronen 2001). The artist can only represent one lifeless viewpoint but there are clues that enable the viewer to appreciate that there are alternative angles from which to examine the scene portrayed by 'stepping inside' the picture itself.

SOCIAL CONSTRUCTIONISM

Social constructionists are detached from the traditions of rationalism and empiricism, challenging the six themes that constitute Shotter's (1993) description of reason:

- The use of analysis to view the world and the belief that systematic observation will reveal the natural order of things
- That language is a code, understood by members of the society, linking words to things
- That there is symbolic representation of knowledge from observation, for example as formulae or classification systems
- That the world has a pre-existing order that can be discovered
- That individuals have the resources to make discoveries
- That new knowledge can be forged without reference to previous understandings.

Instead, social constructionists are attached to ideas around there being no necessary arrangement of words that map out an independent world – 'The terms by which we understand our world and our self are neither required nor demanded by what there is' (Gergen 1999, p. 47) – and that an unlimited number of descriptions are possible. Similarly, 'we could use our language to construct alternative worlds in which there is no gravity or cancer' (Gergen 1999, p. 47).

Consider for example, how people come to be schizophrenic. We know that many people hear voices (Romme & Esher 1989, 1993, Romme et al 1992) without ever being so described. The important point here is that the description 'schizophrenic' arises within the relationship between psychiatrist and voice-hearer. **In the same way, what we conceptualize as nursing support is the product of the relationship between the nurse and individual within a particular context.**

Gergen points out that how we describe the world within one social group can be reduced to nonsense in another situation. So just as some plants become weeds and some animals become pests (depending upon the perception or process of knowing), the nature of support is viewed differently (depending upon perception, context, etc.). Of course, this idea is disturbing for some as it suggests that our world is neither real nor solid, and this can lead to accusations of relativism (Holdsworth 1997). However, the constructionist approach can encourage people to think differently about themselves and the world around them. In taking a reflexive stance, we are invited to suspend our existing beliefs, to listen to alternative 'takes' on reality and to wrestle with a plurality of perspectives. Acceptance of diverse accounts of the world may lead us towards a departure from dichotomous thinking, good–bad, right–wrong, supportive–unsupportive.

COORDINATED MANAGEMENT OF MEANING

In 1976 W. Barnett Pearce introduced a new theory of communication based on social constructionist ideas. Pearce and Cronen (1979) further advanced this theory and, in doing so, created the original form of CMM. **One of the important ideas in CMM theory is that the social world is not found but created and that, for that reason, there is a plurality of possible worlds (Pearce 1999).** Consequently, there is a strong focus upon communication processes, since they constitute our knowledge of ourselves and of the world in which we live. Whereas the ideas and practices associated with the Enlightenment movement tend to place the function of communication as that of transmitting messages, the ideas and practices of CMM place communication as shaping our world. So for example, people who live in different cultures or even histories do not merely communicate differently but experience different ways of being human through communicating differently (Pearce 1999).

Coordinated management of meaning offers practical ways with which to examine interactions and the meanings created within them. It aids exploration of:

- what is conjointly created (*coordination*)
- the processes by which we tell ourselves and others stories in order to interpret the world around us and our place in it (*coherence*)
- the recognition that one perception of reality obscures another (*mystery*).

Within CMM there is also recognition that 'Human beings treat messages as if they were multiply wrapped in layers of meaning' Pearce (1999, p. 35). Pearce and Cronen (1979) define these 'layers' as hierarchies that depict the levels of context within which communication is enacted. Frequently there are four 'layers', these being episode, relationship, self (or self-concept) and culture, although there can be further levels in any given instance. The word 'hierarchy' in CMM relates to levels of, rather than importance of, the context.

The different 'layers' can change and shift position during any communication. For example, the concept of self is dependent upon cultural beliefs in a particular episode. To summarize, CMM is a tool for looking at communication and emergent meaning in detail. With regard to nursing support, a CMM-driven description would identify how the meaning of support arises: a) within a social setting, b) between one or more individuals, and c) during an episode of communication. **Therefore, what support 'means' belongs to the individuals in that particular episode of communication.**

UNPACKING MEANING

'"Unpacking" the meaning of messages is a typical CMM-ish activity' (Pearce 1999, p. 33). It is being employed here in order to help better understand how different meanings of support are created in situations or, put another way, how different episodes are able to construct a meaning of support. This summary from a case study described by Ibrahim (1998, p. 797) works as an example:

Case study 17.1

Example of a strange loop

Cindy, a 20-year-old woman, is admitted to the inpatient eating disorder unit of a psychiatric hospital. She gives a history of being a good student; delaying college plans because of her mother's illness. She attended exclusively to her mother, ate very little and became gradually more isolated from her family and friends. A nursing assessment reported: Height 5'2", Weight 58 pounds (50% of her ideal body weight). She is hypotensive and anaemic. She is placed on therapeutic bed rest to conserve energy and she is prescribed high-calorie supplements. Cindy unwillingly complies with bed rest, although she sees herself as being fatigued and has no issue with her weight or diet. She is soon to be discovered exercising.

The term 'naming' distinguishes between a word (and the thing that it stands for) and 'using' the word is concerned with the context and the intentions of the person using it. In the above episode of communication, the nurse is using the word 'ideal' within the context of a psychiatric hospital and with the intention of implying that there is a normal body weight for a person's height and that Cindy is below it. Cindy's response, together with the interpersonal pattern produced, is referred to as 'calling'. In this scenario, Cindy's instructions are to take bed rest and supplements. She complies (unwillingly); thus a dominant/submissive relationship is created. The reason for Cindy's reaction could be due to 'oughtness' and the 'must do' and 'must not do' perceptions that she has taken on board during her social development.

'Oughtness' is significant in relation to how we see others and ourselves and therefore how we act both individually and in concert. Cindy believes that she must do as people in authority tell her and she must not be selfish. In this episode, she feels obligated towards caring for her mother and following the nurse's instructions. Her use of exercise, however, is an indication of the conflict that exists both within her and within the relationship she has with the nurse. This is a tension between the stories lived conjointly with others and the stories told in order to make sense of those lived. Cindy tells a story of caring exclusively for her mother and consequently being fatigued, but the story lived is one of isolating herself and not eating. She may have stories that she is currently not able to tell – *unknown stories* – or that she does not want to tell – *untold stories*. She may even have stories that she has told but that have not been heard – *unheard stories*.

A useful technique to identify a pattern of social practice is to write down the person's cultural/personal rules of communication, rather like writing a recipe for cooking. Some of Cindy's rules might be:

- It is important to be a good person
- To be a good person you must do as people in authority say
- To be a good female it is important to be thin
- It is a female role to take care of the family and home.

Table 17.2 summarizes the 'layers' of context for both Cindy and the nurse within a structure of dependency (hierarchy) appropriate to each.

The information from the table can be represented simplistically using symbols. The symbol ⌐ originates from G. Spencer Brown in *Laws of Form* (1969) and is adopted by CMM to represent 'in the context of'. The symbol ≠ indicates an exclusive disjunction or non-compatibility. And → means compatibility or coordination.

A STRANGE LOOP

Within certain episodes of communication, rules are applied without tension ('charmed loop'); however, in other episodes difficulties arise ('strange loop'). For example, within the context of the hospital Cindy is unable to both 'do as she is

Table 17.2   Layers of context

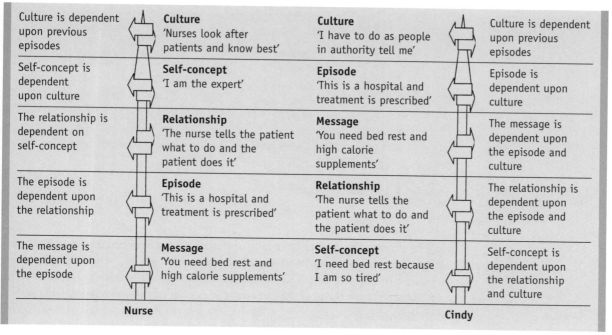

	Nurse	Cindy	
Culture is dependent upon previous episodes	**Culture** 'Nurses look after patients and know best'	**Culture** 'I have to do as people in authority tell me'	Culture is dependent upon previous episodes
Self-concept is dependent upon culture	**Self-concept** 'I am the expert'	**Episode** 'This is a hospital and treatment is prescribed'	Episode is dependent upon culture
The relationship is dependent on self-concept	**Relationship** 'The nurse tells the patient what to do and the patient does it'	**Message** 'You need bed rest and high calorie supplements'	The message is dependent upon the episode and culture
The episode is dependent upon the relationship	**Episode** 'This is a hospital and treatment is prescribed'	**Relationship** 'The nurse tells the patient what to do and the patient does it'	The relationship is dependent upon the episode and culture
The message is dependent upon the episode	**Message** 'You need bed rest and high calorie supplements'	**Self-concept** 'I need bed rest because I am so tired'	Self-concept is dependent upon the relationship and culture

told' and 'remain thin' because both she and the nurse have rules (including 'ought-ness') that conflict, creating tension (strange loop; Fig. 17.1). **Although the nurse views her own actions as being supportive, Cindy does not: she feels obliged to do as the nurse requests and is therefore forced into exercising in secret.**

Having demonstrated disagreement (regarding the meaning of support) with the use of a strange loop, the following example is intended to show shared meaning (of support) by using a 'charmed loop'.

Case study 17.2

Example of a charmed loop

> David has advanced motor neurone disease and is deteriorating rapidly. He has expressed a wish to die at home with his family rather than being admitted to the local hospital. Sam is a Macmillan nurse who expresses 'support' for David's wishes.

Earlier on in the chapter, we introduced the idea of coordination as being what is conjointly created within an episode of communication. Both Sam and David have their own set of rules that govern their behaviour and, although these rules are different, it is possible that they can be coordinated with each other. Coordination occurs when, during the interaction, we move from sense-making to 'lived story'. By taking a closer look at Sam's beliefs in relation to David's request, we see an example of a 'charmed loop' (Fig. 17.2), where the relationship of the words and the context in which they are spoken have shared meaning.

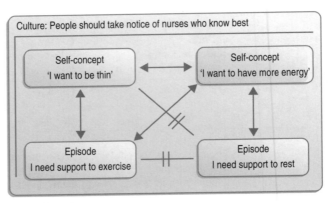

Figure 17.1 A strange loop

The different meanings created in communication between people exist simultaneously at different contextual levels. For example, what Cindy finds supportive at one point she may not find supportive at another. This third example is being used to reveal how the episode can alter the person's meaning of nursing support.

Case study 17.3
The importance of episode

> Jane visits the Baby Clinic with her baby and the health visitor weighs the baby. The health visitor informs Jane that her baby is underweight and therefore needs to see a doctor. Jane feels anxious about this – she thought her baby was doing well.
>
> **Jane**
> **Episode** – Baby Clinic – baby underweight
> **Culture** – A nurse knows best
> **Relationship** – I am here to be advised by the expert
> **Self-concept** – I am a bad mother if I ignore the nurse.
>
> **Nurse**
> **Episode** – Baby Clinic – baby underweight
> **Culture** – I am trained and have access to expert knowledge
> **Relationship** – I am here to advise the patient on what is best
> **Self-concept** – I must be open and honest

In this episode, tension exists between Jane and the nurse, and so Jane feels unsupported. The nurse's information does not make sense in relation to the 'wholeness' of Jane's understanding about her baby (Fig. 17.3). An additional episode, where Jane sees her doctor, will affect this meaning of support. If the doctor informs Jane that her baby is well, she may experience confirmation that she is a good mother and that the nurse has been unsupportive of her. This could negatively influence her relationship with the nurse. However, should the doctor

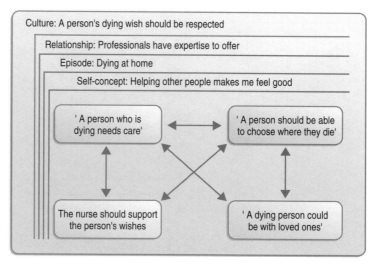

Figure 17.2 A charmed loop

discover and treat a problem that has gone unnoticed, Jane might feel supported by the nurse's actions and their relationship might grow and develop. (Of course, Jane's views about doctors set an additional context for her interpretation of the 'wellness judgement'.)

Unfortunately, nurses are not fortune-tellers in that they can not predict an exact outcome; however a nurse can be open to the possibility of alternative endings.

CREATING SHARED MEANING

Of course, nurses have to operate from their own 'stories told' about well-being, health, illness and care. Yet, they can be open to the possibility of different meanings instead of taking a fixed position with each individual person, who is situated in their own particular context. The idea that nursing support has different meanings in use can influence the interaction of nurses in a positive way. Rather than assuming that something is supportive and offending an individual (perhaps alienating them completely) there is realization about the complexities of interaction and its impact upon people receiving care. Pearce (1999) uses the term 'gamemastery' to define this adaptive form of communication. In ambiguous and unstable episodes, such as when the nurse is unsure as to what support to give, gamemastery allows the nurse to be creative so that clarity and stability can occur. The aim of nursing is therefore towards creating a shared meaning of support, which requires a collaborative and flexible approach. So, for example, how the health visitor might have approached the issue of weight gain would have been to work *with* Jane.

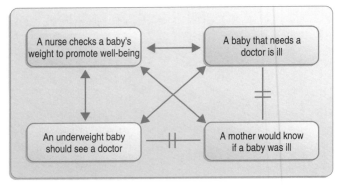

Figure 17.3 Relationship between Jane and her nurse

- 'How has your baby been recently?'
- 'Jane, your baby's weight is below this line here – this information is intended as a guide to help us to understand your baby's weight – what do you think about it?'
- 'Everything about your baby seems fine – but her weight is below the standard scales.'
- 'Would you like your baby to see the doctor?'

CONCLUSION

The examples in the text highlight the fact that the request for a nurse to offer someone 'nursing support' is not as simple or straightforward as it would seem. There are a number of ways for the nurse to respond depending upon the process of knowledge being applied. The nurse could assume a fixed position in relation to support (there is an ideal weight and a nurse must support a person to achieve it). This prevents the nurse from seeing other possibilities (the person is comfortable with his/her weight). This will ultimately impact upon the relationship and effectiveness of support offered.

The application of whole systems thinking enables the nurse, in the first instance, to be aware that there are other possibilities, and then to discover what those possibilities are. By acknowledge this ambiguity about support the nurse can work with the individual to create a meaning in use, i.e. a coordinated understanding of what is supportive to that person. CMM as a method helps to demonstrate the complexities of communication and the different meanings that individuals create given context and previous experience. CMM is therefore a method available to nurses to help them to reflect upon their own practice, examining patterns of communication and assumptions made, as an alternative to seeking the essence of nursing support.

REFERENCES

Allen RE (ed) 1990 Oxford paperback dictionary. Oxford University Press, Oxford

Ashby WR 1952 Design for a brain. John Wiley, New York

Bateson G 1972 Steps to an ecology of mind. Intertext, London

Brown GS 1969 Laws of form. Cognizer Press, Portland, OR

Chinn PL, Kramer M 1993 Theory and nursing: a systematic approach, 3rd edn. CV Mosby, St Louis, MO

Collins Concise Dictionary 2002 Collins Concise Dictionary. Harper Collins, Glasgow

Cronen V 2001 Practical theory, practical art, and the pragmatic-systemic account of inquiry. Communication Theory 11: 14–35

Gergen K 1999 An invitation to social construction. Sage, London

George JB 1995 Nursing theories. Appleton & Lange, London

Hardy ME 1974 Theories: components, development evaluation. Nursing Research 23: 100–107

Holdsworth N 1997 Commentary: postmodernism and psychiatric nursing. Journal of Psychiatric and Mental Health Nursing 4: 309–314

Ibrahim K 1998 Psychosocial needs of the older adult. In: Varcolis EM (ed) Foundations of psychiatric mental health nursing, 3rd edn. WB Saunders, Philadelphia, PA

McKenna HP 1997 Nursing theories and models. Routledge, London

Morse JM, Hupcey JE, Mitcham C et al 1996 Concept analysis in nursing research: a critical appraisal. Scholarly Inquiry for Nursing Practice 10: 253–277

Mwaluko GS, Ryan TB 2000 The systemic nature of action learning programmes. Systems Research and Behavioural Science 17: 393–401

Norris C 1982 Concept clarification in nursing. Aspen Systems, Rockville, MD

Pearce WB 1976 The coordinated management of meaning: a rules based theory of interpersonal communication. In: Miller GK (ed) Exploring interpersonal communication. Sage, Beverly Hills, CA, pp. 17–36

Pearce WB 1999 Using CMM 'the coordinated management of meaning'. Seminar, 4 Aug 1999. Pearce Associates, San Mateo, CA, p. 12

Pearce W, Cronen VE 1979 On what to look at when studying communication: a hierarchical model of actor's meanings. Communication 4: 195–220

Peplau H 1952 Interpersonal relations in nursing. JP Puttnam, New York

Polit D, Hungler B 1987 Nursing research: principal methods. JB Lippincott, Philadelphia, PA

Rodgers BL 1989 Concepts, analysis and the development of nursing knowledge: the evaluation cycle. Journal of Advanced Nursing 14: 330–335

Romme M, Escher A 1989 Hearing voices. Schizophrenia Bulletin 15: 209–216

Romme M, Escher A 1993 Accepting voices. MIND, London

Romme M, Hoing A, Noorthoom E, Escher A 1992 Coping with hearing voices: an emancipatory approach. British Journal of Psychiatry 161: 99–103

Shotter J 1993 Conversational reality. Sage, London

Von Bertalanffy L 1940 The organism considered as a physical system. Reprinted in von Bertalanffy L 1968 General systems theory. Braziller, New York

Walker K, Avant K 1995 Strategies for theory construction in nursing. Appleton & Lange, London

Wilson J 1966 Thinking with concepts. Cambridge University Press, London

A concept analysis of therapeutic touch

Jim Campbell

EDITORIAL

Leaving the jokes about psychiatric/mental health nurses never wanting to touch a patient to one side, it is hard to imagine nursing without involving touch at all. Given that nursing is a practice-based discipline and that practice is the *alpha and omega,* touch of some form or another will be an inevitable part of each nurse's career. We are reminded, in Jim's chapter, that there are various forms of touch (and touching) within nursing and, furthermore, that the category 'therapeutic touch' is still further divided into different interpretations. We will not belabour the obvious need for nurses to be clear about which form of therapeutic touch they are referring to whenever they use this term. The empirical literature in this area consistently shows that: a) nurses have to touch patients a lot, b) most touch is concerned with performing some kind or form of intervention, c) therapeutic touch (not the form of therapeutic touch referred to in Jim's chapter as 'touch as technique') is underutilized and d) patients, in the main, find such therapeutic touch immensely helpful.

However, the editors are unaware how much attention is given to touch and therapeutic touch within nursing curriculums, which rather begs the questions of how we teach students when and how to use touch. The first question is perhaps the more difficult to answer since providing formulaic and causal models of when to touch are problematic at best. Nevertheless, it needs to be acknowledged that, hitherto, insufficient attention may have been given to touch within nursing programmes. This may in part account for the fact that some of the practices of touching patients are usually to perform a task rather than as a form of comfort and/or communication. Further explanations are likely to include the influence of culture on the norms and practices of touch (e.g. the greater comfort that some cultures gain than others with regard to being tactile.) There may well be psychodynamic explanations too (e.g. early formative experiences of physical closeness and touching) and, in considering issues of touch, one needs to be mindful of Argyle's work on proxemics (personal body space and the concomitant degree of comfort we each have when this space is compromised). What is clear is that therapeutic touch remains an immensely powerful and yet significantly underutilized nursing intervention. In the experience of the editors, on occasion, therapeutic touch was the only and most powerful intervention available at certain moments (e.g. gently holding a person's hand as they cried).

INTRODUCTION

> *It is often thought that medicine is the curative process. It is no such thing; medicine is the surgery of functions, as surgery proper is that of limbs and organs. Neither can do anything but remove obstructions; neither can cure; nature alone cures. Surgery removes the bullet out of the limb, which is an obstruction to cure, but nature heals the wound. So it is with medicine; the function of an organ becomes obstructed; medicine, so far as we know, assists nature to remove the obstruction, but does nothing more. And what nursing has to do in either case, is to put the patient in the best condition for nature to act upon him.*
>
> *Nightingale [1860] 1969, p. 133*

Nightingale's statement quoted above indicates that nursing is concerned with optimizing the healing process of nature, by providing the patient with the most comfortable caring environment in order to let nature take its course. In 'modern-day' nursing, many nurses seem to be so concerned with 'miracle' drugs, medical equipment, high-technology hospitals and getting everything done that they have forgotten Nightingale's edict. This is not to apportion blame or to say that the nurse is at fault here. Medical science has been revolutionized since the days of Florence Nightingale in the 19th century. With the improvement of hospital conditions and growth in medical assessments and interventions, the concept of nursing and what it is 'to nurse' have changed dramatically. Yet from the genesis of nursing to the present day, the fundamental importance is the same: the nurse cares for human beings. **The fundamental 'human' needs of the patients are still the same and so the basic importance of comfort, presence, trust, reassurance, support and touch are still just as essential within nursing as they were in Nightingale's day.**

Alongside fundamental, basic needs are the nursing skills that have been used to help meet these needs. Arguably, therapeutic touch is one of these basic, fundamental skills that nurses have always had and needed to care for the patient effectively. Perhaps, the naming of this process of touch has changed since Florence Nightingale's time, yet the actual experience is still the same. The feeling of being cared for by or through touch existed long before the creation of 'formal' nursing systems and practices and is one of the fundamental needs that any human has. When people hurt themselves they rub the area to soothe the pain. When a baby cries, the guardian holds the baby to comfort the child, in order to show them that they are loved and cared for. And this process creates a connection between them; a communication that one cares for the other. Similarly, within nursing in virtually all settings, touch can be used to comfort. From holding a patient's hand during a medical procedure to caring for a patient who is critically ill, touch can communicate a presence, comfort, love, support, trust and reassurance.

It is all well and good stating this; however, what do we mean when we use the term therapeutic touch and what is its significance and uses in nursing? Perceiving therapeutic touch as a concept assists in the latter part of this enquiry, because a concept 'promotes the organization of experience, facilitates communication among individuals, and enables the cognitive recall of phenomena' (Rodgers 1989, p. 330). The employment of concept analysis enables the enquirer to 'refine and define a concept that has originated in practice, research or theory' (McKenna 1997, p. 57).

A variety of authors within nursing have provided different frameworks to carry out concept analyses in order to clarify the meaning and understanding of the concept (Walker & Avant 1983, Chinn & Jacobs 1983). In the context of this chapter, the form of concept analysis advocated by Rodgers (1989) will be used to consider the concept of therapeutic touch. This position sees the dynamic nature of the concept as important, as it changes through context and time. It rejects the traditional essentialist concept analysis approach as concepts change, develop and grow. In order to clearly distinguish essentialist and evolutionary concept analysis, they are described in some details in the following two sections.

ESSENTIALIST CONCEPT ANALYSIS

The essentialist or analytical philosophical position involves defining the concept by its significant attributes in order to find the 'essence' of the concept. These attributes or essences are viewed as the conditions required for the formation of the concept, irrespective of its dynamism and the interrelationship it has with other concepts. These attributes can be thought of in two ways. Rodgers and Knafl (2000) were interested in the differing definitions of the term 'concept' made by nurses and the role of these different viewpoints in the development of knowledge. They described the emergence of two philosophical positions of thought around these diverse definitions, dispositional and entity theories. The dispositional view perceives a concept as habits or abilities that can result in particular mental or emotional behaviours. In contrast, the entity viewpoint of a concept describes a concept as an entity, or form, or body within a system, focusing on the concept as a physical entity in its own right.

Many of the current concept analyses look at concepts as physical entities. Consequently, analysis has taken on an empirical framework, trying to find the characteristics of the concept, the distinct boundaries that form or construct the concept. Once found, these characteristics would take on the 'true value' of the concept, with its various elements that construct it. They would not change with time, with application or use; they would remain rigid with the defined boundaries. The approaches to concept analyses of Chinn and Jacobs (1983), Smith and Medin (1981) and Walker and Avant (1983) are all examples that take on this framework in an attempt to find the true essence of the concept.

EVOLUTIONARY CONCEPT ANALYSIS

Rodgers argues that, as nursing is a discipline that is dynamic and involves different interrelationships, to perceive a concept as rigid with defined boundaries does not capture its true nature. Rodgers' idea is that, through use, application and socialization, a concept becomes associated with a particular set of attributes that can define it. Concepts become publicly marked by certain actions, behaviours and linguistic markers; however, as society is changing so will these attributes change over time or across situations. Therefore, to define a concept by a fixed set of attributes or essence does not accommodate its fluidity, especially in relation to nursing.

The evolutionary view, therefore, considers the concept's position within other concepts and its role or usefulness within this network. For example, therapeutic touch within nursing does not exist as a separate entity. It exists within a network of surrounding concepts within the nursing role. Its use can vary across all patients and all environments. Its application and experience are very much unique to the situation and individual. One person's experience of therapeutic touch is different from another's. To define therapeutic touch by a set of fixed attributes or essence would be defining it from one particular point of view and miss the other attributes, experiences or views of what it is. Instead, the evolutionary view defines a concept by different clusters of attributes compiled from the different experiences of the concept. This allows the concept to be defined by its different attribute clusters rather than by one set of attributes.

This idea of Rodgers' fits with a social constructionist world view that people construct their world through language in different social settings. People construct reality between them as a result of their own interactions. Through daily interlocutions between people in the course of social life, versions of knowledge and reality become fabricated that are ways of making sense of all aspects of the human experience (Gergen 1999). Rodgers argues that the philosophical position of entity theorists does not take this idea of social construction into account. These concept analyses do not reflect the true nature of society and the world around us. Rodgers argues that other concept analyses have fallen into the framework of positivism and forgotten the context-dependent nature of knowledge in the search for truth. So, for Rodgers, the positivist ideal 'persists in the approach to analysis currently employed in nursing' (Rodgers 1989, p. 331).

So, to recap, Rodgers views concepts from an evolutionary perspective, drawing on the work of Price, Rorty, Toulmin and Wittgenstein. Rodgers (1989, p. 332) states: 'Through socialization and repeated public interaction, a concept becomes associated with a particular set of attributes that constitute a definition of the concept'. The analysis of a concept allows it to be used more effectively, which in turn can result in it subsequently changing. Instead of the attributes forming the concept by fixed, rigid boundaries, the attributes appear in clusters: 'Through the process of application, an existing concept may be continually refined... as a result, the concept may be enhanced in its explanatory or descriptive powers, and may thereby offer a greater contribution to the attainment of intellectual ideals' (Rodgers 1989, p. 333).

With this continual socialization, repeated public interaction and refinement, the concept can often become vague and unclear, with its application becoming lost or forgotten. This often results in the concept's purpose and application to knowledge being blurred, uncertain and ambiguous. The use of concept analysis can help clear this, allowing future applications to be clearer. The concept of therapeutic touch within nursing is a good example. Although it is viewed by many as important, its role and application are often unclear. This results in the concept of therapeutic touch within nursing being quite uncertain and ambiguous.

Analysing the concept of therapeutic touch by Rodgers' approach is seen as the most effective way to explore its variety of uses, applications and changes over time. The aim is 'identifying clusters of attributes that may change and are not necessarily limited to fixed and rigid interpretations' (August-Brady 2000, p. 5). However, if the nature of therapeutic touch was less fluid, more fixed and not within a nursing context an essentialist framework might have been considered.

The chosen form of concept analysis involves a number of stages, as listed in Box 18.1.

STAGE 1: THERAPEUTIC TOUCH AS A CONCEPT OF INTEREST

My interest in the concept of therapeutic touch developed from my training in therapeutic massage, which has an underlying basis of therapeutic touch.

Box 18.1

Rodgers's concept
analysis (1989)

1. Identify and name the concept of interest
2. Identify surrogate terms and relevant uses of the concept
3. Identify and select an appropriate realm (sample) for the date collection
4. Identify the attributes of the concept
5. Identify the references, antecedents and consequences of the concept, if possible
6. Identify concepts that are related to the concept of interest
7. Identify a model case of the concept

This training was the beginning of further study and the development of interest in the concepts of therapeutic touch, healing and holistic approaches to care. Through reading a variety of nursing research, the concept of therapeutic touch has been explored at a variety of different levels and it has become clear that therapeutic touch can have different meanings from person to person.

The idea of touch being used in healing dates back to 15000 years ago, evidenced in cave drawings. Early eastern philosophical, religious literatures and Greek mythology all refer to touch as a form of healing (Wright & Sayre-Adams 2001). Many have taken this idea to another level, to include the perception of therapeutic touch as a specific form of a therapy. However, depending from which domain it has been introduced, discussed and constructed, it could have very different meanings. For example, for me, having been trained in therapeutic massage, therapeutic touch is within the process of massage. This is the way I was introduced to the concept, talked about it and experienced it. This is the way the concept of therapeutic touch has been socially constructed for me. However, from a more specific nursing angle, from a holistic/complementary, alternative domain, therapeutic touch is a type of energy healing, using 'hands-on and energy based techniques to balance and align the human energy field' (Umbreit 2000, p. 105).

STAGE 2: SURROGATE TERMS AND USES

Concepts are often referred to by different, or surrogate, terms. Most authors distinguish two types of touch within nursing: necessary touch and non-necessary touch. Necessary touch within nursing is touch that is essential for nursing tasks, e.g. washing, dressing, moving, etc. Non-necessary touch is the opposite and it is this form of touch that we are concerned with in relation to therapeutic touch. There are a number of different surrogate terms that distinguish these two forms of touch, demonstrating the vast use of terms that refer to therapeutic touch, including 'expressive touch' (McCann & McKenna 1993), 'non-procedural touch' (Mitchell et al 1985), 'affective touch' (Lane 1989) and 'caring/social touch' (Adomat & Killingworth 1994).

These forms of touch vary, depending upon the environment, the situation and the particular perception of the nurse who uses it. For example, when working with older people, especially people with dementia, the nursing literature uses the term 'expressive touch' (Kim & Buschmann 1999). In comparison, from a complementary therapy perspective, working with people in palliative and cancer settings, it is described as 'massage touch' (Boissonade 2004). Where nursing is combined with complementary therapy, therapeutic touch is perceived as a particular therapy of healing touch, in which nurses do not actually touch the patient's body, instead moving their hands over the body (Wright & Sayre-Adams 2001). Finally, a nurse asked for the meaning of 'therapeutic touch' could describe the actual experience of feeling 'touched', which can be seen as therapeutic, for example by humour, music, art or eye contact (Perry 1996).

STAGE 3: SAMPLE SELECTION

The concept of therapeutic touch has relevance in diverse settings. With this in mind, a search was undertaken for a selection of articles from a number of different discipline databases. The search was carried out on the electronic databases, MEDLINE, CINAHL, ASSIA and the British Nursing Index. In order to keep the articles to a manageable number, only articles from nursing journals were selected. According to Rodgers (1989) 30 articles should be the minimum sample. In keeping with this, 35 articles were selected.

STAGE 4: ATTRIBUTES

The analysis of the data in Rodgers's (1989) framework generally follows the procedure of thematic analysis. This process involves identifying major themes or attributes within the literature and then organizing and reorganizing the similar points within these themes until a 'cohesive, comprehensive, and relevant system of descriptors is generated' (Rodgers & Knafl 2000, p. 5).

The analysis of the articles of therapeutic touch led to the distinction of a number of themes or attributes. Specifically, these were non-verbal communication, therapeutic experiences, the benefits of therapeutic touch and the combination of therapeutic touch with other nursing skills. Within almost all the literature analysed, therapeutic touch was referred to as a form of communicating, non-verbally, feelings of being cared for, comforted and supported. In addition, it allowed the nurse to build a nurse–patient relationship of trust and reassurance through this non-verbal connection. The use of therapeutic touch was highlighted as a useful benefit for nurses across many nursing environments, including caring for the older person (McCann & McKenna 1993, Wright & Sayre-Adams 2001), caring for patients with dementia (Kim & Buschmann 1999), in acute care settings

(Umbreit 2000), caring for children (Mitchell et al 1985), in intensive care (Adomat & Killingworth 1994) and in palliative care (Perry 1996).

Further analysis of the data resulted in these themes being reorganized into three groups, to form a complete list of attributes. Each of these is discussed in further detail below.

THERAPEUTIC TOUCH AS COMFORT

When we are touched, a connection is created from outside ourselves with someone else in the relationship. Touch has been shown to be vital for humans: they touch and are touched all through their lives (Sung 2001). Touch gives reassurance, it gives warmth, it gives comfort and it tells the person they are not alone. Within nursing, Routasalo (1999) found that the use of touch therapeutically helped people who were behaving aggressively in nursing homes, by comforting and relaxing them, and is a good intervention for nurses to use. Kim and Buschmann (1999) found similar results in a study for people with dementia. With the addition of a gentle voice to touch, the patient's episodes of anxiety and dysfunctional behaviours decreased over time.

Hewitt (2002) carried out a study to look at the therapeutic use of touch in patients undergoing medical procedures, which can often be dehumanizing and uncaring. The study found that touch has a calming effect and helps the patient feel comforted and valued: 'the simple act of holding a patient's hand during medical procedures bridges the technical and human dimensions of critical care' (Hewitt 2002, p. 81). Touch used therapeutically, therefore, allows the nurse to communicate to the patient that they care through offering comfort.

THERAPEUTIC TOUCH AS COMMUNICATION

In nursing, 'touch may be the most important of all non-verbal behaviours' (Gleeson & Timmins 2004, p. 8). Indeed, non-verbal communication is a common theme that runs through many of the papers on therapeutic touch. Therapeutic touch communicates reassurance, warmth and comfort; it communicates to the patient that they are cared for. In particular, for patients who have senses impaired by sedation or are semiconscious, touch is a valuable tool. For example in post- and preoperative care a nurse, by holding a patient's hand, lets them know they are there. This can be seen across many different nursing tasks, e.g. making a patient's bed while they are lying in it. One nurse makes the bed while the other holds the patient on the side of the bed to 'convey the reassuring message to that patient that she is being looked after' (Routasalo 1996, p. 08).

Therapeutic touch as a form of non-verbal communication is very apparent in the literature describing nursing care for older people, especially those with dementia (Gleeson & Timmins 2004). Often, these patients have lost their ability to communicate effectively through cognitive impairments and the use of touch can form part of this lost communication, demonstrated in research to improve their emotional well-being (Kim & Buschmann 1999).

Therapeutic touch does not have to be skin-to-skin contact to communicate. Summers (1992) described an experience as a student nurse being with a dying man. As she was unsure what to say to this patient, she sat with him in silence with a presence communicated of 'being with' him. Perry (1996) explored this non-physical touch in relation to eye contact, in regard to nursing, when caring for their patients. Looking at patients through 'soft eyes' (Sundin & Jansson 2003) allows the nurse to communicate from and to the heart: 'To me touching is critical. It communicates empathy, caring, affections, concern… all of this is transferred through touches with your hands and touches with your eyes' (Perry 1996, p. 11).

THERAPEUTIC TOUCH AS A TECHNIQUE

Within the nursing literature, the term 'therapeutic touch' refers to a form of therapy that involves aligning the human energy field as a kind of 'energy healing' whose benefits have been demonstrated in a variety of nursing practices on physical, mental, emotional and spiritual levels. For the purpose of this chapter, this form of therapeutic touch will not be addressed, as I feel it is different to the form of therapeutic touch being discussed. However, it will be addressed further in the related concepts section of the concept analysis.

Massage is the main form of therapeutic touch that requires actual touch and that nurses can use as a therapy. Massage, is probably one of the oldest forms of human art. It has been described as the 'manipulation of the soft tissues of the body given by a therapist, nurse or carer who has been properly trained' (Boissonade 2004, p. 28). It has a number of benefits, including helping the client feel relaxed, both physically and mentally, increasing mental alertness and helping all the physiological systems, e.g. stimulating the muscular system, neurological system, digestive system, respiratory system and endocrine system. Studies have shown that massage can help arthritis, Parkinson's disease, strokes, migraines and poor sleep patterns (Boissonade 2004).

A similar form of massage that incorporates therapeutic touch and that nurses use is Tellington touch. Tellington touch involves nurses massaging parts of the patient's body with circular movements while retaining a mindful presence and openness. By focusing on the breath, practitioners are able to keep their awareness on the patient's body. Some research investigating the use of Tellington touch found that, for patients undergoing venepuncture, Tellington touch allowed the client to feel relaxed and cared for (Wendler 2002).

STAGE 5: REFERENCES, ANTECEDENTS AND CONSEQUENCES

Rodgers (1989) described the importance of identifying the references, antecedents and consequences of the concept, as they provide additional information and might allow the reader to understand more clearly what the concept is and what it is not.

The purpose of the references within this particular framework of concept analysis is to identify the range of situations, events or phenomena that the concept can be considered in. As already described in this chapter, therapeutic touch can be effective across many different nursing settings, from caring for children to caring for elderly patients, from patients undergoing medical treatments to critically ill patients. However, before touching the patient therapeutically, the nurse needs to carry out an assessment to check whether using it is appropriate within the proposed setting. The criteria for this assessment will be discussed below, as an antecedent.

An antecedent of the concept as described by Rodgers (1989) is the 'events or phenomena that are generally found to precede an instance of the concept' (Rodgers 1989, p. 34). In this context, the antecedent is what the nurse needs to consider prior to touching the patient therapeutically. **The main area highlighted in the literature is whether the patient feels comfortable being touched therapeutically by a nurse.** This is affected by a number of components, including how long the nurse has known the patient, what sex the nurse is in relation to the patient, the age of the patient and the condition of the patient (Wendler 2002). The nurse will need to assess how touch would affect the person, especially considering the condition they are in. For example if the patient is acutely unwell, the nurse needs to decide whether therapeutic touch would be helpful and safe for the patient. The nurse needs to be aware of these issues and on what zone the nurse feels comfortable with the patient.

Nurses need to be aware of the needs of the patient and, if they seem uncomfortable being touched, to respect the patient. In a study by Wendler (2002, p. 8) a patient said, in relation to a nurse's touch: 'I believe there will always be some anxiety involved when a stranger touches you'.

The consequences of a concept are the occurrences that follow after the concept is enacted. In relation to therapeutic touch, as already illustrated in this chapter, a variety of positive gains are achieved for the patient and some for the nurse. These include a feeling of being cared for, feeling comforted, soothed, relaxed and reassured. For the nurse the consequence of therapeutic touch is the connection with the patient and the ability to help the patient feel comfortable, cared for and supported. It creates a connection between the nurse and patient, which allows the building up of trust and a nurse–patient relationship.

STAGE 6: RELATED CONCEPTS

The main concept related to therapeutic touch is the concept of 'healing touch'. Within the nursing literature, a large number of studies describe therapeutic touch as 'healing touch'. This concept has grown from America from the complementary therapy branch of nursing, in which the hands do not actually touch the body. Instead, the nurse unblocks the patient's energy, allowing healing from pain and traumas to take place. Although there is a large debate over the effectiveness of this form of therapy, as it cannot be evaluated scientifically, there are a vast number of examples within the literature describing its effectiveness. Other complementary therapies within nursing can be related to therapeutic touch, including *reiki* and acupuncture.

STAGE 7: MODEL CASE

The model case of the concept as described by Rodgers (1989) is a significant part of the concept analysis because it pulls together the other parts of the framework, presenting a clearing understanding. By providing the model case in an everyday example, the concept is enhanced, resulting in a clearer understanding of how it can be used within practice. It takes the form of a hypothetical case, although this case draws on several 'real' experiences and illustrates a clinical or real-life event (McKenna 1997).

Case study 18.1
A model case of therapeutic touch

> Mrs Martin had been in a car accident with her husband and son. She had experienced fractures to both her legs; however her husband, who had been driving, had only just regained consciousness after a number of days of being in hospital. Unfortunately, their son had died in the accident. Mrs Martin wanted to be the person to break the news to her husband that their son had died. The nurse pushed Mrs Martin, who was in a wheelchair, into Mr Martin's room; she knew what a big ordeal this was going to be for the two of them. As she stopped the wheelchair next to Mr Martin's bed, the nurse placed her hand on Mrs Martin's shoulder, just for a moment, to communicate comfort and reassurance to Mrs Martin and to convey that she would be thinking about her in the next few minutes, as she told her husband of their son's death. The nurse turned and left the room.

CONCLUSION

Within this chapter the concept of therapeutic touch has been analysed as an essential concept in nursing. The use of Beth Rodgers' framework of concept analysis was specifically used as it allows for the dynamism and interrelationships that exist within nursing. This has allowed me to clarify the meaning of therapeutic touch and to help the reader to understand its uses and significance within nursing. In addition, points have been illustrated with examples and research studies, demonstrating that therapeutic touch is an essential fundamental skill in nursing and is used in virtually all situations and areas of nursing. The discussion around necessary touch for nursing duties/tasks and non-necessary touch demonstrates the fluid nature of therapeutic touch in different situations and the use of language in accordance to social construction theorists.

Therapeutic touch allows the nurse to comfort patients on a caring level, connecting with them on a humanistic level away from the medical procedures and techniques that are often experienced. In addition, therapeutic touch allows the nurse to communicate non-verbally a variety of feelings to the patient, including warmth, reassurance and trust. Therapeutic touch can also be used more formally as a named technique, such as massage or healing touch, to help the nurse in a variety of physical, emotional and spiritual aids.

Although large parts of nursing have changed since Nightingale's times, the fundamental use of touch as a human tool to care for oneself and each other is still apparent. Nursing would almost be lost without the ability to touch the patient on a therapeutic level and touch is used almost instinctively by nurses to show that they are 'there for' the patient. With nursing becoming more reliant on medication and medical procedures rather than nature, the use of therapeutic touch should become a more valued nursing skill, which is very much a part of the natural process of humanity rather than a technical approach.

REFERENCES

Adomat R, Killingworth A 1994 Care of the critically ill patient: the impact of stress on the use of touch in intensive therapy units. Journal of Advanced Nursing 19: 912–922

August-Brady M 2000 Flexibility: a concept analysis. Nursing Forum 35: 5–13

Boissonade E 2004 The caring touch: advantages of massage therapy. Nursing and Residential Care 6: 228–231

Chinn PL, Jacobs JK 1983 Theory and nursing: a systematic approach. CV Mosby, St Louis, MO

Gergen kJ 1999 An invitation to social construction. Sage, London

Gleeson M, Timmins F 2004 Touch: a fundamental aspect of communication with older people experiencing dementia. Nursing Older People 16: 18–21

Hewitt J 2002 Psycho-affective disorder in intensive care units: a review. Journal of Clinical Nursing 11: 575–584

Kim EJ, Buschmann MT 1999 The effect of expressive physical touch on patients with dementia. International Journal of Nursing Studies 36: 235–243

Kolcaba K, Kolcaba R 1991 An analysis of the concept of comfort. Journal of Advanced Nursing 16: 1301–1310

Lane PL 1989 Nurse–client perceptions: the double standard of touch. Issues in Mental Health Nursing 10(1): 1–13

McCann K, McKenna HP 1993 An examination of touch between nurses and elderly patients in a continuing care setting in Northern Ireland. Journal of Advanced Nursing 18: 838–846

McKenna H 1997 Nursing theories and models. Routledge, London

Mitchell PH, Habermann-Little B, Johnson F et al 1985 Critically ill children: the importance of touch in a high-technology environment. Nursing Administration Quarterly 9: 38–46

Nightingale F [1860] 1969 Notes on nursing: what it is, and what it is not. Dover Publications, New York

Perry B 1996 Influence of nurse gender on the use of silence, touch and humour. International Journal of Palliative Nursing 2: 7–14

Rodgers BL 1989 Concepts, analysis and the development of nursing knowledge: the evolutionary cycle. Journal of Advanced Nursing 14: 330–335

Rodgers BL, Knafl KA 2000 Concept development in nursing. WB Saunders, Philadelphia, PA

Routasalo P 1996 Non-necessary touch in the nursing care of elderly people. Journal of Advanced Nursing 23: 904–911

Routasalo P 1999 Physical touch in nursing studies: a literature review. Journal of Advanced Nursing 30: 843–850

Smith EE, Medin DL 1981 Categories and concepts. Harvard University Press, Cambridge, MA

Summers S 1992 A long night. Nursing Times 88(19): 47

Sundin K, Jansson L 2003 'Understanding and being understood' as a creative caring phenomenon – in care of patients with stroke and aphasia. Journal of Clinical Nursing 12: 107–116

Sung C 2001 The conceptual structure of physical touch in caring. Journal of Advanced Nursing 33: 820–827

Walker LO, Avant KC 1983 Strategies for theory construction in nursing. Appleton-Century-Crofts, Norwalk, CT

Wendler MC 2002 Tellington touch before venipuncture: an exploratory descriptive study. Holistic Nursing Practice 16: 51–64

Wright S, Sayre-Adams J 2001 Therapeutic touch and the older person: healing and connecting. Nursing and Residential Care 3: 174–176

Umbreit AW 2000 Healing touch: applications in the acute care setting. AACN Clinical Issues 11: 105–119

A concept analysis of therapeutic relationships

Mary Chambers

EDITORIAL

A book focusing on the concepts of nursing without including a chapter on therapeutic relationships would be analogous to a collection of classical music without including Mozart; something integral would be missing. Nursing is without question an interpersonal endeavour framed by the relationship that exists and is developed between patient and nurse. Yet all too often only cursory attention is given to the incredibly complicated practice of therapeutic relationship formation. The complexity of what, at face value, is often seen to be a straightforward and simple activity is rarely referred to. How often is it spelled out how nurses can form relationships with patients who possess a personal value set and philosophy antagonistic to the nurse's own? Similarly, how often is it simply assumed that, given attendance at one short course on basic interpersonal skills, students will have the knowledge, self-awareness, techniques and attitudes necessary for relationship formation? And more worryingly for the Editors, how often is the pivotal process of relationship formation given far less attention in nursing curricula, both theoretical and clinical attention, than is given to physical skills, technological tasks and the more visible, overt interventions?

> In all the years the Editors have been working with students through the medium of reflective journals, it is extremely rare for students to focus on how they established a therapeutic relationship with a patient as an example of a 'critical incident'. Mary's chapter not only reminds us of the importance of this but also points out the paradox that these processes still retain a degree of mystery and vagueness. Noteworthy questions remain, particularly around the domain of empirical referents. While many nurses, particularly expert nurses, would be able to describe their intuitive felt-sense when a relationship is established, as a scientific academy we currently lack the sophisticated instruments to 'measure' the depth or degree of the relationship. Clearly this is an area where a great deal more research is needed.

INTRODUCTION

Interpersonal and therapeutic relationships are at the centre of nursing work. The relationship that exists between nurse and patient can often provide the energy and be the catalyst, the motivation and the source of strength to continue with treatment or face difficult, sometimes life-threatening situations. Therapeutic relationships can often be taken for granted or their full potential not be realized on either the part of the patient or the healthcare professional. As part of my socialization into 'general' nursing I learned that it was important when answering examination questions to begin each clinical practice answer with 'screen the bed and inform the patient'. Similarly, in psychiatric nursing I learned that the 'catch phrase' was 'establish a good nurse–patient relationship'. These statements were important for successful examination results and for the documentation of care planning, beyond which they appeared to have no apparent further clinical or therapeutic relevance. Often such behaviours or sentiments were not enacted in the clinical environment. A clear chasm existed between what appeared to be the espoused values of educators and clinicians and the clinical reality.

On reflection, neither teaching nor clinical staff challenged or explored this ritualistic, somewhat thoughtless behaviour. No one ever questioned what a nurse–patient relationship was. There was no guidance as to how I would recognize such a relationship or its potential in terms of facilitating patient recovery. I knew instinctively that such a relationship was a good thing, as it felt right to get on well with patients. However, getting on well with someone is quite different from having a therapeutic relationship with that person. **Getting on well with an individual is a necessary component of the therapeutic process but in itself insufficient to facilitate personal discovery, growth, self-acceptance and/or recovery from mental health problems.**

It was not until I started practising as a nurse behaviour therapist that I began to appreciate the meaning, power, potential and significance of the nurse–patient relationship. During therapeutic engagement with patients I began to recognize the importance of negotiation, honesty, equality, trust, professional competence and power as necessary components that facilitate patients to achieve their desired goals or outcomes from therapy. I also began to appreciate the 'faith' patients placed in the competence of the therapist as well as the desire to 'please'. In the context of behaviour therapy, patients confronted their fears and carried out behaviour of which they were 'terrified', an achievement enabled through the therapeutic relationship, which was a supporting, facilitating force. This relationship enabled an understanding of the lived experience of the patient and an opportunity to realize the espoused values of the therapeutic relationship in practice.

Therapeutic relationships are not exclusive to the domain of nursing but are integral to all helping relationships regardless of professional affiliation. Such relationships exist in a variety of forms across the caring communities. However, the discussion in this chapter draws upon the literature from the domain of psychiatric/mental health nursing.

Whilst 'therapeutic relationships' may have different meanings, there does appear to be a consensus, and increasingly so, that such a relationship is critical to therapeutic outcome and survival from and of the experience of having mental health problems (Barker 1999). There would appear to be a further consensus that this relationship consists of various processes and attributes, some of which will be highlighted in subsequent sections. How these elements are recognized, respected and utilized is influenced by the philosophical perspective, experience and perceptions of both nurse and patient.

This chapter is concerned with deepening our understanding of therapeutic relationships. While I recognize that there are a variety of approaches to concept analysis each with strengths and limitations, I have chosen Walker and Avant's (1995) approach. However, this approach is not being adhered to in its strictest form and is used more as a loose structure. Accordingly, the remainder of this chapter is organized tentatively around the seven stages suggested by Walker and Avant (1995):

1. Select a concept
2. Determine the aims and purpose of the analysis
3. Identify all uses of the concept that you can discover
4. Determine the defining attributes
5. Construct a model case
6. Identify antecedents and consequences
7. Define empirical referents

I will next address uses of the concept and then attempt to explore some of the defining attributes by way of comparing the differences between social and therapeutic relationships. Making a comparison between social and therapeutic relationships in this manner will make explicit the differences between the two types of relationship and facilitate the process of defining the key attributes of therapeutic relationships. This comparison will highlight some defining attributes, but not all; others will be addressed in a later section.

USES OF THE CONCEPT 'THERAPEUTIC RELATIONSHIP'

Much discussion has taken place in the psychiatric/mental health nursing literature around the concept of therapeutic relationships. There is, however, a shared belief as to its importance in facilitating patient recovery or adjustment to mental illness. Many authors (e.g. Peplau 1952, Porter 1992, Forchuk 1994, Hall 1997, Chambers 1998, Speedy 1999, Cutcliffe 2000) consider therapeutic relationships to be the backbone of psychiatric/mental health nursing. Although frequently used, the term is not always defined; it is taken for granted that it is universally understood, with a shared meaning. Yet the definitions or descriptions that are available include some but not all of the same elements.

Lauder et al (2002), for example, consider therapeutic relationships to be the cornerstone of nursing practice for those experiencing threats to their health, including but not restricted to those with mental illness; therapeutic relationships enable patients to cope more effectively with threats to their health. When looking at the aims of the therapeutic relationship, Forchuk and Reynolds (2001) assert that they are about initiating supportive interpersonal communication in order to understand the perceptions and needs of the other person, empowering the other person to learn or cope more effectively with their environment, and a reduction or resolution of their problems. Stuart (2001, p. 15) adds:

> *... the therapeutic (nurse–patient) relationship is a mutual learning experience and a corrective emotional experience for the patient. It is based on the underlying humanity of nurse and patient with mutual respect and acceptance of cultural differences. In this relationship the nurse uses personal attributes and clinical techniques in working with the patient to bring about insight and behavioural change.*

Whereas Riley et al (2003, p. 93) state that 'therapeutic relationships are about 'patients' disclosure of personal and occasionally painful feelings with the professional at a calculated emotional distance near enough to be involved but objective enough to be helpful'.

These examples from various authors have different perspectives as to the nature and uses of therapeutic relationships. However, there are common features such as supporting individuals through periods of stress and promoting learning, personal growth and self-exploration in an environment of respect and trust.

DIFFERENCE BETWEEN SOCIAL AND THERAPEUTIC RELATIONSHIPS

Social relationships centre on the disclosure of personal information and intimacy, in a situation where both parties enjoy equal opportunities for spontaneity and where both sets of needs can be met (Riley et al 2003). **There is no requirement or expectation that one party will be instrumental in bringing about a change in the life chances of the other. This is in contrast to the requirements of a therapeutic relationship, which is devoted to individuals in the experience or distress of 'mental illness' and aimed at how best to facilitate understanding, adjustment or recovery from and through the experience.** Social relationships have no set plan and are not surrounded by any formal negotiation, whereas therapeutic relationships set the conditions for the introduction of 'therapeutic techniques' or 'treatment modalities'. A social relationship is concerned with the equivalent disclosure of daily living issues such as personal, social, moral, ethical, local, national and international concerns as they impact on the lives of individuals and communities. It is neighbourhood 'chit-chat' and 'party talk' and an important part of community 'togetherness'.

The boundaries surrounding social relationships are societal, in contrast to a therapeutic relationship where professional boundaries are established. However, within nursing literature there is much debate as to the utility of such boundaries. For example, Riley et al (2003) speak of the necessity of a 'calculated emotional distance'. In a therapeutic relationship Hem and Heggan (2003) question whether or not nurses should 'be themselves'. They point out that studies have demonstrated that patients want nurses be human – friendly, available and receptive – and that patients want to be listened to. Hem and Heggan (2003) use the work of Beech and Norman (1995), Pejlant et al (1995) and Cleary and Edwards (1999) to illustrate this point. However, Ramos (1992) found that too much emotional involvement on the part of nurses was unhelpful for both nurse and patient.

This is the opposite view to that of Jackson and Stevenson (2000), who want nurses to share personal data with patients. These authors seem to suggest that sharing on the part of the nurse leads to a more equitable relationship, as otherwise only the patient will be sharing information. Sometimes psychiatric/mental health nurses want to create distance, as described by Bray (1999). Bray found that, because of the emotional demand placed on nurses working with those experiencing psychological disorders, they found it necessary to create a physical distance from patients. Hem and Heggan (2003) state that there may be a lack of congruity between nurses' views of professionalism and what patients really want from them. There are also some tensions within the literature about the nature of the therapeutic relationship: for example, uncertainty surrounds whether or not different levels of distance are required depending on age, gender or client group. There does seem to be a view that, early in a relationship, both the emotional and physical distance are greater in order to facilitate the development of a therapeutic relationship and reduce patient anxiety.

Further clarity is required as to whether or not the degree of distance remains constant throughout the relationship. It seems reasonable to suggest that distance will change depending on the nature of the work taking place within the relationship and also the stage or duration of the relationship. Some authors, for example, Jackson and Stevenson (2000), make it clear that the nurse is not the patient's friend but that a friendship should exist. And Keltner et al (2003) state that the nurse and patient should be viewed as a whole that operates within an environmental context. It could be concluded therefore, that there is no clear consensus about the nature of distance other than that there should be one.

From a practitioner's perspective, despite the emotional distance, the stress of managing a therapeutic relationship is different (and could be argued greater) than that of managing a social relationship. The nature of what is disclosed places demands on the personal resources of professionals; hence the importance of clinical supervision to enhance coping capacity (Chambers & Long 1996, Cutcliffe et al 2000). This requirement for clinical supervision is a further difference between social and therapeutic relationships.

Social relationships, as outlined by Riley et al (2003), do have some therapeutic value, but at a superficial or surface level, and they also provide the foundation for therapeutic relationships to be nurtured. In the absence of a therapeutic relationship a social relationships is the lowest level required when carrying out physical caring or procedural nursing tasks. For those less experienced in the skill and art of therapeutic relationships, combining the social relationship with a task can help to reduce anxiety for the practitioner and perhaps also for patients. The task acts as a focus and distraction from engaging in more exploratory 'personal' or catalytic work.

In task-focused interactions (like many others) the nurse or healthcare professional holds the balance of power. Focusing on a task can make the interaction easier from a professional perspective and can help to create the climate for a therapeutic relationship to develop. The task-focused interaction itself may do little to enhance the therapeutic performance of the practitioner or promote therapeutic outcomes for the patient. However, dealing with a task, for example, dressing a leg ulcer or completing an application form for financial assistance, can add to psychological well-being and hence facilitate recovery. Even when therapeutic relationships have been established, task-focused interactions may have a greater role to play in patient recovery than is currently acknowledged. Perhaps they are what patients need at different points as they journey through their experience or when therapy is particularly challenging and there is a need to retreat (Stein-Parbury 2000). Patients have the right to choose which form of relationship best suits their needs at any one time. As Vuokila-Oikkonen et al point out (2004, p. 130): 'therapeutic interaction means that the relationship between the nurse and the patient is based on the patient's needs and is meaningful for the patient.'

In the context of a social relationship and social communication, confidentiality of material is understood to have certain respectful, personal boundaries. How those boundaries are appreciated or prized is up to individuals. In contrast, ethical guidelines and data protection laws determine therapeutic disclosure. Social relationships allow for the exchange of personal information in a manner not possible within a therapeutic relationship, where there is less 'give and take'. Some disclosure may be beneficial to the therapeutic process, but nothing too personal.

Highlighted within this discussion are defining attributes of negotiation, distance and boundaries, disclosure, confidentiality with a passing reference to power. The following section will highlight other defining attributes of the therapeutic relationship.

OTHER DEFINING ATTRIBUTES OF THERAPEUTIC RELATIONSHIPS

As previously stated, therapeutic relationships are necessary in all nursing and the foundation of all helping relationships, especially in psychiatric/mental health nursing. Each therapeutic relationship is different by virtue of its individual, dynamic nature but there are commonalities, and these may be regarded as key or defining attributes. This section will concentrate on some of the most fundamental of those commonalities.

TRUST

Trust forms the basis of a therapeutic relationship and as such is one of the most important attributes. Without trust the relationship is superficial, with little personal involvement of either the client or the carer (Ralston 1998). Trust develops from creating an ambience of openness, honesty, warmth, acceptance and understanding through 'presence', as outlined by Heron (1990). A sense of genuineness, humanness, ordinariness and concern are conveyed to the patient when these qualities are reflected in both verbal and non-verbal behaviour – in other words the person feels valued as a fellow human being.

Engaging in trusting open relationships and demonstrating humanness can highlight a practitioner's vulnerability, which is a human quality. Both patients and nurses may feel vulnerable at different times, something that needs to be recognized and not dismissed. Hem and Heggan (2003) point out that nurses are reluctant to acknowledge vulnerability. They also state that there is potential to devalue vulnerability in the context of professionalism and also the possibility that its importance can be romanticized. Through openness, honesty, warmth, sincerity and ordinariness the practitioner becomes an almost transparent ingredient of congruence that Rogers (1975) considered an essential part of the therapeutic relationship. In the formation of trust it is essential that practitioners keep all promises and appointments made, including respect for the confidentiality of shared material. Patients must know that some information may need to be shared and the conditions under which this will take place; agreement needs to be sought in advance. In some instances, in order to retain trust, a contractual relationship may be required and signed by both parties.

RESPECT

Therapeutic relationships differ in terms of focus, length, depth and degree of closeness. Regardless of this, they need to be grounded in respect for the patient/client. According to Wilson and Kneisl (1992) the behaviour of some people with mental health problems would indicate loss of self-respect, for example, lack of attention to personal hygiene, physical self-harm or begging. Therefore they believe that 'a relationship in which the person can experience a sense of dignity and receive messages of respect is of inestimable value' (Wilson & Kneisl 1992, p. 31). For Stuart and Laraia (2001, p. 866), respect is "an attitude of the nurse that conveys caring for, liking and valuing the patient. The nurse regards the patient 'as a person of worth' and accepts the patient without qualification."

Conveying the message of respect to a person can be accomplished in a number of ways as part of the therapeutic relationship; for example by ensuring that all conversations take place in private, keeping to any timetable set, being 'present', listening and validating material that is disclosed. Honesty and genuineness play a key role in conveying respect, even when the information shared may be difficult for the patient/client.

Sometimes practitioners will be challenged by the views of patients; nevertheless, it is necessary to respect them. As Egan (1985, p. 37) pointed out: 'respect to be effective cannot remain a mere attitude but must be expressed in behavioural ways in the helping encounter. Skilled helpers are genuine and do not hide behind professional roles. They are spontaneous and open, remaining human being to the human being with whom they are working.'

Respect is a necessary condition for an empathic relationship, as the patient needs to feel valued and understood for the relationship to develop.

EMPATHY

Empathy is the ability to recognize and understand the patient's feelings and point of view objectively. According to Riley et al (2003, p. 93), 'empathy expressed verbally and non-verbally conveys caring, compassion and concern for patients but never implies that the nurse can fully experience patients' feelings'.

Empathy is about getting into the shoes of the other person and trying to see things – emotions and experiences – from their perspective where possible. Listening is an important element in the empathic process. It is critical to 'hear' what the patient is saying, verbally and non-verbally. Information disclosed by the patient needs to be validated in order to demonstrate respect and empathy and increase understanding of the patient's feelings. This validation can only take place if the practitioner has 'heard' what the patient has said and demonstrated through a catalytic form of intervention (Heron 1990). Beech and Norman (1995) found that patients perceived listening as more important than what was said to them and that the giving of undivided attention formed an important aspect of that listening process.

According to Stuart (2001), empathy is the ability to enter into the life of another person and to accurately perceive their current feelings and their meaning. Stuart (2001, p. 35) goes on to say that:

> *... empathic understanding consists of a number of stages if patients allow nurses to enter their private world – nurses need to be receptive to this communication; nurses must understand the patient's communication by putting themselves in the patient's place; nurses must step back into their own role and communicate understanding to the patient but it is not necessary or desirable for nurses to feel the same emotions as the patient.*

Stuart (2001) also states that the research on empathy indicates its importance in the therapeutic process (e.g. it is related to positive clinical outcome), that the ideal therapist is first of all empathic and that empathy is correlated with self-exploration and self-acceptance. This view adds to that of Reynolds (1998), who believes that where empathy is less evident patients will perceive care as impersonal, leading to reduced opportunity for emotional support, consequently impacting on clinical outcome. Unconditional positive regard (Rogers 1975) and genuineness form part of the empathic process. It is through the practitioner conveying these messages to patients that they can begin to internalize them, consequently impacting on their sense of self and who they are. When this process takes place the patient is on the way to developing new coping strategies and onwards to acceptance, adjustment and/or recovery.

POWER

Power is a potent force that explains a good deal about the nature, operation and patterns of interpersonal behaviour (Wilson & Kneisl 1992). Within a therapeutic relationship the patient may be deemed to have less power than the professional, given that 'knowledge' is considered to be power. However, patients too have personal power as only they have the individual experience and experiential knowledge of their mental health problem. Further, they retain the power to choose what information to share and what to withhold and can choose to resist engagement.

Nevertheless, there is still a tendency to perceive power as negative; however, it should be remembered that in the context of therapeutic relationships power can be exercised through empathy and respect and used positively to promote self-discovery. As Price and Mullarkey (1996) point out, power can be a healthy dynamic tool in the therapeutic relationship.

Rightly or wrongly, society invests power in professionals. There is an associated perception that professionals are cold and detached, and, indeed, some are. Other associated characteristics include control, superiority and inflexibility, none of which is conducive to a therapeutic relationship because of the barriers they create. **Language is the most influential way in which professionals exercise power, for example by overuse of jargon and/or medical terminology, leading to**

alienation. In therapeutic relationship the use of common, everyday language is important, fitting in with the attributes of humanness and ordinariness.

Within nursing literature there are tensions as to the balance between professionalism and humanism; in my view they are not mutually exclusive. Barker (1999) points out that professionalism has always been associated with power and, as nursing strives for greater professionalism, it runs the risk of extending its power base and disempowering individuals. Hem and Heggan (2003) suggest that there may be a lack of congruity between nurses' views of professionalism and what patients really want from them. They go on to state that the ideal of the friendly professional (Jackson & Stevenson 2000) who balances intimacy and distance is too harmonic a notion and that it may be too difficult to expect individuals to be both human and professional. It would be very difficult, in my opinion, to be professional without being 'human'.

It is not possible to fully explore the tensions around being human and professional here; however, it is important to note that they do exist. There is little doubt that in therapeutic relationships there is a need to balance power and humanism and that this can be a challenge. Exploring and managing that balance can form the practitioner's agenda for clinical supervision and self-reflection and adds to the dynamic nature of therapeutic relationships and to the personal growth and development of practitioners.

ANTECEDENTS AND CONSEQUENCES OF THERAPEUTIC RELATIONSHIPS

In this context an antecedent is an event or incident that precedes the development of a therapeutic relationship and the consequences are the outcomes of such a relationship. Therapeutic relationships do not exist in a vacuum: they are influenced by a variety of antecedents, including environment, the communication process and the preconceptions of key participants, in this instance patients, carers and professionals. A therapeutic interaction is a conversation with a purpose that aims to explore, understand, interpret and appreciate what for the individual patient is causing distress, in order to facilitate assessment of need and negotiation of approach and to plan for interventions to promote development and recovery. Developing such a relationship is a highly skilled activity requiring the practitioner to be 'present' and focused and not distracted by extraneous activity.

The appropriate interpersonal and physical environment plays a key role in facilitating the development of therapeutic relationships. Much has already been written about the environment, so what is presented here is simply a brief reminder as to its importance and contribution to the development and maintenance of the therapeutic relationship. Environmental factors play a key role in either facilitating or hindering communication, consequently the therapeutic relationship. Nurses and others need to remember the importance of ensuring an environment conducive to privacy (no personal communication in a public place), a quiet area. Peplau demonstrated this very well during her earlier work at Greystone

Park Hospital New Jersey 'where she took patients into broom cupboards and stairwells – anywhere which might allow the necessary space and privacy to serve as the natural boundaries for intersubjective discourse' (Barker 1999, p. 6).

Attention to space is important (Riley et al 2003). An environmental layout with low levels of noise and few interruptions can do much to reduce patient and nurse anxiety, facilitating communication and consequently the therapeutic process.

It is well documented that communication is a two-way process between two or more individuals where knowledge and information is shared. In this discussion, communication is being considered as an antecedent and central to the development of the therapeutic relationship. Communication is about transmitting a message from one person – a sender – to another person – a receiver – through verbal, written and non-verbal behaviour. According to Burgoon et al (1996) and others, in order to enhance communication high levels of social competency involving, for instance, voice modulation, eye contact and posture, are important. Accepting the importance of social competency for therapeutic relationships, it is important that practitioners are sufficiently skilled to manage and engage in such relationships. If accounts in the literature around problems of engagement are taken as indicative (Beech & Norman 1995, Breeze & Repper 1998, Cutcliffe 2000, Secker et al 2004), then the conclusion could be reached that currently the level of skill is not high.

High levels of social competency may not in themselves be sufficient as preparation for responding to challenging situations and the development of therapeutic relationships. It is easy to specify mechanistically and identify core components of the communication process; however, being able to determine the appropriate combination of interpersonal skills, knowledge, experience and personal characteristics required to develop such relationships is much less simple. As each relationship is different it is difficult to predict and specify the 'mix' of personal characteristics, interpersonal competencies, professional skills and knowledge required for developing a therapeutic relationship. Each situation and therapeutic interaction is unique, generating a different synergy between participants. Therefore, despite high levels of social competency and therapeutic skill, some communications and interactions will remain challenging with the outcome less than might be expected or desired.

Other elements impacting on the development of therapeutic relationships include personal experiences, gender, culture and the values, beliefs and world views of those involved. These factors and others can lead to preconceptions that impact upon the relationship. Such preconceptions have been outlined by Peplau (1952) and referred to by Forchuk (1994). Peplau was of the view that both nurse and patient have preconceptions that will influence how they get to know each other and consequently the development of the therapeutic relationship. Forchuk (1994) found this to be the case in a study involving patients with long-term mental illness. She determined that preconceptions exist early in evolving relationships (Orientation Phase; Peplau 1952), tend to be positive (this could be a misconception, as it is unlikely that practitioners will admit to or suggest any other type) and remain stable over time, and that nurse and patient need to be aware of their own stereotypes.

Stereotypes and perceptions, not to mention 'reality', can present challenges for the development of therapeutic relationships, for example when working with individuals convicted of serious crime. (This situation may be confounded if the nurse or health professional has had personal experience of crime.) It could be deduced from the literature that developing a therapeutic relationship is relatively easy provided the various steps are worked through (Schwecke 2003, Forchuk 1994). However, appreciating the importance of developing a therapeutic relationship and achieving it can be quite different.

Having outlined three important antecedents supporting the development of therapeutic relationships, a further aspect is the relationship itself. Before a therapeutic relationship can develop there must firstly be a social relationship. The respective individuals need to get to know each other and form an alliance before engaging in anything resembling a therapeutic relationship. The linear progression of that relationship is difficult to predict. Peplau (1952) did suggest that therapeutic relationships consisted of key phases: orientation, working (subphases of identification and exploitation) and resolution, suggestive of a developmental process. However, Forchuk (1994), describing Peplau's theory, states that phases can fluctuate with movement in between. This would indicate that linear development does not always happen but rather that the process of engagement determines the therapeutic relationship.

Having looked at antecedents it is necessary to consider the consequences of therapeutic relationships. A therapeutic relationship can be an emotional rollercoaster for both patient and practitioner, bringing out the best in both but also exposing the vulnerable. As a result of this experience there will be outcomes for patient and practitioner. Some will be in common, for example learning, personal growth and development; others will be individual and different. According to Reynolds (1998), the definition of therapeutic relationships proposed by Kalkman (1967) is useful to measure the successful ingredients of helping relationships.

> Relationship therapy refers to a prolonged relationship between a nurse therapist and a patient during which the patient can feel accepted as a person of worth, feels free to express himself without fear of rejection or censure, and enables him to learn more satisfactory and productive patterns of behaviour.
> Kalkman 1967, p. 226, cited in Reynolds & Cormack 1992, p. 154

Using this definition as a basis to consider the outcomes of therapeutic work would suggest that patients should be enabled to engage in a process of self-discovery and to better understand and manage their coping mechanism, leading to an enhanced sense of self. A greater self-understanding will promote the necessary self-confidence and self-esteem to resume their previous role in society or to develop or adjust to something different, depending on which is more appropriate. Individual capacity for the resumption or development of relationships should be enhanced, again reinforcing self-belief and the potential for greater autonomy and independence. **Both the patient and the practitioner should have increased self-awareness and be able to expand quadrant 1 of the Johari window. Such an outcome could be used as evidence of a successful therapeutic relationship. For the practitioner an indicator may be that hope had been inspired and that the patient is able to see their life chances more positively (Cutcliffe 2004).**

EMPIRICAL REFERENTS

Therapeutic relationships are the core activity of psychiatric/mental health nursing and, because of their tacit nature, difficult to describe (Meerabeau 1995). According to Meerabeau (1995), tacit knowledge only becomes explicit when we rely on our awareness of it to attend to a second activity; it is a hallmark of skilled practice but also a feature of many everyday activities (Meerabeau 1995, p. 33). This description aptly covers therapeutic relationships, and their intangible nature, and creates challenges in terms of empirical enquiry and outcome measurement. Despite this, attempts have been made to measure some aspects, such as empathy (Reynolds 1998), as well as the therapeutic relationship itself. Lauder et al (2002) point out that research is starting to provide evidence of the value of therapeutic relationships.

According to Horvath (2000) the results of the various studies looking at the theoretical hypothesis set out by Rogers (1975) support the hypothesis that a good therapeutic relationship correlates with positive outcome:

> *Specifically it was found that it was not the objectively measured level of the therapist's empathy, congruence, or unconditional positive regard per se that had the most powerful impact on the therapy outcomes rather it was the client's perception of these qualities that foretold the success of the helping process.*
>
> *Horvath 2000, p. 166*

In this same paper Horvath refers to a meta analysis conducted earlier by Horvath and Symonds that examined the results of the first 15 years of investigations into therapeutic relationships. They found that the quality of the alliance is a robust predictor of therapy outcomes; that the alliance is evident as early as the third session of therapy and that the results hold reasonably constant across various treatment approaches, client groups and clinical diagnosis. It appears that there is some empirical evidence in support of the therapeutic relationship as a predictor of treatment outcomes and that this body of knowledge is growing.

CONCLUSION

Therapeutic relationships are a recurring theme across the caring community and especially in psychiatric/mental health nursing. While their importance is recognized in facilitating patient recovery or adjustment to mental illness, the term is not always defined. It is taken for granted that the concept is universally understood, with a shared meaning. From loosely using Walker and Avant's approach to concept analysis it was possible to explore a number of key attributes, for example boundaries and distance, trust, respect, empathy and power. Three key antecedents were considered to be environment, communication and preconceptions. Outcomes for both patient and practitioner were considered to be learning, personal growth and development and increased self-awareness. Patients would have an enhanced sense of self and enhanced coping capacity, with the potential to engage with society in a manner appropriate to them. In terms of empirical referents, while there is some evidence as to the power of the therapeutic relationship there remains much yet to be understood in terms of empirical research.

REFERENCES

Barker PJ 1999 The philosophy and practice of psychiatric nursing. Churchill Livingstone, Edinburgh

Beech P, Norman I 1995 Patient's perceptions of quality of psychiatric nursing care: findings from a small-scale descriptive study. Journal of Clinical Nursing 4: 117–123

Bray J 1999 An ethnographic study of psychiatric nursing. Journal of Psychiatric and Mental Health Nursing 6: 297–305

Breeze JA, Repper J 1998 Struggling for control: the care experiences of 'difficult' patients in mental health services. Journal of Advanced Nursing 26: 1301–1311

Burgoon JK, Buller DB, Woodal WG 1996 Nonverbal communication; the unspoken dialogue, 2nd edn. McGraw-Hill, New York.

Chambers M 1998 Interpersonal mental health nursing: research issues and challenges. Journal of Psychiatric and Mental Health Nursing 5: 203–211

Chambers M, Long A 1995 Supportive clinical supervision: a crucible for personal and professional change. Journal of Psychiatric and Mental Health Nursing 2: 311–316

Cleary M, Edwards C 1999 'Something always comes up': nurse-patient interaction in an acute psychiatric setting. Journal of Psychiatric and Mental Health Nursing 6: 469–477

Cutcliffe JR 2000 Mental health fit for purpose? Promoting the human side of mental health nursing. British Journal of Nursing 9: 632–637

Cutcliffe JR 2004 The inspiration of hope in bereavement counselling. Jessica Kingsley, London

Cutcliffe JR, Butterworth T, Proctor B 2000 Fundamental themes in clinical supervision: national and international perspectives of education, policy, research and practice. In:

Cutcliffe JR, Butterworth T, Proctor B (eds) Fundamental themes in clinical supervision. Routledge, London

Egan G 1985 The skilled helper: models, skills and methods for effective helping, 2nd edn. Brooks/Cole, Monterey, CA

Forchuk C 1994 Preconceptions in the nurse–client relationship. Journal of Psychiatric and Mental Health Nursing 1: 145–149

Forchuk C, Reynolds W 2001 Guest editorial – interpersonal theory in nursing practice: the Peplau legacy. Journal of Psychiatric and Mental Health Nursing 5: 165–166

Hall JM 1997 Packing for the journey: safe disclosure of therapeutic relationships with abuse survivors. Journal of Psychosocial Nursing 35: 7–13

Hem MH, Heggan K 2003 Being professional and being human: one nurse's relationship with a psychiatric patient. Journal of Advanced Nursing 43: 101–108

Heron J 1990 Helping the client: a creative practical guide. Sage, London

Horvath AO 2000 The therapeutic relationship: from transference to alliance. Psychotherapy in Practice 56: 163–173

Jackson S, Stevenson C 2000 What do people need psychiatric nurses for? Journal of Advanced Nursing 31: 378–388

Kalkman M 1967 Psychiatric nursing. McGraw-Hill, New York

Keltner NL, Schweeke LH, Bostrom CE 2003 Psychiatric nursing, 4th edn. Mosby, St Louis, MO

Lauder W, Reynolds W, Smith A, Sharkey S 2002 A comparison of therapeutic commitment, role support, role competency and empathy in three cohorts of nursing students. Journal of Psychiatric and Mental Health Nursing 9: 483–491

Meerabeau L 1995 The nature of practitioner knowledge. In: Reed J, Proctor S (eds) Practitioner research in health care. Chapman & Hall, London

Pejlant A, Asplund K, Norberg A 1995 Stories about living in a hospital ward as narrated by schizophrenic patients. Journal of Psychiatric and Mental Health Nursing 2: 269–277

Peplau HE 1952 Interpersonal relations in nursing. JP Putman, New York

Porter S 1992 Institutional restrains upon education reforms; the case of mental health nursing. Nurse Education Today 12: 452–457

Price V, Mullarkey K 1996 Use and misuse of power in the psycho-therapeutic relationship. Mental Health Nursing 16: 16–17

Ralston R 1998 Communication: create barriers or develop therapeutic relationships. British Journal of Midwifery January 6: 8–11

Ramos MC 1992 The nurse-patient relationship; theme and variation. Journal of Advanced Nursing 17: 496–566

Reynolds WR 1998 A study of the effects of an empathy education programme on registered nurses' empathy. Unpublished PhD, Open University, Milton Keynes

Reynolds W, Cormack D 1992 The primary focus of psychiatric nursing. In: Reynolds W, Cormack D (eds) Psychiatric and mental health nursing: theory and practice. Chapman & Hall, London

Riley JB, Keltner BR, Schwecke LH 2003 Communication. In: Keltner BR, Schwecke LH, Bostrom S (eds) Psychiatric nursing, 4th edn. Mosby, St Louis, MO

Rogers C 1975 Empathic: an unappreciated way of being. Journal of Counseling Psychology 5(2): 2–10

Schwecke LH 2003 Nurse patient relationship. In: Keltner BR, Schwecke LH, Bostrom S (eds) Psychiatric nursing, 4th edn. Mosby, St Louis, MO

Secker J, Benson A, Balfe E et al 2004 Understanding the social context of violent and aggressive incidents on an inpatient unit. Journal of Psychiatric and Mental Health Nursing 11: 172–178

Speedy S 1999 The therapeutic alliance in advanced practice in mental health nursing. In: Clinton M, Nelson S (eds) Advanced practice in mental health nursing. Blackwell Science, Oxford

Stein-Parbury J 2000 Patient and person: developing interpersonal skills in nursing, 2nd edn. Harcourt, Sydney

Stuart GW 2001 Therapeutic nurse–patient relationship. In: Stuart GW, Laraia MT (eds) Principles and practice of psychiatric nursing, 7th edn. Mosby, St Louis, MO

Stuart GW, Laraia MT 2001 Principles and practice of psychiatric nursing, 7th edn. Mosby, St Louis, MO

Vuokila-Oikkonen P, Janhonen S, Vaisanen L 2004 'Shared-rhythm cooperation' in cooperative team meetings in acute psychiatric inpatient care. Journal of Psychiatric and Mental Health Nursing 11: 129–140

Walker LO, Avant KC 1995. Strategies for theory construction in nursing, 3rd edn. Appleton & Lange, Norwalk, CT

Wilson HS, Kneisl CR 1992 Psychiatric nursing, 4th edn. Addison-Wesley, Menlo Park, CA

Towards an understanding of trust

Wendy Austin

EDITORIAL

Whether we as practitioners are conscious of it or not, we are often being tested out by our patients. These implicit (and sometimes overt) tests are a necessary part of the interpersonal process of nursing. It is through 'passing these tests' that our patients learn that they can trust their nurse; that they can establish that we as practitioners are trustworthy. An emerging and growing literature alludes to these processes and attempts to make them more visible. This literature has started to illustrate that, as practitioners, we need to be aware that these dynamics of establishing trust may be more important with certain people and with particular patient groups than with others. This appears to be the case with, for example, individuals who have had a previous experience where their trust has been 'broken'; where the individual feels they have been 'betrayed', e.g. bereaved patients, patients with a history of abuse. In these situations the patients are more than likely to be suspicious of forming a close trusting relationship again for fear of this new trust being broken too.

As we are reminded in Wendy's chapter, the development of trust within interpersonal relationships can be an iterative, cyclic process and it can inversely require a 'leap of faith'. Interpersonal relationships within certain clinical scenarios allow for the gradual establishment of trust – relationships, for example, that perhaps exist over a longer time line (e.g. some counselling/therapy helping relationships can exist for years). Trust in these situations is often built up and established over time. At the same time, emergency or 'acute' healthcare situations often require an instantaneous degree of trust – or, to paraphrase, a leap of faith – on the part of the patient (e.g. someone presenting to the Accident & Emergency room). Accordingly, there may be a great deal more we could learn about trust by examining the trust building dynamics in these very different but related clinical scenarios. Final questions that come to mind here are: How does one know when (enough) trust has been established? Is the interpersonal work of creating an atmosphere of trust ever 'finished' in patient–nurse relationships? How does one measure trust? Wendy's chapter helps us reflect on these important questions, among others, and similarly indicates that our understanding of trust is, as yet, far from complete.

INTRODUCTION

For all of us trust is the most everyday thing.

O'Neill 2002

Trust is an essential aspect of being human that shapes the way we experience the world. Every relationship we have involves it or its absence. Although most of us feel that we know what is meant by trust, we find it difficult to define. Philosophers seem to share that difficulty as, until recently, they have been rather silent on the subject (Baier 1994, Pellegrino et al 1991). Trust may be a neglected area of study also because, despite its importance (or because of it), we are only vaguely aware of trust in the everydayness of our lives. 'We inhabit a climate of trust as we inhabit an atmosphere and notice it as we notice air, only when it becomes scarce or polluted' (Baier 1994, p. 98).

In this chapter, we take notice of trust and explore it as a phenomenon. The reader will not find a concept analysis in the sense that trust is clearly defined, its conceptual boundaries demarcated, preconditions specified or outcomes described (Gift 1997); rather, it is a reflection on trust as a *thick concept*.

A thick concept is what Bernard Williams (1985, p. 129), in discussing the language of moral philosophy, describes as 'a union of fact and value, a concept whose application is determined by what the world is like. Thick concepts (such as courage and jealousy) are action-guiding.' They give us access to our social reality in what they reveal about human interaction (Levering 2002). Understanding thick concepts can give us insight into how to live, how to make sense of what we are doing and how to act and behave toward others. Consideration of the fact and value of trust can give us greater insight into nursing practice. It will help us consider what it means to assert 'Nursing requires a trusting relationship' (George 1995, p. 358) or that, in our practice environments, 'Nurses must support a climate of trust' (Canadian Nurses Association 2002, p. 17).

The chapter begins with an anecdote that is used to explore aspects of trust. Trust in healthcare is then considered, including nurses' conceptions discovered in the nursing literature.

AN EXPERIENCE OF TRUST

In September 2002, in my city, Edmonton, Canada, there was a terrible apartment fire. One resident, his back and hair on fire, plunged to his death as he jumped from the fourth floor. A woman living on the same level was saved when she jumped to the waiting arms of a group of professional football players (the North American variety). 'They had their hands out ready for me. I felt I was going to be safe, and I am.' One of the players said later, 'We knew we had to catch her, to break her fall' (Mulen & Cryderman 2002, p. A1).

This brief but eventful episode reveals aspects of trust as we live it. We can readily imagine the situation: a woman standing at a window of a burning building facing the realization that she must jump or be burned alive. Beneath her lies the body of a neighbour who has fallen to his death. For her and for those gathered outside the flaming building, her predicament is terribly apparent. Suddenly, a group of men run forward. They have, in a moment, decided that they must and can help. The woman at the window sees them and their hands reaching out to catch her. She wonders at her chances of being caught and, thinking that she will be safe in these strong, skilled hands, jumps.

Many times and in many ways, we trust '*because we have to*' (Solomon & Flores 2001, p. 41, original italics). As the woman trusts those hands to catch her, we trust that we will be safe in our beds at night, that the water from our taps is drinkable, that our physician is qualified to do her job and that the driver of the car behind us is licensed and without a death wish. We must bestow trust if we are to live in the world. Niklas Luhmann (1979), a sociologist, suggests that trust is a human way of dealing with complexity. The world is so complex and full of possibilities, he argues, that confronting it in the absence of trust would be almost beyond human endurance. There is a mental disorder, paranoid personality disorder, in which the afflicted person lives with a pervasive sense of distrust and suspicion (Kaplan & Sadock 1998). It is a fearsome thing to have such a disorder, to be constantly afraid that one is surrounded by deception.

The philosopher Knud Løgstrup (1997, p. 8) believes that 'It is a characteristic of human life that we normally encounter one another with natural trust. This is true not only in the case of persons who are well acquainted with one another but also in the case of complete strangers.' It is only in special circumstances, he says, that we distrust a stranger in advance; this trust, believes Løgstrup, is a part of what it means to be human.

Trust is the 'reliance or resting of the mind on the integrity, veracity, justice, friendship, etc., of another person; a firm reliance on promises or on laws or principles' (Thatcher & McQueen 1984, p. 899). As a word, trust shares the same base as true, meaning firm, certain and to believe, to be persuaded (Skeat 1993).

Our need for trust speaks to our essential vulnerability as humans. To survive, we must rely or depend on one other. Reliance is the 'ground of trust' (Thatcher & McQueen 1984, p. 709) and to live well we must come to understand when and upon whom we can rely. We learn basic trust as an orientation to the world in infancy, according to the child psychoanalyst, Erik Erikson (Crain 1980). This orientation is either enhanced or undermined through life experience. Annette Baier (1994) relates the story of a boy whose father had him climb to a high place and stood with outstretched arms. His father, however, did not catch him, but let him fall. When the father was asked why by the hurt child, he replied 'So that from now on you will know no-one is to be trusted.' Our 'trusting impulse' is shaped by our personality and experiences (Sztompka 1999). Erikson believes that we need experiences of mistrust if we are to be discerning in our trust (Crain 1980). Trust always involves risk and the possibility that the trusted person will not act as desired (Luhmann 1979). In that sense, to trust is always a bet, a gamble (Luhmann 1979, Sztompka 1999). To trust authentically, rather than blindly or naively, is to be mindful of that (Solomon & Flores 2001).

Although the woman in the window literally has no choice but to jump, she pauses to consider her chances: 'I felt I was going to be safe.' What is involved in such a calculation? Of what are we cognisant when we assess the risk of trusting? Trust, according to Baier (1994), is an expectation of another's goodwill (p. 99). When we trust we accept our vulnerability to the other's potential lack of goodwill or even ill-will. The woman assesses good intent in the actions of her rescuers: they are volunteers and she can see in their faces that they want to catch her. We trust in appearances, 'we would go mad if we did not and could not' (Baier 1994, p.159). Even though we know appearances can be false, consider how we trust uniforms, badges and credentials; even though they can be faked (Baier 1994) we often have to rely upon them (Baier 1994, Weber & Carter 2003). The woman cannot be totally certain that her rescuers will not, at the last moment, stand back and let her fall or pull back to protect themselves. In trusting their goodwill, however, she expects they will not.

According to Luhmann (1979), familiarity supports trust, but it can support distrust too. The woman recognizes the men below her; they are not complete strangers to her. Because she knows who they are, she has confidence that they have the competence to catch her (Baier 1994). They have good ability, both in skill and strength. After all, some of them are professional 'catchers'. All the goodwill in the world will not help if those trusted are without the ability to carry out what is expected.

Reputation can be a basis for initial trust (Weber & Carter 2003). What others say about us can be evidence of our character and abilities. Nurses, for example, have a good reputation with the public and as a group are seen as highly trustworthy (Ulrich 2001, CNEWS 2004). Recently, nurses' trust rating has been slightly surpassed by another uniformed group, firefighters. The 11 September 2001 images of firefighters running into the burning towers as others rushed out to safety has given great credence to their reliability as a group. They have a high degree of what Buchanan (2000) terms 'status trust'. Distinct from 'merit' trust, which attaches to individuals on the basis of their specific capacities and behaviour, status trust attaches to a person identified as a member of a particular profession. The woman told reporters she thought, 'They'd better catch me or it's going to be a bad season.'

Predictability is a source of trust (and distrust). Knowing what we can expect, or should not expect, from someone is an important element in our decision to trust. We are less confident in trusting strangers as we are necessarily more uncertain whether they can and will act as we desire (Weber & Carter 2003). Onora O'Neill (2002) in the BBC Reith Lectures for 2002, *A Question of Trust*, asserted that knowing whether someone is conscientious or not is more crucial to trust than having their goodwill. We may be wiser to withhold trust from those neglectful of their responsibilities, even if they wish us well (2003).

Trudy Govier (1998) says that our judgement regarding the degree of trust or mistrust that is warranted is based on the evidence we have and the level of our vulnerability. Actions that seem particularly relevant to trusting seem to be truth-telling, respect for property, sincerity (as opposed to hypocrisy), promise-keeping, keeping confidences, reliability, dependability, competence (as pertinent to context) and concern for others (Govier 1998). Our evidence may be based largely upon presentation (Luhmann 1979). We may be basing our response on what is socially visible about other persons, what these persons have made known about themselves. It is necessary to be aware that our first impressions might be wrong and be open to reconsider our evidence. Consistent trustworthiness becomes important; Sztompka (1999, p. 97), in fact, terms consistent trustworthiness the 'meta-cue for trust'.

THE 'SHADOW SIDE' OF TRUST

With trust, there is always the possibility of disappointment. This is probably the reason that, when a person demands 'trust me', it has an effect opposite to its intent. Such a plea heightens our awareness of the need for trust and the risk it involves. Trust comes into our conscious awareness when something in our environment or in our relationship changes or is at odds with our normal expectations of things. For instance, the water supply of a Canadian city becomes contaminated and people die. In our own city, thousands of miles away, we pause before drinking a glass of water and wonder if we should switch to drinking only the bottled kind. Our physician makes a diagnostic error, one she recognizes when her prescribed treatment is ineffective. We have less confidence in her new diagnosis and consider getting a second opinion. The driver in the car behind us, is following so close that we switch lanes to get away from him. Trust and distrust are not opposites on a continuum: they co-exist. Trust encompasses distrust (Gilbert 1998, Solomon & Flores 2001) and we trust within constraints (Farrell 2002).

Our circumstances influence our trusting reactions. At times, as with the woman at the window, we have no real choice but to trust. In a medical emergency, for instance, we will place ourselves, with relief, in the hands of a hospital's Emergency Room staff. When the emergency is over, however, we may only trust our health and body to our own physician. A sense of our own vulnerability may make us more cautious, more hesitant, even if we take an essentially trusting stance in the world. Consider what happens when a stranger approaches as we are walking down the street. If it is daytime on a familiar, busy street, we may respond easily to a request for directions or for spare change. If it is at night on a deserted street, we may respond by walking quickly away when someone approaches. If we were once robbed when walking down such a street, we might start to run. Although trust occurs in the present, the past and future is there as well (Meize-Grochowski 1984, Hams 1997, Govier 1998).

The trust that one has learned over many years and contexts can be destroyed in a moment. Baier (1994) uses the analogy of a web to illustrate how a single betrayal can destroy trust: as with a web, disrupting one part can ruin the entire web.

Betrayal is the shadow side of trust (Farrell 2002). It is trust abused. 'Abused trust is trust that is turned against the person who does the trusting' (Løgstrup 1997 p. 9). A common, contemporary experience, travelling by plane, has radically changed since 11 September 2001. Every fellow traveller has become a potential terrorist. It is now routine to remove our shoes and hand them to airport security to be checked for explosive devices. (This morning my newspaper has a Bizarro cartoon showing a disgruntled passenger putting his shoes back on at airport security. The security officer is saying to him 'Stop complaining, just be thankful the shoe bomber didn't hide it in his shorts.' (Piraro 2003, p. R6)) This and other signs of reduced trust, like being unable to leave our doors unlocked or needing to be escorted to our car in the employee parking lot, may seem minor inconveniences. Thomas (1996), a philosopher and political scientist, argues, however, that the everyday lessening of trust fundamentally affects our humanity. Trust, he believes, involves a positive attitude toward others and a change in that attitude can lead us to a moral numbness that will ultimately affect how we care (or do not care) about one another.

Bauman (2003) notes that Løgstrup's conception of trust came before experiences in the Second World War impacted his image of the world. Bauman believes that today's generation may find Løgstrup's idea of a trustworthy world far-fetched and at odds with their reality. Bauman goes to 'reality TV' for his examples. He finds in popular shows like *Survivor*, *Big Brother* and *The Weakest Link* the message: Trust No One. This message reverses Løgstrup's conclusion to 'we normally encounter one another with natural suspicion' (Bauman 2003, p. 88). It supports, rather, the verdict of the philosopher Hobbes, that *homo homini lupus* ('man is to man a wolf').

Man may be perceived as not so trustworthy as other species, as well. Govier (1998), in her work on trust, tells the story of Charles Russell and Maureen Enns, Canadian researchers who catalogued the lives of Siberian grizzly bears and worked to prove that grizzlies and humans could peacefully share the same territory. They kept safe in bear encounters by acting unprovocatively and speaking softly. Govier concludes from their story 'that animals can be the objects of our trust' (p. 15). Unfortunately, when the researchers returned to Siberia in 2003, they discovered that all the sturdy bears had been slaughtered. It appears that the bears trustingly approached their killers (Mitchell 2003).

Our sense of trust is deeply influenced by our underlying assumptions regarding human nature. It is also shaped by the general attitude toward trust that exists within our society. In societies in which suspicion or distrust is the general stance, a sense of solidarity is eroded. A society that experiences a loss of trust in leaders, institutions (e.g. educational, religious) and systems (e.g. judicial and monetary) becomes unstable (Lewis & Weigert 1985). As a social good, when trust is damaged or destroyed everyone suffers (Bok 1978). As I write this, the government of Canada is responding to a report by the Auditor-General that identifies serious financial wronging. The Prime Minister is pledging to overhaul the way the government works and 'restore trust in the parliament' (Yourk 2004). He is said to be purging the top echelons of Canada's Crown corporations (LeBlanc 2004). As the Prime Minister obviously recognizes, the maintenance of trust is integral to the functioning of the complex systems that make up a society (Gilbert 1998). Health care is one of the most important and crucial of these systems.

TRUST IN HEALTHCARE SYSTEMS

Valemar Lopes de Moraes was a 39-year-old Brazilian man who went to his local clinic complaining of an earache. On that day at the clinic, a vasectomy was scheduled for Aldemar Rodrigues. When the nurse called for 'Aldemar', Valemar thought he was being called and responded. A vasectomy was performed on him. He did not question or protest about the procedure because he thought his earache had become something more serious (Globe and Mail 2003, p. A14). For Valemar the clinic staff, the nurses and physicians, were professionals who would do their best to heal whatever was wrong with him. He didn't question their actions as they were the experts. His trust in them was implicit.

Valemar's level of trust in healthcare professionals is not far removed from that once expected of all patients. Chalmers Clark (2002, p. 14), writing about trust in medicine, notes: 'Not so long ago the question of trust in the medical profession simply did not arise. Doctors functioned in a quasi-ecclesiastic atmosphere of patient awe and confidence.'

The relationship between professionals with their patients is a fiduciary one. *Fiduciary* comes from the Latin *fidere*, 'to trust' (Barber 1998). A promise to be trustworthy seems necessary: the lives, health and safety of the public can be significantly affected by the services professionals offer.

To need trust is obvious when one enters the healthcare system. One must entrust oneself to physicians, nurses, laboratory technicians, administrators, researchers, and manufacturers. One trusts that surgical techniques, sterilization, drug administration or any therapeutic intervention will be safely carried out. In a qualitative study on healthcare relationships, nurse researchers Thorne and Robinson (1988, p. 783) found that patients enter such relationships with 'an almost absolute trust in the professionals who would provide care'. Valemar, although worried that his earache is more serious than he thought, silently endures his treatment for it. Whether or not it is realistic to do so, patients like Valemar trust that entering the system means that there are competent hands reaching out to them and that there is good intent toward them, or at least no ill intent. They remain trusting until that trust is called into question.

In the report of the Institute of Medicine's Committee on the Quality of Healthcare in America (Kohn et al 2000), it is estimated that 44 000–98 000 deaths occurred in 1997 that were due to medical mistakes. This number is greater than the number of deaths due to motor vehicle injuries, AIDS or breast cancer in that year (Rosenthal & Sutcliffe 2002).

Unfortunately, the trust of every patient in Thorne and Robinson's study was shattered. The researchers describe how blind faith became impossible for patients once they had insight into the working of the healthcare system. Some still maintained that particular healthcare professionals were worthy of absolute trust, although they came to distrust these professionals' discipline as a whole.

Edmund Pellegrino (1991, p. 77), a physician and ethicist, described in *Ethics, Trust and the Professions* how trust in the medical profession had deteriorated as patients came to perceive physicians as more interested in their money than in them. He identified the commercialization of medical care, its depersonalization and the legalistic atmosphere surrounding it as problems creating a situation in which 'wariness replaces trust'. An ethics of distrust, he claims, is arising in which professionals and those whom they seek to help assume a self-protective stance, and look to spell out strict contractual obligations. Farrell (2002) described three nurses' experiences of trust, mistrust and betrayal during a transitional time of reorganization in their facility. She noted that fatigue, overload and confusion prevented usual trusting relationships from occurring and mistrust arose. One of her informants related how nurses felt betrayed when they were excluded from decisions that affected their work life.

Health professionals, under increasing pressure to uphold the institutional goal of curtailing costs, may find themselves in conflict with their duty to their patients (Caulfield 2002). As health care is increasingly conceived as a market commodity, a market ethos (*caveat emptor*, 'buyer beware') is replacing an ethos of trust. For example, does one fully trust one's nurse knowing that she will receive a bonus for achieving one's early discharge? Gail Mitchell (2002), a nurse administrator and scholar, finds that research values and priorities, along with market values, are eroding public trust and raising the question: 'Whose interests are being served?' Mitchell notes that some nurses are pressured to enlist patients as research participants only to find that the patients suffer because of the research protocol. Edson (1999), in her Pulitzer-Prize-winning play *Wit*, has superbly dramatized this issue. Now a movie, this work brings the questions 'Who is being served by research?' and

'Can I trust the good intentions of healthcare organizations?' to a wider audience. The nurse character in *Wit* reveals how nurses are distressed as institutional constraints and nurses' lack of power within the organization make them less able to protect their patients' interests in the way they believe they should. Research on moral distress supports this contention (Austin et al 2003).

Mallick (2003, p. F3), in her 'As If' column in *The Globe and Mail*, described how she was alerted to possible dangers of the system by an anonymous letter in a newspaper from a nurse 'warning readers that Canadian hospitals are so bad that you must never leave a family member unaccompanied. You must be there to speak for them, check their medication and keep them comfortable and clean'. Mallick goes on to tell what happened during her mother's hospitalisation in a large city hospital. She came to agree with the anonymous nurse through her interactions with 'Dr Pain' and 'Nurse Sneer'. She found these professionals to be dismissive and patronizing. She believes it was her anger at the care her mother was receiving (or not receiving) that brought 'Nurse Angel' on to the scene. This nurse took measures that instantly relieved her mother's pain. She writes that Nurse Angel had both 'compassion (goodwill) and an innate talent for his job (competence)' (Mallick 2003, p. F3).

Patients and families tend to trust or not trust on the basis of caring behaviours: the caregiver makes eye contact, listens without interruption and seems to value what patients have to say about their own condition. These behaviours have great significance in promoting trust, even though such behaviours can be counterfeit rather than genuine (Buchanan 2000). (Hillel Finestone and David Conter (1994) have proposed that medical training should include an acting curriculum.) Mallick appreciates the caring and skilful behaviour of 'Nurse Angel' but remains suspicious that it was only her own outrage that brought him to the bedside of her mother. Physician and professor of law Gregg Bloche begins his cogent examination of *Trust and Betrayal in the Medical Marketplace* (2002) with his mother's story: her refusal to be a good hospice patient and her fight for treatment. He acknowledges that anecdotes may make bad policy but that stories of breaches of trust are proliferating.

NURSES STUDYING TRUST

As the ethos of trust within the healthcare sphere becomes more scarce and polluted, nurses are increasingly researching trust. Nurses began studying trust utilizing trust measures. A widely used psychometric scale devised by a psychologist is Rotter's Interpersonal Trust Scale (ITS; Rotter 1967). It measures the expectancy that the word or promise (verbal or written statement) of an individual or group will be relied upon. Rotter envisions trust as a psychological trait dependent on social learning. Distefano et al (1981) found that patient satisfaction at a psychiatric hospital correlated with results on Rotter's scale. Beard (1982) used Rotter's scale and found significant relationships between interpersonal trust, life events and the risk factor of diastolic blood pressure, body mass index and exercise. Luster (1984) used the scale to study team nursing and total patient care but found no significant differences, concluding that Rotter's scale could not specifically measure patients' trust of the nurse.

Nurse researchers have studied trust, as it is experienced in particular clinical settings. Trojan and Yonge (1993) interviewed home care nurses and elderly clients as a means of exploring the process of developing a trusting relationship. They identified four phases through which nurses and clients moved: initial trusting, connecting, negotiating and helping. Hams (1997, p. 352) studied trust in a coronary care setting, asking colleagues about their personal concept of trust. The general theme of their answers was 'being a friend and providing nursing care beyond minimal expectation'. Hams defines trust as 'a *willingness* to engage *one self* in a *relationship* that has *reliance* upon either a person(s) or thing(s), with an *expectation* that vulnerability may arise from either the trustee's or truster's *performance*. The primary aim, however, is to provide *empowerment* to both parties' (Hams 1997, p. 353, original italics). She identifies the antecedents of trust as reliability, perception of competence, past experience, trustworthiness of the trustee, risk and expectation of positive consequences. Consequences of trust are expected benefits, unanticipated results and formation of a stable or varying level of trust.

Trust evolved as a theme in Bricher's (1999) phenomenological study of paediatric nurses' experiences. In describing nurses' experience of trust with children, she found that nurses held trust as important but acknowledged that breaking trust can be essential to complete procedures. Nurses described 'keeping faith' with children (be honest, let them know what is going on, genuine liking and respect for children) and sharing the self (not being detached, using touch). Some nurses noted that parents at times blocked trusting relationship between the nurse and child (e.g. 'the nurse will give you a needle if you don't behave'). A need for trusting relationships with parents was recognized. 'What appears almost unrecognized is the fragility of the trusting relationship and the time and patience expended in building trust' (Bricher 1999, p. 11).

Meize-Grochowski (1984, p. 564) asked nursing colleagues to define trust and found a recurring theme in their definitions to be 'confidence in someone or something'. Dependability, consistency, and predictability were also used. Johns (1996), critical of trust discourse in nursing literature as based on vague conceptualizations or the work of other disciplines, analysed trust as it occurs in nurse–patient relationships and the work environment. Using Walker and Avant's (1995) method of concept analysis, she found trust to be both process and outcome. As process, trust is a sequential step model with feedback. As outcome, it is a snapshot of process that is captured in time. Johns's process model has four steps: assimilation of information (regarding competence, reliability, relevant prior experience, risk, potential benefits), decision-making, trust relationship (willingness to assume vulnerability) and consequences of trusting (feedbacks to the first step).

Hupcey et al (2000) advanced the conceptualization of trust by examining patients' perspectives of establishing and maintaining trust in healthcare providers.

Using grounded theory methods, they found 'meeting expectations' to be the core variable linking developing and maintaining trust. Although patients had difficulty describing trust and the factors that made them trust or distrust healthcare providers, the majority trusted the institution and its providers on admission and felt the same way when discharged. Patient outcomes did not seem to impact trust. Trust was dynamic: those moving toward distrust when expectations were not met changed course through positive interactions. These researchers found that trust could be generalized, going beyond a single relationship, and that global trust was extended to the system as a whole. They discovered, in fact, that nurses were blended into faceless caregivers in the patients' perceptions, even when they stood out. Patients with unmet expectations were distrustfully vigilant and looked for negative evidence of the system's failure. Unlike Meize-Grochowski (1984), these researchers found trust to be a robust rather than a fragile state. Given their findings, realistic expectations on entry into the system seem particularly important to the establishment and maintenance of patients' trust. The researchers concluded that trust is 'the willing dependence on another's actions for an identified need that cannot be met without the assistance of another. Trust is limited to the area of need and is subject of both overt and cover testing' (Hupcey et al 2000, p. 240).

Adding Carl Mitcham to their team, Hupcey et al (2001) further explored trust with a criteria-based evaluation of its maturity across medicine, psychology, sociology and nursing. They determined trust to be scientifically ambiguous and immature as an interdisciplinary concept. Based on this analysis, they used techniques of concept development with the literature as data to advance the concept of trust toward greater maturity. An expanded interdisciplinary definition came to light. Trust:

> ... emerges from the identification of a need that cannot be met without the assistance of another and some assessment of the risk involved in relying on the other to meet this need. Trust is a willing dependency on another's actions, but it is limited to the area of need and is subject to overt and covert testing. The outcome of trust is an evaluation of the congruence between expectations of the trusted person and actions.
>
> *Hupcey et al 2001, p. 290*

Recently Peter and Morgan (2001) have considered the promise of a trust approach to nursing ethics, grounded in the work of Annette Baier (1985, 1994). They emphasize that trust relationships can not be idealized and that the vulnerability and potential for evil (e.g. abuse of power) inherent in such relations must be recognized. They conclude that incorporating Baier's feminist approach offers a means of addressing political dimensions while retaining core values such as care and commitment.

Peter and Morgan make a key point in asserting that trust is often conceptualized within nursing as morally unproblematic. As a clinical professor in a forensic psychiatric setting, I experienced the difficulty of guiding nursing students in meeting the complex, competing demands of caring relationships in a 'secure environment,' an environment that meets Løstrup's notion of a special circumstance (Austin 2001). The deep and multifaceted aspects of trust become highly apparent in such a setting, with its mandate to confine psychiatric patients who have broken the law. These patients may be perpetrators of awful crimes such as arson, murder, rape and child abuse. Nurses must be mindful of that and of their professional responsibilities in terms of custody, as well as of healing and change. Students can have particular difficulty addressing trust issues if they come prepared with only a simplistic, unidimensional conceptualization of trust. Their education fails them if it does not move them toward a deeper understanding of this essential aspect of being human.

Being a nurse is, in some sense, making a moral claim. We profess to use our specialized knowledge and skills for the public's best interest in a trustworthy way. Grounded in the public trust is the privilege of self-regulation, allowing nurses to set and enforce regulations for entering the profession and to establish and monitor the standards governing our practice. To be worthy of this privilege, it seems imperative that we become highly attuned to the fact and value of trust, as it is manifested within ourselves, within our relationships with patients and colleagues and within our healthcare institutions. The work toward understanding trust has more than begun, but there is much to learn before we grasp the way it shapes our everyday existence.

REFERENCES

Austin W 2001 Relational ethics in forensic psychiatric settings. Journal of Psychosocial Nursing 39: 12–17

Austin W, Bergum V, Goldberg L 2003 Unable to answer the call of our patients: mental health nurses' experiences of moral distress. Nursing Inquiry 10: 177–183

Baier A 1985 What do women want in a moral theory? Nous 19: 53–65

Baier A 1994 Moral prejudices: essays on ethics. Harvard University Press, Cambridge, MA

Barber K (ed) 1998 The Canadian Oxford Dictionary. Oxford University Press, Oxford

Bauman Z 2003 Postmodern ethics. Blackwell, Oxford

Beard MT 1982 Trust, live events and risk factors among adults. Advances in Nursing Science 4: 27–43

Bloche G 2002 Trust and betrayal in the medical marketplace. Stanford Law Review 55: 919–954

Bok S 1978 Lying: moral choice in public and private life. Pantheon Books, New York

Bricher G 1999 Paediatric nurses, children and the development of trust. Journal of Clinical Nursing 8: 451–458

Buchanan A 2000 Trust in managed care organizations. Kennedy Institute of Ethics Journal 10: 189–212

Canadian Nurses Association 2002 Code of ethics for registered nurses. Canadian Nurses Association, Ottawa

Caulfield T 2002 Malpractice in the age of healthcare reform. In: Caulfield T, von Tigerstrom B (eds) Health care reform and the law in Canada: meeting the challenge. University Press of Alberta, Edmonton, Alberta

Clark C 2002 Trust in medicine. Journal of medicine and philosophy 27: 11–29

Craine W 1980 Theories of development: concepts and applications. Prentice-Hall, Englewood Cliffs, NJ

CNEWS 2004 Poll released on trustworthiness. CNEWS 15 February

Distefano MK, Pryer MW, Garrison JL 1981 Clients satisfaction and interpersonal trust in the communication process. Psychological Bulletin 68: 104–120

Edson M 1999 Wit. Dramatists Play Service, New York

Farrell M 2002 Trust during times of turbulence: three nurses' perspectives Nursing Administration Quarterly 26: 20–25

Finestone H, Conter D 1994 Viewpoint: acting in medical practice. Lancet 344: 801–802

George GB (ed) 1995 Nursing theories: the base for professional practice, 4th edn. Appleton & Lange, Norwalk, CT

Gift A 1997 Clarifying concepts in nursing research. Springer, New York

Gilbert T 1998 Towards a politics of trust. Journal of Advanced Nursing 27: 1010–1016

Globe and Mail 2003 Valemar and Aldemar. The Globe and Mail 22 August: A14

Govier T 1998 Dilemmas of trust. McGill–Queens University Press, Montreal, Quebec

Hams SP 1997 Concept analysis of trust: a coronary care perspective. Intensive and Critical Care Nursing 13: 351–356

Hupcey J, Penrod J, Morse J 2000 Establishing and maintaining trust during acute hospitalizations. Scholarly Inquiry for Nursing Practice 14: 227–242

Hupcey J, Penrod J, Morse J, Mitcham C 2001 An exploration and advancement of the concept of trust. Journal of Advanced Nursing 36: 282–293

Johns J 1996 A concept analysis of trust. Journal of Advanced Nursing 24: 76–83

Kaplan HI, Sadock BJ 1998 Synopsis of psychiatry: behavioural sciences/clinical psychiatry, 8th edn. JB Lippincott, Baltimore, MD

Kohn LT, Corrigan JM, Donaldson MS (eds) 2000 Committee on Quality of Health Care in America, Institute of Medicine. To err is human: building a safer health system. National Academy Press, Washington, DC

LeBlanc D 2004 Martin's housekeeping sweeps out the BDC Vennat. The Globe and Mail 13 March

Levering B 2002 The language of disappointment: on the language analysis of feeling words. Phenomenology and Pedagogy 10: 38–52

Lewis JD, Weigert A 1985 Trust as a social reality. Social Forces 63: 967–985

Løgstrup K 1997 The ethical demand. University of Notre Dame Press, Notre Dame, IN

Luhmann N 1979 Trust and power. John Wiley, New York

Luster D 1984 The effects of nursing care system on trust development. Unpublished Master's thesis, University of Nevada, Reno, NV

Mallick H 2003 Dear Doctor: you call this health care? The Globe and Mail 8 November

Meize-Grochowski R 1984 An analysis of the concept of trust. Journal of Advanced Nursing 9: 563–572

Mitchell G 2002 Self-serving and other-serving: matters of trust and intent. Nursing Science Quarterly 15: 288–293

Mitchell A 2003 Alberta researchers reeling from grizzly bear slaughter. The Globe and Mail 26 July

Mulen C, Cryderman K 2003 Esks save woman as two jump to flee highrise fire: fatal fall, miracle catch. Edmonton Journal 23 September: A1

O'Neill O 2002 A question of trust. Cambridge University Press, Cambridge

Pellegrino E 1991 Trust and distrust in professional ethics. In: Pellegrino E, Veatch R, Langan J (eds) Ethics trust and the professions. Georgetown University Press, Washington, DC

Pellegrino E, Veatch R, Langan J (eds) 1991 Ethics, trust and the professions: philosophical and cultural aspects. Georgetown University Press, Washington, DC

Peter E, Morgan KP 2001 Explorations of a trust approach for nursing ethics. Nursing Inquiry 8: 3–10

Piraro D 2003 Bizarro. The Globe and Mail 22 August

Rotter J 1967 A new scale for the measurement of interpersonal trust. Journal of Personality 35: 651–665

Rosenthal M, Sutcliffe K (eds) 2002 Medical error; what do we know? What do we do? Jossey-Bass, San Francisco, CA

Skeat W 1993 The concise dictionary of English etymology. Wordsworth Reference, Ware, Hertfordshire

Solomon R, Flores F 2001 Building trust in business, politics, relationships and life. Oxford University Press, Oxford

Sztompka P 1999 Trust, a sociological theory. Cambridge University Press, Cambridge

Thatcher VS, McQueen A (eds) 1984 The new Webster encyclopedic dictionary of the English language. Avenel Books, New York

Thomas L 1996 Becoming an evil society: the self and strangers. Political Theory 24: 271–294

Thorne S, Robinson C 1988 Reciprocal trust in health care relationships. Journal of Advanced Nursing 13: 782–789

Trojan L, Younge O 1993 Developing trusting, caring relationships: home care nurses and elderly clients. Journal of Advanced Nursing 18: 1903–1910

Ulrich B 2001 A matter of trust: public continues to regard nurses highly in honesty and ethics. Newsweek 17 December

Walker L, Avant K 1995 Strategies for theory construction in nursing, 3rd edn. Appleton & Lange, Norwalk, CT

Weber LR, Carter AI 2003 The social construction of trust. Kluwer Academic/Plenum Publishers, New York

Williams B 1985 Ethics and the limits of philosophy. Harvard University Press, Cambridge, MA

Yourk D 2004 Ottawa will never be the same, Martin vows. The Globe and Mail 17 March

A concept analysis of vulnerability

Jude A. Spiers

EDITORIAL

Nurses are likely to encounter what are described as 'vulnerable populations' or 'vulnerable people' during their nursing careers. Even a cursory examination of the associated literature of healthcare ethics would indicate that some populations (and therefore individuals belonging to these populations) have been termed 'vulnerable' (e.g. children). Furthermore, certain individuals are given the designation 'vulnerable' as a result of being in a certain state (e.g. someone with compromised cognitive abilities). However, as we are reminded in Jude's chapter, the idea of a fixed state of 'vulnerability', bestowed upon someone because they belong to a particular population or culture or encounter a certain lived experience, may not be the most helpful conceptualization; it fails to account for the individual nature of vulnerability. As with many of the concepts examined in this book, vulnerability is a term that has a tacit meaning based on an assumption of a common world view. To a large extent, this meaning is drawn from the lay definition, of the potential for harm or danger. On closer inspection, 'vulnerability' has a wide range of meanings, perspectives and applications, from statistical susceptibility and sensitivity to experiential phenomena.

People can often be in what would no doubt be regarded by many as 'vulnerable' situations without necessarily feeling vulnerable. The first editor can attest to such a situation; many is the time during his mountaineering and rock climbing that he has been in what would be regarded as extremely physically exposed and vulnerable situations. However, during these times he experienced no sense of being vulnerable; only a sense of concentration and fun. Inversely, patients may be in vulnerable situations but may lack the insight or information and therefore don't feel particularly vulnerable (e.g. a patient who insists on trying to get out of bed one day post myocardial infarction).

What begins to become clear is that arbitrary predetermined assessments of vulnerability will do little to adequately inform appropriate nursing care; furthermore any assessment of vulnerability must include the patient's awareness and sense of their own vulnerability. There are a number of additional issues that arise from Jude's chapter, including those concerned with the skills and abilities that nurses need in order to work with people who are feeling vulnerable. While we have some evidence to underpin this practice (e.g. help create a sense of trust and safety), exactly how nurses can help facilitate this in different situations is unclear. It is unlikely that there will be one 'best' way to help all vulnerable patients. Given the individualistic nature of vulnerability, it is likely that any 'interventions' will require an individualized approach.

INTRODUCTION

The notion of vulnerability is an essential concept that nurses use in the daily course of their professional work. We are careful to be sensitive to and respect the vulnerability of our patients or clients. We are aware of the vulnerability of specific population groups to particular environmental or social risk factors. Occasionally we even recognize our own vulnerability as we negotiate difficult and complex relationships, interactions and therapeutic interventions with patients, their families and co-workers. Despite a number of critical publications about vulnerability (Rose & Killien 1983, Chenitz 1989, Aday 1993, Lessick et al 1992, Phillips 1992, Savage & Conrad 1992, Stevens et al 1992, Demi & Warren 1995, Rogers 1997, Rogers & Henson 1997, Spiers 2000), as well as two entire nursing journal issues devoted entirely to research related to vulnerability (the *Western Journal of Nursing Research* volume 14, issue 6 (1992) and the *Journal of Perinatal and Neonatal Nursing* volume 6, issue 3 (1992)), there is little consensus about its attributes or dimensions beyond agreement that vulnerability is an important concept underlying nursing.

As a common word in colloquial usage, it is appropriate for vulnerability to have a range of meanings. It does, however, pose a problem for the discipline of nursing, as ordinary language often lacks the structure necessary for a scientific discipline and the scientific usage may need to be differentiated from the everyday usage (Aday 1994). In the professional arena, it is increasingly evident that there are negative implications and consequences both for the persons labelled as vulnerable and for the organization of nursing services when the emic and etic perspectives of vulnerability to danger are not congruent.

In this chapter I will describe my work in clarifying the concept of vulnerability using Morse's approach (Morse 2000). Using this theoretical concept clarification, a skeletal framework was developed to investigate vulnerability in healthcare relationships using video-based qualitative ethology (Hupcey et al 2000). This project advanced the concept further toward maturity, although some aspects remain unclear.

PHASE 1: THEORETICAL CONCEPT CLARIFICATION

The concept of vulnerability became a focus of inquiry because, in my earlier work, vulnerability in some form kept emerging as an important, yet vague concept. For example, underlying concepts of trust and respect was acknowledgement of the notion of personal vulnerability, and respecting vulnerability was an important aspect in the development of the nurse–patient relationship. However, *how* vulnerability was recognized, constructed and responded to in interpersonal interaction was not understood. As with other fundamental concepts in interaction, such as trust (Morse et al 2002), vulnerability appeared to be treated only as a component of the interaction or relationship; so as a concept it was not well demarcated. The concept clarification explored the full range of meaning and uses of the term vulnerability in the caring disciplines. Only articles with a main focus on vulnerability in reference to the human condition were selected.

It became quickly clear that there were many 'lay' meanings of the term; it was used interchangeably with 'risk' and 'harm'; it was used in a variety of contexts from a variety of perspectives; and it pertained to both consideration of large numbers of people as a whole and the nature of the relationship between individuals. However, there was little agreement about the definition and structural features among the disciplinary perspectives. Although the body of literature was enormous in volume and adequate in quality, the literatures were not well integrated toward an interdisciplinary consensus in meaning. Therefore, the next step was to clarify vulnerability, conceptually, through a critical analysis of the literature.

CONCEPT CLARIFICATION

The goal here is to ask critical questions of the data/literature. I used the literature as data and initially used critical questions (Schwartz-Barcott & Kim 2000) to guide the process:

- What are the different perspectives of vulnerability?
- What disciplinary perspectives are apparent?

- What is the essential nature of vulnerability?
- What are the different dimensions of vulnerability?
- How is vulnerability identified?
- Is vulnerability an objective or subjective phenomenon?
- What role does it play in the determination of equality and need in healthcare provision?
- How does the balance between an individual's external context and internal needs influence the determination and experience of vulnerability?
- What is the relationship between risk and vulnerability?
- What implications do vulnerability-as-a-group and vulnerability-as-an-individual have?
- Is vulnerability unilateral, bilateral or reciprocal – and determined by whom?
- Are there types or kinds of vulnerability?
- What are the ramifications and/or manifestations of vulnerability? (From Spiers 1999, with permission of Blackwell Publishing.)

This process involved individual analysis of articles as well as consideration of each discipline's perspective. Processes of constant comparison and contrast were used to uncover the assumptions and dimensions underlying different conceptualizations of vulnerability and to clarify the structural features of the concept.

THE ROOTS OF VULNERABILITY

The common meaning of vulnerability comes from the Latin root of 'wound' (*vuln-*). Vulnerability is defined as a 'state or quality of being vulnerable' (Brown 1993). Vulnerable means 'to be able to be physically or emotionally hurt' and 'liable to damage or harm, especially from aggression or attack' (Rogers 1997). This definition incorporates two distinct possibilities. One is the susceptibility and possibility of harm and the other is a state, perception or feeling of potential harm. The determination of vulnerability can be differentiated by whether the assessment is objectively or subjectively derived (Rose & Killien 1983). An objective assessment views the person as they actually are while subjective assessment derives from the self-concept. These represent two different approaches to the identification of harm; as an external or *etic* (Stevens et al 1992) assessment of liability or risk and an internal, *emic*, experience of threat. It is this locus of evaluation that appears to reveal the essential meanings of vulnerability and helps tease out a related concept, that of risk.

EXTERNAL EVALUATIONS OF LIABILITY AND RISK

Generally, 'vulnerability' is used to refer to liability to be hurt (MacMullen et al 1992, Demi & Warren 1995), which embraces the assumptions of susceptibility or potentiality for harm (Phillips 1992). **In other words, vulnerability is a synonym for being at risk.** Population groups are labelled as vulnerable because they are known to be at greater risk of poor health than the greater population because of their 'socioeconomic status, their minority status, or other stigmatizing status' (Demi & Warren 1995). Groups often defined as vulnerable include the elderly, fetuses, children, the poor, people with chronic illnesses, people from minority cultures and members of captive populations, such as prisoners and refugees (Saunders & Valente 1992). The etic perspective has its origins in epidemiology and defines vulnerability on the basis of demographic characteristics that assign to particular individuals or groups a higher relative probability of health or social problems (Demi & Warren 1995). Generally, these characteristics refer to deficits that are assumed to increase social dependence (Ferguson 1978). For example, the elderly, based on demographic characteristics, are at greater risk of harm such as falls.

Etic views are based on three primary assumptions (Ferguson 1978):

- Vulnerability describes people who are less able to function adequately in socially desirable ways
- Function is based on normative social values so that harm can be objectively assessed
- Socially sanctioned intervention is necessary and desirable.

The values of a particular society determine the nature of deficient functioning. For example, many Western societies value independence and self-sufficiency. Thus, a commonality of the homeless, mentally ill, poor, people with disabilities and the frail elderly is lack of self-sufficiency. Immigrants or minority groups may also be considered deficient if they are unable to function independently in the dominant culture because of language difficulties or values that prevent them from accessing mainstream societal institutions (Muecke 1992). In other cultures, of course, independence and self-sufficiency may not be valued as a normative assumption, and thus these same groups may not be labelled as vulnerable.

Identification of deficient functioning, however, does not usually provide sufficient cause for social intervention or even the label of vulnerability. There must be a balance between the need for intervention and the rights and autonomy of those seen as dependent (Ferguson 1978). Thus a condition of *objective harm* is required to determine which individuals or groups are identified as vulnerable and to defend this determination of need for intervention. This is achieved by societal authoritative, professional or legal definitions of the level of endangerment that warrants intervention. Such definitions are based on the relative risk of harm of a particular group compared to the larger society.

Endangerment is the term usually used when referring to objective harm. It is an euphemism that incorporates the ideals of objective determination of danger and social responsibility for minimizing that danger. For example, children are defined as nutritionally vulnerable and in need of nutritional interventions based on factors such as age, weight and height compared to international standards (World Health Organization 1983). Intervention is justified when endangerment or threat of objective harm can be proved.

The third assumption is that there is social sanction for intervention based on an assessment of deficit or endangerment status relative to objectively determined standards (Rogers 1997). Certain groups in the society are specifically sanctioned to determine those at risk on the basis of assumptions of normative social functioning and need (Ferguson 1978). **These assumptions point to a definition of vulnerability as the universally present relative risk of potential or actual harm from external judgements of endangerment, functional capacity and socially sanctioned need for intervention.** Risk is quantifiable so there is a normatively defined threshold beyond which the individual has a greater likelihood of developing health-related deficits (Lessick et al 1992).

Defined as relative risk, vulnerability is located within an epidemiological framework that is largely driven by biomedical views of pathology and illness (Lessick et al 1992). These assumptions give rise to a number of attributes of vulnerability-as-relative-risk:

- *Endangerment*, which refers to internal or external threats, exposure factors, or liabilities that inhibit functioning and thus place the person at a higher relative risk of objective harm.
- *Functional capacity*, which refers to the ability to deal with the threats and to compensate for deficits in functioning (Ferguson 1978). An individual's position along this continuum of relative risk of harm represents the balance between these two attributes. Vulnerability is the culmination of internal and external normative deficits that make people susceptible to illness.
- *External recognition of the increased susceptibility to harm*. Individuals' awareness of their own vulnerability is irrelevant to the label of vulnerability because of the need for objective assessment (Ferguson 1978).
- *Observable and measurable behaviour*. Human functioning is considered to be the expression of vulnerability because it reflects the balance or imbalance between endangerment and capabilities. Behaviour that is functionally effective indicates that the person is successful in adjusting to the environment. Ineffective behaviours point to an imbalance in assets and liabilities (Lessick et al 1992). Consequently, assessment of the potential for harm does not rely on personal perception but on normative comparison of behaviours with those of the larger group. Emotional vulnerability may be regarded as a covariant or intervening issue rather than a key determinant of vulnerability (Aday 1993, 1994).
- *Universality*. Every person is potentially at risk. Levels of vulnerability are dynamic because one's threshold is flexible. Vulnerability refers to a threshold of factors beyond which harm is a likelihood. Yet, vulnerability tends to be a dichotomous condition. An individual or group is either vulnerable or not vulnerable based on the criterion of objective harm. Within these categories, individuals are assumed to be homogeneous (Phillips 1992).

LIMITATIONS OF THE ETIC APPROACH TO VULNERABILITY

This 'higher than normal risk of endangerment' view of vulnerability is commonly employed in social policy. It is possible to determine normative standards and predict risk on a population basis. However, researchers are finding that vulnerability as normative deficit alone is inadequate to predict individuals' health outcomes (Werner 1996). For example, it is inadequate to explain phenomena of interest to nursing, such as addiction, that do not fit easily on the deficit–capacity balance (Muecke 1992). The etic approach can be a hindrance in understanding self-conceptualizations of health, threat or quality of life by those labelled etically as vulnerable because the subjective view is not privileged, only the expert and 'objective' evaluation. This approach to vulnerability has unintentionally become a source of stereotyping groups on the basis of functional deficits rather than strengths or experiential qualities. To gain access to public resources, people must often promote themselves as members of a group with some weakness that makes them dependent.

The segregation of person from environment by locating vulnerability intrapersonally, as a personal attribute or behaviour or a genetic predisposition, discounts environmental endangerment beyond individual control. There can be a tendency to 'blame the victim' rather than the social structures creating or maintaining situations in which persons are vulnerable (Stevens et al 1992). Finally, the right to intervene creates difficulties when the views of need and intervention differ between those evaluating the situation and those experiencing the situation. Often, the people seen to require intervention do not have the power to decide on those interventions. Whether they perceive that they need help is irrelevant.

Nursing has a particular social sanction to help those who are suffering (Morse 1997) but this mandate is conceptualized with facilitative and cooperative principles rather than paternalistic principles. Contemporary nursing researchers advocate helping clients to articulate their own perceptions and realities rather than imposing externally defined conditions and interventions upon them. Nonetheless, the etic perspective has largely been adopted and has persisted in nursing (Lessick et al 1992, Rogers 1997) despite recognition that arbitrary boundaries between person and environment do not facilitate investigation of their interrelationships. The priority public health and epidemiology has in the nursing literature is a partial explanation. However, the assumptions underlying etic views of vulnerability are not congruent with contemporary humanistic nursing ideology. The etic view of vulnerability is more accurately defined as relative risk. This term acknowledges the epidemiological perspective from which it originates.

EXPERIENTIAL STATE OF THREAT AND FEAR OF HARM

It is rare to find nursing scholars who have defined vulnerability as a state of being threatened, a feeling or fear of harm (Black & Weiner 1992, Rich 1992). The foundation of vulnerability as an experiential quality of life refers to individuals' 'experiences of being unprotected and open to damage in threatening environments' (Stevens et al 1992, p. 758) and is an emerging perspective. In this approach, vulnerability is based on the experience of exposure to harm through challenges to one's integrity. This perspective places vulnerability in a psychosocial–cultural context. An advantage of viewing vulnerability as challenges experienced by the person is that it avoids regarding vulnerability as an inevitable consequence of the person's gender, socioeconomic status, race, marital status, health status or occupation (Stevens et al 1992). This allows a broader perspective because the focus is on the realities of everyday lives.

ASSUMPTIONS UNDERLYING EMICALLY DEFINED VULNERABILITY

The primary assumption of emic vulnerability is that vulnerability is manifested as lived experience. It is the individual, who, based on their self-perceptions and discernment of challenges to self and of the available resources to withstand such challenges, defines vulnerability. These perceptions may have origins in socially determined values of performance and function but these are always filtered through personal values and realities. People may 'rationally' consider themselves to carry risk factors but, unless they perceive that some aspect of their self integrity is threatened and they do not have the capacity to respond to the threat, they do not experience vulnerability.

The second assumption is that people have a sense of themselves, their private and public selves, constituted as objects and uniquely perceived. People have the cognitive capacity to imagine their selves and their subjective experience (Morse 1997). A third assumption of the emic perspective is that vulnerability is universal, not because aggregate risk is reflected in individual risk but because the potential for danger from challenge to some aspect of integrity is an existential human condition. The fourth assumption is that vulnerability can only be determined from the perspective of the person experiencing it, just as quality of life can only be determined by the person experiencing it (Parse 1996). **Vulnerability must be described from the person's perspective and it is not quantifiable.**

ATTRIBUTES OF EMIC VULNERABILITY

In the emic approach, vulnerability has four primary attributes:

- Integrity
- Challenge
- Capacity for action
- Multidimensionality.

Integrity refers to the person's sense of soundness in the various dimensions of her or his life. Integrity is challenged when something has the potential to disrupt that conceptualization. People have a unique sense of integrity not only on the personal level but also as a couple, as a family, or as a community.

The second attribute of emic vulnerability is the presence of a *challenge*. Vulnerability is experienced when there is a perceived challenge to integrity with a corresponding uncertainty about the ability to respond adequately. Challenge refers to some perceived force requiring a response, and it also implies a potential for growth (Phillips 1992). It is not necessarily negative and should not automatically be construed as a negative threat.

Capacity for action refers to the individual's perceived ability to withstand, integrate or cope with the challenge. The terms 'strengths', 'assets' and 'functional ability' are not applicable here. Capacity for action draws upon resources, strengths and assets but it is the ability as perceived by the individual rather than an imposed standard.

The fourth attribute of *multidimensionality* reflects the fact that vulnerability varies from one person to another and from one experience to another. Experiences of vulnerability may be multiple, simultaneous or cumulative. A consistent dimension of the experience is the presence of challenge. If there are different challenges to different aspects of integrity, the individual may experience these as individual happenings, as accumulative and undifferentiated whole. However, the significance here is not in estimating the total level of vulnerability but in identifying what aspects of integrity are challenged.

A fifth dimension of vulnerability is *power*, or the extent to which a challenge directs or constrains action, and the extent to which the person perceives the potential for change. Power is particularly important in interpersonal relationships, because power differentials may constrain one person's ability to express vulnerability. Perceptions of power may differ between individuals and this results in different experiences of vulnerability.

The sixth attribute of the mutuality of vulnerability embraces the notion that threat to one's sense of integrity is a *universal experience* even though, for example, in interpersonal interaction the threat and the dimension of self implicated may be different for each person.

IMPLICATIONS OF EMIC APPROACHES TO VULNERABILITY

From an emic perspective, vulnerability is not defined by a preset number or category such as age, gender or education. Risk may still be pertinent to emically experience vulnerability but of priority is the *individual's experience* of that risk. Relating vulnerability to a dimension of lived experience makes it more difficult to ascertain any direct impact on health and illness; rather, as a dimension of quality of life, it may have more indirect or hidden consequences. The emic view provides a framework for understanding how people integrate and manage multiple challenges in their daily lives and how their choices about prioritizing and selectively attending to challenges are manifested in quality of life. As nursing most frequently occurs at an interpersonal level, it would seem that vulnerability as experienced threat to integrity would be the most productive approach.

PHASE 2: DEVELOPING THE SKELETAL FRAMEWORK

The next step was to engage in fieldwork to further clarify the concept. My goal in the fieldwork phase was to refine the concept with ongoing empirical observation. As my interest was in vulnerability as an interpersonal phenomenon in nursing,

I chose a site and participants in which vulnerability was most likely to be manifested: home-care nursing. (For a more detailed description of the study, the reader is referred to Spiers 2002.) This study was based on the strategies of qualitative ethology for video-based research as described by Bottorff (1994), using very in-depth observation and inquiry with 10 nurse–patient dyads. In the inductive phase of identifying patterns of behaviour, analysis was guided by the assumption that vulnerability could occur as a nursing concern in nursing interactions. Evolving analysis shaped this assumption to represent vulnerability as a unilateral or mutual challenge to the sense of personal integrity (Spiers 2000).

RESULTS

Identifying instances of vulnerability, responses to vulnerability and the interactional outcomes emerged as the analysis proceeded through various layers of interpretation of what was going on during the home-care activities. Initially, I needed to identify the kinds of interactional context in which there was a potential for vulnerability and the communicative means by which it was addressed. The nurses and patients were brought together for highly defined nursing needs (e.g. teaching, monitoring, wound care, health assessment and caregiver support). Their interaction created contexts in which their cooperative work was strengthened. **Vulnerability was an interactional phenomenon manifested in these contexts.**

These interpersonal contexts of vulnerability were interdependent as they functioned at different levels in the interaction. They could be either a goal or a means to a goal. For example, nurses and patients might actively work toward increasing the friendliness of a relationship out of genuine liking for the other. Or, friendliness could be a means to reach another goal, for example forging an amicable relationship in which each person recognizes the other's sincerity in their regard and desire to develop a shared understanding of the patient's situation. This in turn could facilitate the initiation of discussion around a taboo topic, something that, if not mitigated by the level of amicable regard, would exacerbate the patient's vulnerability. The six interpersonal contexts of interaction (Tables 21.1, 21.2) were deliberately and strategically negotiated, and they fluctuated in intensity and importance in response to the flow of events in the home-care visits.

Having identified the context of interaction, I then identified instances of threat to those contexts. In other words, it was challenges to the cooperative intent and work within each of these contexts that illuminated occurrences of actual or potential vulnerability.

DEVELOPING THE SKELETAL FRAMEWORK

I used the notion of face to represent the social identity that the nurse and patient wish to claim in the relationship (Brown & Levinson 1987). Face has been identified as another term for vulnerability (Watts 1989). Threats to face

Context I: Territoriality	This involved negotiating shared public space in the patient's home to facilitate caregiving activities
Context II: Perceptions of well-being and progress	The goal here was to create a significant degree of consensus in perception of the patient's current and projected state of well-being and treatment plans
Context III: Negotiating amicable working relationship	Nurse–patient dyads negotiated and maintained a friendly sense of collaboration bound by the therapeutic relationship, in which each person recognized the individuality of the other beyond the immediate demands of the caregiving activities. This fostered a sense of sincerity and friendliness that was therapeutically driven. Nurses used this knowledge of the patient's situation to tailor care, whereas patients used it to feel comfortable in raising sensitive issues and to express their appreciation (or otherwise)
Context IV: Synchronizing role expectations	Nurses and patients had different types of expertise and knowledge, and both needed to recognize and negotiate role boundaries and expertise and to evaluate performance within those roles. This was essential work associated with determining relative autonomy, collaboration or dependence in caregiving decisions
Context V: Negotiating knowledge	This included obtaining and providing information or advice within an interpersonal context in which nurses and patients had to explore each other's existing competency, find appropriate ways to offer new information without imposing or demeaning, affirm correct knowledge or identify and supplant incorrect information
Context VI: Sensitivity to taboo topics	This was the context in which participants were able to raise and negotiate taboo topics, which could range from pain tolerance to issues of private habits or personal fears

With permission from Spiers 2002, pp. 1037–1038.

occurred when the communicative action called into question their claimed identity (Tracy 1990). Face became a metaphor for vulnerability because vulnerability referred to a sense of threat to some aspect of personal integrity of self-presentation that each person cooperated in managing during the interaction (Spiers 2000). To this end, face work theory, as conceptualized by Brown and Levinson (1987) and the subsequent modifications by Lim and Bowers (1991), and Wood and Kroger (1993), were used to frame the notion of intra- and interpersonal vulnerability.

The interactional and behavioural elements within each communicative context were reanalysed to identify how they illuminated type of face/vulnerability,

Table 21.2
The communicative contexts of home-care nurse–patient interaction

Context	Established by	Challenges
Territoriality	Negotiating shared space	Withdrawing permission
	Reaffirming negotiated space	Space unprepared, inappropriate, non-existent Entering private areas without announcing intent Uninvited advice on use of space Environmental evaluation and changes for N's safety and comfort
Shared perceptions	Seeking participation/ opinion	Incongruent perceptions
	Checking consensus	Challenging the other's views Assuming or imposing views Misinterpreting message Excluding P or answering for P Failing to attend/be engaged
Amicable working relationships	Maintaining exclusivity of relationship	Assuming interchangeability of Ns
	Maintaining privacy of visit	Intrusion by others in person/phone
	Getting to know each other	Placing boundaries on familiarity
	Showing liking, respect, familiarity	Rejecting/deflecting/redirecting compliments
	Being engaged	Inattention
Role synchronization	Being interested in P's context	Different goals in role boundaries, expectations, performance
	Coordinating P, N and Dr role activities	Challenging role boundaries
	Letting P know that N acts on medical orders	Asserting autonomy
	Role performance	Inability to fulfil expectation
	Supporting, positive appraisal	Challenging role performance through criticism
	Pain management	Inappropriate stoicism
	Congruent approaches to expressing, perceiving, understanding, evaluating pain	Non-congruent approach to pain Doubting accuracy of P's information N personalizing infliction of pain Imposing beliefs about treatment efficacy Feeling helpless

Table 21.2

The communicative contexts of home-care nurse–patient interaction—cont'd

Context	Established by	Challenges
Knowledge	Integrating information to immediate situation	Incongruent perceptions of need for knowledge: N perceives P doesn't have or doesn't understand
	Balancing information with social talk	Importance of information requires reinforcement regardless of patient knowledge
	Structured and unstructured teaching	
Sensitivity to taboo topics	Perceiving which areas are sensitive	Embarrassment indicated by withdrawal or inadequate responses
	Minimizing embarrassment	

N = nurse; P = patient; Dr = physician

the nature of the threat to face, and the ways in which that threat was responded to, mitigated, resolved or exacerbated. It was particularly important to identify those areas of congruence and incongruence between the original face work conceptualization and face-as-vulnerability that emerged in the data analysis. This pointed to the formulation of vulnerability as it occurs within the healthcare interaction rather than as it is conceptualized by face work theorists in ethno-linguistics.

ANALYSIS AND INTEGRATION OF FINDINGS

The field work phase enabled me to verify the notion of vulnerability in interaction and to see actual instances of situations in which vulnerability was at issue. It developed and refined the tentative structure I identified during the theoretical concept analysis. What then are the structural features of vulnerability within the interpersonal context?

Attributes

- Vulnerability is at issue whenever people are invested in protecting their own, and other people's, sense of self-identity.
- Vulnerability is a universal experiential aspect of quality of life that is experienced in contexts of threat to sense of personal integrity or preferred social identity. Thus, in nursing interactions, it is a mutual factor at work in the encounter. All participants in an interaction are involved in perceiving, imagining and assessing actual or potential face vulnerabilities and threats.
- Vulnerability occurs within a psychosocial–cultural context within interpersonal interaction.
- Vulnerability is not a personal assessment of the resources in comparison to threats. However, it is an emic phenomenon. The internal structures of

vulnerability – the relative valuing of different types of integrity/self-presentation, and the power relationship between people, are more important in determining vulnerability than any eternal scheme. Although face as vulnerability may ultimately be idiosyncratically determined, it is also influenced by extrapersonal determinants such as social distance, power, intimacy, mood and the interactional competence of others.

- Vulnerability is defined by basic human wants or desires related to social identity and self esteem that can potentially be harmed in social intercourse. These are culturally, socially, idiosyncratically influenced.
- Vulnerability is closely related to the concept of self-disclosure, which is one way of describing how people manipulate boundaries to reveal and protect various aspects of themselves. Self-disclosure always involves self-presentation at some level because it is a sensitive business (Holtgraves 1990).
- Awareness of vulnerability often does not take place at a conscious level of experience. The conventions in language and interaction enable people to draw from a large repertoire of communication strategies to avoid or mitigate threats to integrity in such a way that the result is not conceptualized consciously.
- Risk is an associated concept that frequently functions with vulnerability. However, it refers to assessment of threat based on external perceptions rather than existential ones.
- Addressing vulnerability in interaction is relational work that occurs in conjunction with, and often facilitates, the accomplishment of instrumental goals.

Preconditions

- Individuals have a sense of the type of image they would like to present in public and are interactionally competent in cooperating to negotiate that presentation.
- Individuals are willing to imagine the face needs or vulnerabilities of others within the particular social context and have the interactional competency to negotiate face or vulnerability concerns.

Boundaries

- Vulnerability is a feature of interpersonal interaction. For, although there may be an intrapersonal sense of vulnerability (idiosyncratically derived), it is only within the interpersonal encounter that these claims can be negotiated.
- The concept of risk comes into play when consideration of threat is based on endangerment, functional capacity and observable behaviour rather than on the experiential phenomenon.
- Risk and vulnerability are often both implicated. However, risk is an external evaluation, whereas vulnerability is existential.

OUTCOMES

The potential for vulnerability is a universal feature of human interactions. However, the interactional skills used by people in interaction avoid or mitigate any conscious sense of vulnerability. Successful negotiation of dimensions of vulnerability in interaction result in each person in the encounter feeling that their sense of self presentation or image has been successfully presented and accepted. When this does not occur, by mistake or design, the outcomes are communication breakdown and individual experience of alienation, exclusion, isolation, embarrassment, discomfort and frustration.

CONCLUSION

A concept analysis of vulnerability was important because although it seemed to be a foundation of nursing practice, in that it was widely regarded as having profound influences on nursing outcomes, its characteristics and boundaries were vague and largely confused with a related concept, that of risk. In the first phase of analysis, there was primary consideration of the state of science surrounding the concept of vulnerability. If the concept of risk was delineated, the concept of vulnerability was unclear and thus inappropriate for use in research or practice. Using the literature as data was the first step in a process of clarifying the conceptual attributes through an inductive analysis of the literature. This analysis was guided by critical questions to further illuminate the characteristics and assumptions of the concept of interest. A series of questions regarding the differentiation of emic and etic perspectives helped fill in the theoretical gaps identified in the analysis. This was only possible because the data consisted of insights presented in the multidisciplinary literature rather than conjecture and there was an adequate and appropriate data set available in the various caring disciplines (Morse et al 2002).

This theoretical analysis allowed the emergence of a tentative form of the concept, or skeletal framework, to emerge – vulnerability as an existential human experience related to the negotiation of self-image and presentation in interpersonal interaction. Yet significant gaps in understanding persisted. The attributes were not well defined. Therefore, this theoretical analysis served as an important preliminary step that illuminated questions for further study. Qualitative fieldwork was used to identify and describe the interpersonal contexts in which vulnerability was at issue, the behaviours involved in expressing and negotiating vulnerability and the outcomes of those behaviours. This exhaustive investigation of vulnerability in interaction revealed the attributes of the experience of vulnerability and provided the basis of an analytic framework for understanding vulnerability.

However, as with any study, there are limitations. As I progress in my research, I am talking components of vulnerability in interaction to explore further in order to build a fuller model of vulnerability.

REFERENCES

Aday LA 1993 At risk in America: the health and health care needs of vulnerable populations in the United States. Jossey-Bass, San Francisco, CA

Aday LA 1994 Health status of vulnerable populations. Annual Review of Public Health 15: 487–509

Black K, Weiner S 1992 Platelet vulnerability in the fetus/neonate with neonatal autoimmune thrombocytopenia. Journal of Perinatal and Neonatal Nursing 6: 47–63

Bottorff JL 1994 Development of an observational instrument to study nurse–patient touch. Journal of Nursing Measurement 2: 7–24

Brown L (ed) 1993 The new shorter Oxford English dictionary: on historical principles, 4th edn. Clarendon Press, Oxford

Brown P, Levinson SC 1987 Politeness: some universals in language. Cambridge University Press, Cambridge

Chenitz WC 1989 Managing vulnerability: nursing treatment for heroin addicts. Image – Journal of Nursing Scholarship 21: 210–214

Demi AS, Warren NA 1995 Issues in conducting research with vulnerable families. Western Journal of Nursing Research 17: 188–202

Ferguson EJ 1978 Protecting the vulnerable adult: a perspective on policy and program issues in adult protective services. Institute of Gerontology, University of Michigan/Wayne State University, Ann Arbor, MI

Holtgraves T 1990 The language of self-disclosure. In: Robinson WP (ed) Handbook of language and social psychology. John Wiley, Chichester, pp. 191–207

Hupcey J, Penrod J, Morse JM 2000 Meeting expectations: establishing and maintaining trust during acute care hospitalizations. Scholarly Inquiry for Nursing Practice 14: 227–242

Lessick M, Woodring BC, Naber S, Halstead L 1992 Vulnerability: a conceptual model applied to perinatal and neonatal nursing. Journal of Perinatal and Neonatal Nursing 6: 1–14

Lim TS, Bowers JW 1991 Facework: solidarity, approbation, and tact. Human Communication Research 17: 415–450

MacMullen N, Dulski LA, Pappalardo B 1992 Antepartum vulnerability: stress, coping, and a patient support group. Journal of Perinatal and Neonatal Nursing 6: 15–25

Morse JM 1997 Responding to threats to integrity of self. Advances in Nursing Science 19: 21–36

Morse JM 2000 Exploring pragmatic utility: concept analysis by critically appraising the literature. In: Knafl KA (ed) Concept development in nursing: foundations, techniques, and applications, 2nd edn. WB Saunders, Philadelphia, PA, pp. 333–352

Morse JM, Hupcey JE, Penrod J et al 2002 Issues in validity: behavioral concepts, their derivation and interpretation. International Journal of Qualitative Methods 1: Article 3. Available on-line at: http://www.ualberta.ca/~ijqm (retrieved 17 Dec 2002)

Muecke MA 1992 Nursing research with refugees: a review and guide. Western Journal of Nursing Research 14: 703–720

Parse RR 1996 Quality of life for persons living with Alzheimer's disease: the human becoming perspective. Nursing Science Quarterly 9: 126–133

Phillips CA 1992 Vulnerability in family systems: application to antepartum. Journal of Perinatal and Neonatal Nursing 6: 26–36

Rich OJ 1992 Vulnerability of homeless pregnant and parenting adolescents. Journal of Perinatal and Neonatal Nursing 6: 37–46

Rogers AC 1997 Vulnerability, health and health care. Journal of Advanced Nursing 26: 65–72

Rogers JK, Henson KD 1997 'Hey, why don't you wear a shorter skirt?' Structural vulnerability and the organization of sexual harassment in temporary clerical employment. Gender and Society 11: 215–237

Rose MH, Killien M 1983 Risk and vulnerability: a case for differentiation. Advances in Nursing Science 5: 60–73

Saunders JM, Valente SM 1992 Overview. Western Journal of Nursing Research 14: 700–702

Savage TA, Conrad B 1992 Vulnerability as a consequence of the neonatal nurse-infant relationship. Journal of Perinatal and Neonatal Nursing 6: 64–75

Schwartz-Barcott D, Kim HS 2000 An expansion and elaboration of the hybrid model of concept development. In: Knafl KA (ed) Concept development in nursing: foundations, techniques, and applications, 2nd edn. WB Saunders, Philadelphia, PA, pp. 129–160

Spiers JA 1998 The use of face work and politeness theory. Qualitative Health Research 8: 25–47

Spiers JA 1999 Redefining vulnerability from emic and etic perspectives. Journal of Advanced Nursing 31: 715–721

Spiers JA 2000 New perspectives of vulnerability using emic and etic approaches. Journal of Advanced Nursing 31: 715–721

Spiers JA 2002 The interpersonal contexts of negotiating care. Qualitative Health Research 12: 1033–1057

Stevens PE, Hall JM, Meleis AI 1992 Examining vulnerability of women clerical workers from five ethnic/racial groups. Western Journal of Nursing Research 14: 754–774

Tracy K 1990 The many faces of facework. In: Robinson WP (ed) Handbook of language and social psychology. John Wiley, Chichester, pp. 209–226

Watts RJ 1989 Relevance and relational work: linguistic politeness as politic behavior. Multilingua 8: 131–166

Werner EE 1996 Vulnerable but invincible: high risk children from birth to adulthood. European Child and Adolescent Psychiatry 5(suppl 1): 47–51

Wood LA, Kroger RO 1993 A manual for coding the politeness of discourse. Unpublished manuscript, University of Toronto, Toronto, Ontario

World Health Organization 1983 Measuring change in nutritional status. Guidelines for assessing the nutritional impact of supplementary feeding programs for vulnerable groups. World Health Organization, Geneva

The evolution of concept analysis – where do we go from here?

John R. Cutcliffe and Hugh P. McKenna

BRIEF BACKGROUND OF THE DEVELOPMENT OF CONCEPT ANALYSIS

In Chapter 1, we pointed out that concept analysis per se (in nursing) is a relatively recent phenomenon. Even though there is historical evidence of 'nursing' dating back many centuries (see Barker 1999 and his reference to the first recorded carers being Celtic monks), and 'modern' nursing is often attributed to Florence Nightingale's work in the mid/late 19th century (Nightingale 1859), the first evidence of academic endeavours geared towards formalized concept analysis in nursing is perhaps Dickoff and James' (1968) seminal work on theory construction and development. In their paper entitled 'A theory of theories: a position paper', these authors posited four levels of nursing theory. These are presented in a hierarchical taxonomy with the 'lowest level' of theory being 'factor isolating theory'. Sometimes referred to as 'naming theory', the product of this intellectual enterprise is the naming, describing and classification of concepts. Or, to rephrase, this process can be thought of as a concept analysis, producing qualitative, descriptive theory (pertaining to the nature of the concept under investigation).

One needs to be mindful of the contemporary criticisms of this work. In particular, Sandelowski's (1997) and Morse's (1996) cogent arguments concerning the inappropriate (and inaccurate) conceptualization of qualitative research as only the preliminary forerunner of a quantitative study. Nevertheless, it needs to be acknowledged that Dickoff and James' contribution has influenced subsequent meta-theorists (see Meleis 1991) and the ways in which these epistemologists think about the development of nursing theory.

Wilson's (1969) approach can also be regarded as influential as it represents the theoretical underpinning of both Walker and Avant's (1995) and Chinn and Kramer's (1995) approach to concept analysis. This approach has been much criticized (see for example Morse 1995, Morse et al 1996a, b), in the main for its linear approach, positivistic (overly quantitative) nature and oversimplistic procedures. However, even a cursory examination of the relevant literature would reveal that there are a great number of concept analysis papers that have used this approach. Accordingly, there is considerable evidence that attests to the contribution this approach has made. More recently, two highly significant additional approaches, those of Rodgers (1989) and Morse (1995), have provided a more qualitatively orientated approach. As we pointed out in Chapter 1, within these approaches concepts are regarded as fluid, evolutionary and dynamic. **Notably, Morse's approach was the first one to draw heavily on 'real-life' qualitative data and this represents a significant advancement in the practice of concept analysis.**

Each of these approaches to concept analysis has been criticized, to a greater or lesser extent, and it is fair to say that there is no universally accepted approach. In his own inimitable style Paley (1995), for example, argues that current approaches to concept analysis have, in effect, 'placed the cart before the horse'. Paley's view is that concepts are not the building blocks of theory but the niches created by theory. He argues that the meaning of a term is made specific when it becomes part of a specific theory. Consequently, it is apparent that there are a myriad of approaches to concept analysis, and each approach is not without its detractors and/or critics.

According to Morse et al (1996a), concept analysis is a capacious term, one that encapsulates many processes. They argue that the processes facilitate the unfolding, exploring and understanding of concepts for the purposes of concept development, delineation, comparison, clarification, correction, identification, refinement and validation. Thus, while accepting the limitations of these different approaches, each appears to have enabled scholars to make contributions and enhance our understanding of concepts related to and important to nursing.

Given Morse et al's (1996a) comments, it is heartening to see to that, within this book, the contributing authors' selection of an approach mirrors this capacious, broad view of concept analysis in that a wide range of approaches has been used. Wilsonian approaches, as epitomized by Walker and Avant, have been used in the chapters analysing the concepts of caring, shame and facilitation, and as epitomized by Chinn and Kramer in the chapter analysing dignity. Rodgers' approach to concept analysis was used in the chapters analysing the concept of loneliness, comfort and therapeutic touch. Morse's approach was used for the chapter analysing fatigue. McKenna's approach, which incorporates Morse's approach and Wilson's approach, was used for the analysis of coping. Critical analysis and/or reviews of the literature as a means to unfold, explore and facilitate understanding of the concept, were used in the chapters on empathy, empowerment and hope. The much underexplored and underused approach of phenomenological writing as a means to concept analysis was used in Wendy Austin's chapter focusing on trust. Further, alternative ways to undertake a concept analysis and at the same time expand the scope and boundaries of the practice of concept analysis, were provided by Chris Stevenson and her colleagues in their chapter on support.

Box 22.1
Key issues/questions in
the evolution of the
practice of concept
analysis

- Does the nature of the criticism (and resultant limitations) of an approach to concept analysis mean that the 'findings' have no credibility?
- If one accepts that a concept is a fluid, dynamic entity, what is the value in undertaking a concept analysis at all?
- Given that there are (broadly) quantitative and qualitative approaches to concept analysis, do we need to develop different criteria for critiquing them?
- Exploring the role of 'maturity' in gauging the evolution and development of concepts
- The maturity of the practice of concept analysis per se

While there is clear synchronicity between the approaches to concept analysis and the methods used in these chapters, the practice of concept analysis is not free from unresolved issues and associated debates. This leaves the way open for additional theoretical, epistemological and methodological discussion. Accordingly, we add to this debate by highlighting five questions/issues, which are set out in Box 22.1. The remainder of this chapter will therefore examine some of the criticisms of approaches to concept analysis and then consider each of the questions/issues in turn; concluding with some thoughts on where the practice of concept analysis may go from here.

CRITICISMS OF CONCEPT ANALYSIS

Common and frequent criticisms of approaches categorized broadly as quantitative concept analysis (e.g. those based on Wilson's (1969) approach) include the following:

- This approach posits concepts as characterized by a set of rigid conditions that are both necessary and sufficient to identify an instance of the concept (Rodgers 1989).
- This approach posits concepts as static, unchanging over time or context.
- The use of 'model cases', which are synthetic constructions (e.g. not 'real world' examples), does little to enhance the understanding of the concept.
- The use of a linear, stepwise approach is too reductionist; it adheres to the tenets of positivism and rejects all metaphysical statements and referents (Rodgers 1989). **Accordingly, the dispositional theories of concepts (Wittgenstein 1968) are ignored.**

At the same time, criticisms of Rodgers' (1989) approach include the following:

- If concepts are indeed fluid, dynamic and change over time, then what is the point in obtaining a 'cross-sectional' view of the concept in the present, since tomorrow its use may have evolved through application? Indeed, Rodgers (1989, p. 333) states: 'Through the process of application, an existing concept may be continually refined, or conceptual variations and innovations may be introduced. As a result the concept may be enhanced in its explanatory or descriptive powers, and may thereby offer a greater contribution to the attainment of intellectual ideals.' Thus a concept analysis undertaken today may reveal little about a concept that tomorrow, through application, becomes significant, meaningful and important.

■ According to Paley (1995), Rodgers' approach does not explain many terms. Paley draws particular attention to the process of how the researcher identifies the defining attributes of the concept. Paley claims that it is not clear in Rodgers' writing how the 'common uses' of the concept are determined.

Concomitantly, criticisms of Morse's (1995) approach include the following:

■ In their writing on the 'maturity' of certain concepts, Morse et al (1996b, p. 387) state: 'In a mature concept there will be consensus and consistency with its use among theoreticians, researchers and practitioners'. Yet it is worth considering whether a lack of consensus is necessarily an indication of immaturity. As a concept undergoes original and frequent subsequent analysis, and thus the processes of development identified by Morse et al (1996b), is the product always a higher degree of consistency and consensus? To draw on the concept of hope here as an example, theoreticians, researchers and scholars have studied hope for many years. Specific attempts at the concept analysis of hope have occurred frequently during the last two decades. However, as Cheryl Nekoliachuk succinctly points out in her concept analysis of hope in Chapter 12, conceptual differences regarding hope are inevitable, given the complexity of the concept. These differences can enrich, yet also complicate, understandings about hope. Cheryl goes on to suggest that a complex concept such as hope cannot be simplified to a universal definition or conceptual framework. Thus, it is imperative to situate oneself amid the complexity of perspectives. From this argument one can deduce that, far from achieving consensus and consistency, additional and future attempts to analyse the concept of hope are as likely to add to the complexity as they are to achieve consensus. Furthermore, accepting the view of concepts as dynamic entity, as the concept develops and evolves through application, the once established mature concept (as determined by the scientific community) may then become dissimilar to the contemporary view of the concept.

KEY ISSUES IN THE EVOLUTION OF CONCEPT ANALYSIS

DOES THE NATURE OF THE CRITICISM (AND RESULTANT LIMITATIONS) OF AN APPROACH TO CONCEPT ANALYSIS MEAN THAT THE 'FINDINGS' HAVE NO CREDIBILITY?

We would assert that, as yet, insufficient attention has been paid to this key issue. In essence, the question is: When does a concept analysis become credible? According to Chinn and Kramer (1995), the product of a concept analysis has credibility when it has validity and reliability. It is not surprising that these criteria are suggested, given the alleged positivistic underpinnings of Chinn and Kramer's approach to concept analysis. In essence, they have transplanted the criteria for determining the 'accuracy' of results/findings obtained from a quantitative study and have overlaid these on their approach to concept analysis. As a result, Chinn and Kramer declare that a concept analysis is valid if it is based on multiple examples that are fully representative of the range of meanings of the concept. Similarly, the concept analysis can claim to be reliable if the concept can be consistently recognized using the attributes and indicators that the author has identified.

As commendable as that argument may be, there appear to be a number of issues that could stand further scrutiny and additional questions. For example, how many examples constitute 'multiple' – two, 30, 100? How should the researcher determine whether the concept is fully representative of the range of meanings? Is there an arbitrary time period during which the consistent recognition takes place? Is this consistency with the same 'sample' or with different 'samples'? Is it therefore necessary to undertake a test–retest in order to measure the consistency over time? Whatever the possible value of such an enterprise, there is little evidence of such undertakings in the literature where a concept analysis is reported. Further, this very practice would appear particularly compromised if one accepts the fluid, dynamic nature of concepts. Any 'test' or measure of consistency is likely to indicate that the concept has poor consistency, when in fact, this may simply be showing the evolution of the concept over time, through the iterative process of application.

In light of Chinn and Kramer's (1995) position, it needs to be pointed out that determining when the results/findings of a research study become credible enough to be accepted as an established known remains a contested matter. As we have written elsewhere (Cutcliffe & McKenna 2002), in quantitative research the α levels of significance are considered of crucial importance in determining the credibility and value of the findings. Since Fisher first suggested it, quantitative researchers throughout the world have accepted as the 'gold standard' an $\alpha(p)$ level of less than or equal to 0.01 or 0.05. We continued: 'There is little debate in the nursing research literature as to the suppositions underpinning this numerical line in the sand.' In effect, knowing in the quantitative paradigm is based on a number of unconscious assumptions (McCarl-Nielsen 1990, Angen 2000).' Furthermore, establishing when researchers can assert with empirical confidence that they know when working within the qualitative paradigm is similarly unresolved and remains a matter of much debate (Cutcliffe & McKenna 1999, 2002). Consequently, if confusion still exists around establishing the credibility of results/findings from a research study, it should be of little surprise that confusion still exists around establishing the credibility of a concept analysis.

It is often stated as an axiom that that there is no such thing as a perfect study; a study without limitations (Cutcliffe & Ward 2003). Consequently, it can be seen that the findings from 'imperfect' studies are accepted by scientific communities and are used as underpinning evidence in both further academic/research work and clinical practice. Consequently, we assert, with a degree of empirical confidence, that the same axioms can be applied to a concept analysis. In other words, while there is no such thing as a 'perfect' concept analysis (methodologically speaking), there is always something of value in each concept analysis undertaken; always something we can learn from the analysis.

IF ONE ACCEPTS THAT A CONCEPT IS A FLUID, DYNAMIC ENTITY, WHAT IS THE VALUE OF UNDERTAKING A CONCEPT ANALYSIS AT ALL?

This question may, on first consideration, appear to be something of an oxymoron when it is posed in a book that is explicitly concerned with concept analysis in nursing. However, in asking and addressing the question we believe that additional justification is provided for undertaking a concept analysis. Even some of the approaches to concept analysis that are based on analytical philosophy (e.g. Chinn and Kramer 1995) acknowledge the position that the product of a concept analysis is a tentative product. Dispositional philosophical underpinnings to concept analysis, typified in Rodgers' (1989) approach, clearly posit concepts as evolutionary. Consequently, a concept analysis can then only offer a 'cross-sectional' conceptualization of the concept in the 'here and now'. Thus, if we are seeking a better understanding of the concepts relevant and important to nursing (practice, research and education), is this a futile exercise if 'tomorrow' the concept has evolved beyond our current understanding?

We would suggest that there is immense value in this intellectual enterprise, even given the argument highlighted above. In order to illustrate this value, we draw on the previously stated parallels between concept analysis and qualitative research. In order to articulate this argument it is necessary to point out the key differences in the underpinning philosophy when compared to quantitative approaches. Lincoln and Guba (1985) have pointed out that a variety of adjective labels have been coined to capture the philosophical underpinnings of the qualitative paradigm, including naturalistic, interpretivist, postpositivist and hermeneutic. These approaches each incorporate the view that acknowledges a 'real world' where 'concrete phenomena' exist. Nevertheless, and importantly, the experience of that real world, the symbolic meanings ascribed to it and how one subsequently behaves and acts in it, are determined by a web of factors made up of language, symbol, culture, history and individual situatedness. Consequently, in terms of culture, human behaviour, experience and process, qualitative researchers purport that there is no 'objective truth'. Truth is contextual, temporal, locally located and constructed as a result of shared inter-subjective meanings. Further, the qualitative researcher has no aspirations towards *nomothetic* generalizations: generalizations relating to universal laws and absolute 'truths'. Instead, if they aspire to generalizable findings, they wish to uncover *idiographic* generalizations – or, to rephrase, contextually based truths, essences or universals that are understood in terms of the particulars of various cases. These are generalizations about and drawn from cases (Sandelowski 1997) – generalizations drawn from purposeful samples with experience of the 'case' and thus applicable to similar 'cases', questions and problems, irrespective of the similarity between the demographic group (Morse 1999).

Thus we need to consider the process of establishing the credibility of a concept analysis underpinned by dispositional philosophy; the product being an evolutionary concept. In such cases, the 'truth' (or validity or accuracy) of the concept analysis would not be judged in terms of generalizations about universal application of the concept or absolute 'truths' pertaining to the concept. Instead, just as the findings from a qualitative study are contextual, temporal, locally located and constructed as a result of shared intersubjective meanings, so too is the product of a concept analysis obtained through methods that are underpinned by dispositional philosophy. As Rodgers (1989, p. 336) points out, 'a concept is considered to be an abstraction that is expressed in some form, either discursive or non-discursive. Through socialization and repeated public interaction a concept becomes associated with a particular set of attributes... concepts are publicly manifest through certain behaviours.'

Hence, the 'truth' or validity of such a concept analysis would be based on *idiographic* generalizations of the concept – or, to rephrase, contextually based truths, essences or universals that are understood in terms of the particulars of various concepts, i.e. generalizations about and drawn from cases where the concept is used. Consequently, the concept should have meaning and spontaneous validity (Kvale 1996) for purposeful samples who have experience of the 'concept' and thus find it applicable to similar instances and experiences of the concept in their own lived world.

Accordingly, it can be seen that through the means of idiographic generalization and through the iterative process described by Rodgers, the utility of undertaking a concept analysis is made clear. Practitioners, educationalists and researchers who experience the concept and include it in their day-to-day practice should be able to draw upon the 'case'-related generalization of the concept and thus find meaning (for them) in the analysis. This is an argument supported by both Rodgers (1989) and Toulmin (1972). Indeed, Toulmin declares that, even though the concept is evolutionary and any concept analysis is a cross-sectional representation, it can still have meaning, utility and value if it serves the nurse, educationalist or researcher through its idiographic generalization and practical use.

GIVEN THAT THERE ARE (BROADLY) QUANTITATIVE AND QUALITATIVE APPROACHES TO CONCEPT ANALYSIS, DO WE NEED TO DEVELOP DIFFERENT CRITERIA FOR CRITIQUING THEM?

While, as yet, insufficient attention has been paid to the matter of determining the credibility of a concept analysis, the existing literature, such as it is, provides an equivocal picture. While Rodgers' approach is widely recognized and described as a qualitative approach, she still refers to the need for a 'representative sample', samples drawn (presumably randomly) from computerized data bases and thus, according to Rodgers (1989), the concept analysis is more likely to be representative of the total population. Further, she argues that if the concept analysis is representative of the total population then the credibility of the concept analysis is enhanced. Clearly, these arguments are based on positivistic underpinnings and the desire for nomothetic generalizability. They are driven by the view that the validity is increased if more people support the findings; in other words, if the p value is increased. Rodgers' suggestion of including maximum variation in one's sampling strategy might be more indicative of the historical qualitative methodological orthodoxy that prevailed at the time. Whereas, if contemporary methodological reasoning around the issue of sampling were invoked, perhaps purposeful sampling would be more appropriate, whereby the 'researcher' should access those data and literature that would provide the deepest and richest information available on the concept.

Perhaps there are additional methodologically congruent approaches that might be used for establishing the credibility of a concept analysis. While one might argue that any concept analysis is, by definition (e.g. factor-isolating) descriptive theory and therefore synonymous with qualitative research, we would argue that the philosophical underpinnings and resultant method used in the analysis would be a better determinant for describing the approach as qualitative or quantitative. Consequently, given the existence of Chinn and Kramer's (1995) existing criteria, here we provide additional criteria that might be particularly useful for establishing the credibility of concept analyses that use a qualitative approach.

Possible alternatives include:

- the use of some form of audit trail
- establishing the credibility of the concept by gaining meaning from those who 'use' the concept.

The use of an audit trail

While we acknowledge the substantive argument that highlights the limitations of 'audit trails' in qualitative researcher (Cutcliffe & McKenna 2004), there may be some value in providing a trail of evidence in the form of explanations for methodological decisions (e.g. what literature and other forms of data were accessed and why.

Gaining meaning from those who 'use' the concept

To explain this method in more detail, people who 'use' the concept need to recognize it as it is applied in their world; it has to have meaning and utility for those who are to 'use' the concept. Perhaps, as we have written elsewhere (Cutcliffe & McKenna 2002), this recognition of the concept and its meanings could be brought about by dialogue, explanation and discussion occurring between the person(s) who undertakes the concept analysis and those who the 'use' it in their world. This process is perhaps analogous to Angen's (2000) and Nielsen's (1995) process of evoking an immediate feeling of authenticity, a smile of recognition, providing spontaneous validity. At the very least, this form of validation implies that the person who has undertaken the concept analysis should take care to avoid the alienating role of privileged possessor of expert knowledge and suggests a more cooperative approach between the researcher/analyst and those who 'use' the concept.

Even after undertaking a methodologically congruent examination of the credibility of the concept analysis, we would not suggest that this means that the concept is now 'set in stone'. Given that concepts evolve over time, the analysis of the concept can never seen to be 'complete'. A concept analysis that has a high level of credibility then represents the most complete understanding possible for that situated group who 'use' the concept (in our cases – nurses), at that particular moment in time.

EXPLORING THE ROLE OF 'MATURITY' IN GAUGING THE EVOLUTION AND DEVELOPMENT OF CONCEPTS

According to Morse et al (1996a, p, 387), 'not all concepts have been developed to a level to which they are useful in *quantitative* research [emphasis added]. What we can call a useful concept is "mature", it is well defined, has clearly described characteristics, delineated boundaries, and documented preconditions and outcomes'. These authors then provide four criteria for evaluating the maturity of a concept:

- Is the concept well defined?
- Are the characteristics/attributes identified?
- Are the preconditions and outcomes of the concept described and demonstrated?
- Are the conceptual boundaries delineated?

We have already pointed out the counter-argument vis-à-vis well-defined concepts being synonymous with mature concepts. Nevertheless, this issue warrants further consideration. Perhaps the key question is: When is a concept too immature to be of theoretical and practical value? Accordingly, we will consider each of the four criteria identified by Morse et al (1996a).

Is the concept well defined?

Here we draw on the example of two concepts that have been analysed: caring and therapeutic humour. The concept of caring has been analysed many times. Morse et al (1996a), for example, found five conceptualizations of caring. A concept analysis of therapeutic humour is, by contrast, almost non-existent. As a result, there is far greater epistemological cohesiveness currently for the concept of therapeutic humour than there is for caring. Yet, the depth and extent of analysis for caring perhaps lends support to the idea that the concept is more mature than that of therapeutic humour, in that, arguably, the extensive exploration and analysis of caring indicates that we know more about caring than we do about therapeutic humour. The simple fact that the concept has undergone less analysis obviously explains some of this. Morse et al (1996a) state that a mature concept has definitions (note plural) that are relatively consistent and cohesive. However, this raises other questions, including how consistent the definitions have to be in order for the concept to be regarded as mature and how many individual concept analyses are required before one can even think about determining consistency and cohesiveness. Consequently, further debate is required around this criterion before we can assert that consistency and cohesiveness are clear indicators of the maturity of a concept.

Are the characteristics/attributes identified?

This criterion poses less methodological dissonance but operationalizing it is still not without its associated difficulties. Morse et al (1996a, p. 388) state that 'the test of validity is to ensure that the characteristics selected have maintained contextual relevance and abstract generalizability for each instance in which the concept appears.' This, in our view, is 'asking a lot'; it is placing a great deal of 'epistemological pressure' on any concept, no matter what its current level of maturity. To posit such a test implies that, irrespective of time, place, context or application of the concept, a mature concept should *always* have the conceptual characteristics/attributes present. We would assert that few (if any) concepts that are used in (although not exclusive to) nursing would meet this criterion and that therefore all such concepts are immature. Again, drawing on the concept of hope to illustrate this point, Morse et al (1996a) appear to use the concept as an example of a mature concept. Yet, as previously indicated, there is anything but consensus in the (extensive) literature pertaining to hope or, more importantly, in the existing concept analyses of hope. Indeed, in Part 1 of their six-part series on hope in nursing, published in the *British Journal of Nursing*, Cutcliffe and Herth (2002) stated:

> *Comparison of the above definitions of hope appears to indicate that, although the concept of hope has been discussed in health care literature since the 1960s, it is still difficult to find one definition that encapsulates all that hope is and specifically how it relates to health, disease and healthcare.*

Are the preconditions and outcomes of the concept described and demonstrated?

This third criterion appears to be very much grounded in analytical philosophical views of the nature of concepts. Such a view posits concepts as characterized by a rigid set of conditions that are both necessary and sufficient to identify an instance of the concept. Therefore the preconditions must be present in order for the concept to develop and the outcomes are the results of the use of the concept. Since the concept will not change over time, the preconditions and outcomes are also fixed, thus making it possible to determine the maturity of the concept.

However, if one were to adopt the dispositional philosophical view of concepts, it would appear epistemologically unbecoming to suggest that a concept, no matter how it evolves through future application (Rodgers 1989), must always have the same preconditions and outcomes present in order to be considered mature. Using the concept of hope to exemplify this (like Morse et al 1996a) casts considerable doubt both on a) whether or not hope is a mature concept and b) the validity and utility of this third criterion. To explain these problems, both contemporary and vintage conceptual literature posit alternative views of hope to those proffered by Morse et al; more especially, this literature contradicts the view that for hope to exist there must be a perceived threat. Lynch's (1965) seminal work asserted that hope often remains implicit, ever-present and influences the individual, without the individual necessarily being aware of this presence. Further Erickson (1964), Snyder (1996) and Cutcliffe (1997) all predicate that hope begins as a subconscious process in infants, who hope that their basic physiological and safety needs are met. Consequently, while at the moment we lack the methodological and technological sophistication to determine whether or not these infants are perceiving and subsequently reacting to a threat, current understanding of infants' cognitive developmental abilities would suggest not. A person's awareness of hope increases when they have the need for hope (Cutcliffe 1997), so perhaps here there is commonality with Morse et al's (1996a) view. Thus these differing views, many of which do not have the precondition of a perceived threat, suggest either that hope is not a mature concept (which may be the case) or that this criterion lacks utility.

Are the conceptual boundaries delineated?

The fourth criterion also appears to be very much grounded in analytical philosophical views of the nature of concepts. It clearly has merit since one of the rudiments of any concept analysis is to help determine where one concept ends and another begins. However, if one were to adopt the dispositional philosophical view then even this meritorious process may have limited value. As pointed out previously, dispositional philosophical underpinnings to concept analysis posit concepts as evolutionary and thus any attempt to identify the conceptual boundaries can only offer a 'cross-sectional' view in the 'here and now'. Nevertheless, as with establishing the credibility of a concept analysis, delineating the boundaries of related concepts provides the most complete representation possible for that situated group who 'use' the concept (in our cases – nurses) at that particular point in time.

THE MATURITY OF THE PRACTICE OF CONCEPT ANALYSIS PER SE

It is interesting to note that the 'age' of a concept is not necessarily related to its maturity (Morse et al 1996b). If one accepts this position, then can the same be said about the practice of concept analysis? Does the relatively short period of time in which formal concept analysis has been undertaken in nursing account for the developmental stage of the practice? In our view, it may account for some of it but not all. The fact that concept analysis is still at the developmental stage may be explained, at least in part, because of the limited amount of associated literature (and ensuing debate) that exists. It appears that the practice of concept analysis per se is not often critiqued, examined or debated. Given that the practice of concept analysis has existed in nursing since (at least) 1968, one might expect to see more literature and a higher degree of development.

Consider, for comparison, the case of grounded theory method(ology), which was first published by Glaser and Strauss in 1967, and the now substantial methodological literature that focuses on grounded theory. Indeed, almost a decade ago, such was the interest (and number of papers) that a special interest of the journal *Qualitative Health Research* was dedicated to developments in grounded theory. No such special issue has been dedicated to developments in concept analysis.

As a result, it stands to reason that more attention to the practice of concept analysis is needed. More scholars are needed in order to unravel some of the complexities of and answer some of the questions we have raised in this chapter and, for that matter, in this book. More debate is needed where paradigmatic struggles and epistemological insights occur. In some small way we hope that this book has contributed to this much needed body of literature and we look forward to seeing the future analyses and debates.

REFERENCES

Angen MJ 2000 Evaluating interpretive inquiry: reviewing the validity debate and opening the dialogue. Qualitative Health Research 10: 378–395

Barker P 1999 The philosophy and practice of psychiatric nursing. Churchill Livingstone, Edinburgh

Chinn P, Kramer MK 1995 Theory and nursing: a systematic approach, 4th edn. CV Mosby, St Louis, MO

Cutcliffe JR 1997 Towards a definition of hope. International Journal of Psychiatric Nursing Research 3: 319–332

Cutcliffe JR, Herth K 2002 Hope – a concept at the heart of nursing. Part 1: The origins, background and nature of hope. British Journal of Nursing 11: 832–840

Cutcliffe JR, McKenna HP 1999 Establishing the credibility of qualitative research findings: the plot thickens. Journal of Advanced Nursing 30: 374–380

Cutcliffe JR, McKenna HP 2002 When do we know that we know? Considering the truth of research findings and the craft of qualitative research. International Journal of Nursing Studies 39: 611–618

Cutcliffe JR, McKenna HP 2004 Expert qualitative researchers and the use of audit trails. Journal of Advanced Nursing 45: 126–133

Cutcliffe JR, Ward M 2003 Critiquing nursing research. Quay Books, London

Dickoff J, James P 1968 Symposium on theory development in nursing. A theory of theories: a position paper. Nursing Research 17: 197–203

Erickson EH 1964 Childhood and society, 2nd edn. WW Norton, New York

Glaser BG, Strauss AL 1967 The discovery of grounded theory: strategies for qualitative research. Aldine, Chicago, IL

Kvale S 1996 Interviews: an introduction to qualitative research interviewing. Sage, Thousand Oaks, CA

Lincoln YS, Guba EG 1985 Naturalistic inquiry, Sage, Newbury Park, CA

Lynch WF 1965 Images of hope. Garamony/Trichemah, Baltimore, MD

McCarl-Nielsen J 1990 Feminist research methods: exemplary readings in the social sciences. Westview Press, Boulder, CO

Meleis A 1991 Theoretical nursing: development and progress, 2nd edn. JB Lippincott, Philadelphia, PA

Morse JM 1995 Exploring the theoretical basis of nursing using advanced techniques of concept analysis. Advances in Nursing Science 17: 31–46

Morse JM 1996 Is qualitative research complete? Qualitative Health Research 6: 3–5

Morse JM 1999 Qualitative generalisability. Qualitative Health Research 9: 5–6

Morse JM, Hupcey JE, Mitcham C et al 1996a Concept analysis in nursing research: a critical appraisal. Scholarly Inquiry for Nursing Practice 10: 253–277

Morse JM, Mitcham C, Hupcey JE et al 1996b Criteria for concept evaluation. Journal of Advanced Nursing 24: 385–390

Nielsen HB 1995 Seductive texts with serious intentions. Educational Researcher 24: 4–12

Nightingale F 1859 Notes on nursing (Reprinted: Duckworth 1970)

Paley J 1995 How not to clarify concepts in nursing. Journal of Advanced Nursing 24: 572–578

Rodgers B 1989 Concepts, analysis and the development of nursing knowledge: the evolutionary cycle. Journal of Advanced Nursing 14: 330–335

Sandelowski M 1997 'To be of use': enhancing the utility of qualitative research. Nursing Outlook 45: 125–132

Snyder CR 1996 To hope, to lose, and to hope again. Journal of Personal and Interpersonal Loss 1: 1–16

Toulmin S 1972 Human understanding. Princeton University Press, Princeton, NJ

Walker LO, Avant KC 1995 Strategies for theory construction in nursing, 3rd edn. Appleton & Lange, Norwalk, CT

Wilson J 1969 Thinking with concepts. Cambridge University Press, London

Wittgenstein L 1968 Philosophical investigations, 3rd ed (trans GEM Anscombe). Macmillan, New York

Zimmer L 2004 Qualitative Meta-synthesis: does it violate the interpretive paradigm? Journal of Advanced Nursing, in press

Index